Food Literacy

Globally, the food system, and the relationship of the individual to that system, continues to change and grow in complexity. Eating is an everyday event that is part of everyone's life. There are many commentaries on the nature of these changes to what, where and how we eat and their socio-cultural, environmental, educational, economic and health consequences. Among this discussion, the term 'food literacy' has emerged to acknowledge the broad role food and eating plays in our lives, and the empowerment that comes from meeting food needs well.

In this book, contributors from Australia, China, the United Kingdom and North America provide a review of international research on food literacy and how this can be applied in schools, health-care settings and public education at the individual, group and population level.

These varying perspectives will give the reader an introduction to this emerging concept. The book gathers current insights and provides a platform for discussion leading to further understanding and application in this field. It stimulates the reader to conceptualize what food literacy means to their practice and to critically review its potential contribution to a range of outcomes.

Helen Vidgen has worked as a public health nutritionist in government, civil society and academic organizations for over twenty years. During this time she has been involved in the development of policy, programmes and evaluation. Her PhD thesis defined food literacy and its relationship to nutrition. She continues to work in this and other areas related to the everyday practicalities of meeting nutrition recommendations at the Queensland University of Technology, Australia.

Routledge Studies in Food, Society and the Environment

For further details please visit the series page on the Routledge website:
www.routledge.com/books/series/RSFSE/

Food Literacy

Key concepts for health and education

Edited by
Helen Vidgen

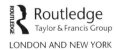

Routledge
Taylor & Francis Group
LONDON AND NEW YORK

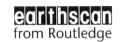

earthscan
from Routledge

First published 2016
by Routledge
2 Park Square, Milton Park, Abingdon, Oxon OX14 4RN

and by Routledge
711 Third Avenue, New York, NY 10017

Routledge is an imprint of the Taylor & Francis Group, an informa business

British Library Cataloguing in Publication Data
A catalogue record for this book is available from the British Library

Library of Congress Cataloging-in-Publication Data
Names: Vidgen, Helen, editor, author.
Title: Food literacy / edited by Helen Vidgen.
Description: London ; New York : Routledge, [2016] |
Includes bibliographical references and index.
Identifiers: LCCN 2015042646 | ISBN 9781138898516 (hbk) |
ISBN 9781138898523 (pbk) | ISBN 9781315708492 (ebk)
Subjects: LCSH: Food habits--Social aspects. | Nutrition--Social aspects.
Classification: LCC GT2850 .F676 2016 | DDC 394.1/2--dc23
LC record available at http://lccn.loc.gov/2015042646

ISBN: 978-1-138-89851-6 (hbk)
ISBN: 978-1-138-89852-3 (pbk)
ISBN: 978-1-315-70849-2 (ebk)

Typeset in Bembo
by Taylor & Francis Books

This book is dedicated to my parents Valentino and Anita (née Gottardo) Valentini, my family and friends, and all the beautiful food moments we have shared together.

Contents

Illustrations

Box

Contributors

Andrea Begley, Senior Lecturer, School of Public Health, Nutrition, Dietetics and Food Technology, Curtin University, Perth, Australia. Andrea is an advanced accredited practising dietitian and has a research background in qualitative research exploring nutrition issues across the lifecycle and food literacy with a particular interest in effective cooking skill interventions. She has been employed at Curtin University since 1996 with responsibility for teaching and research in public health nutrition for postgraduate dietetic and public health students.

Carole Bisogni, Associate Dean for Academic Affairs, College of Human Ecology, Professor, Nutritional Sciences, Cornell University, New York, USA. Carole Bisogni sadly passed away during the writing of this book. With colleagues, she developed several award winning nutrition education programmes for adults and youth using multi-media interventions in schools, supermarkets, and after school programmes. The challenges of this work led her to develop a research programme based in the social sciences so that design and evaluation of programmes could be strengthened by employing social science theories and methods. Bisogni's food choice research reflected her longstanding interest in the ways that people manage myriad influences and goals when they interact with food.

Stephanie Bostic, Graduate Student, Division of Nutritional Sciences, Cornell University, New York, USA. Stephanie is interested in how households conceptualize and manage food and cooking. She earned a Master of Science in Agriculture, Food and the Environment from Tufts University. She is currently a doctoral candidate at Cornell University.

Martin Caraher, Professor of Food and Health Policy, Centre for Food Policy, Department of Sociology, School of Arts and Social Sciences, City University, London, UK. Martin is Professor of Food and Health Policy at the Centre for Food Policy at City University. He has worked on issues related to food poverty, cooking skills, local sustainable food supplies, the role of markets and co-ops in promoting health, farmers markets, food deserts and food access, retail concentration and globalization.

Sandra Fordyce-Voorham, Head of Food and Nutrition, Mentone Girls' Grammar School, Melbourne, Australia. Sandra trained in Home Economics and has been working as a food educator in schools for many years. Her PhD (University of Wollongong) research augments the consultancy work she is currently undertaking in promoting food skills in schools and communities. She is a past President of Home Economics Victoria and Education Chair with the International Federation for Home Economics.

Danielle Gallegos, Discipline Head, Nutrition and Dietetics, School of Exercise and Nutrition Sciences, Queensland University of Technology, Brisbane, Australia. Danielle's research portfolio emphasizes qualitative methodologies in the development, implementation and evaluation of nutrition programmes. Her predominant research interests are food literacy, food security, early childhood feeding and evaluation. The majority of her work has occurred in the development and evaluation of programmes for specific sub-populations, including refugee families, youth in transition and other potentially marginalized groups. All her work has an element of social justice.

Doris E. Gillis, Associate Professor and Chair, Department of Human Nutrition, St Francis Xavier University, Antigonish, Nova Scotia, Canada. Doris draws on her background in public health nutrition and adult education in her current role as a teacher and researcher. Her research centres on health literacy, food security and breastfeeding. She has been involved in several national health literacy research and policy initiatives, including the Canadian Expert Panel on Health Literacy (2006–2008).

Margaret Jastran, Research Support Specialist, Nutritional Sciences, Cornell University, New York, USA. Margaret is a registered dietitian and a research support specialist who has worked on food choice research for close to twenty-five years at Cornell University. She has conducted hundreds of interviews, analysed the qualitative data, and assisted with writing professional papers.

Theresa Wai Ling Lai-Yeung, Assistant Professor, Department of Health and Physical Education, The Hong Kong Institute of Education, Hong Kong, China. She has extensive experiences in teaching and teacher education. Her publications focused on food choice, dietary habits, and implications of food literacy education for health.

Rebecca McKecknie, Lecturer, School of Exercise and Nutrition Sciences, Faculty of Health, Queensland University of Technology, Brisbane, Australia. She worked in community and public health nutrition, specializing in research, for nearly ten years. Her area of expertise is nutritional epidemiology with a focus on the measurement of diet and nutrition related concepts.

Jeffery Sobal, Professor, Nutritional Sciences, Cornell University, New York, USA. Jeffery is a Professor in the Division of Nutritional Sciences at Cornell University. He is a sociologist who uses multiple theoretical perspectives and quantitative and qualitative research methods to study and teach about food choice, body weight, commensality, built food environments, food systems, and family food relationships.

Helen Vidgen, Senior Research Fellow, School of Exercise and Nutrition Sciences, Faculty of Health, Queensland University of Technology, Brisbane, Australia. Helen has worked as a public health nutritionist in civil society, government and academic organizations for over twenty years. During this time she has been involved in the development of policy, programmes and evaluation. Her PhD thesis defined food literacy and its relationship to nutrition. She continues to work in this and other areas related to the everyday practicalities of meeting nutrition recommendations at the Queensland University of Technology.

Heather Yeatman, Professor, Public and Population Health, Head, School of Health and Society, University of Wollongong, Wollongong, Australia. Heather has extensive experience in public health, including food and nutrition policy, food labelling, food education programme evaluations, professional development and research translation. She has held numerous statutory appointments and is President, Public Health Association of Australia (2012–2016).

Preface

Helen Vidgen

I first came across the term 'food literacy' while working as a senior public health nutritionist in the corporate office of our State health department. My role there was as part of a small team of nutritionists who guided State government policy and investment. In 2007 we were conducting a midpoint review of our State's first public health nutrition strategy. This began with a review of existing investment and activity against the plan and was then followed by consultation with key stakeholders. A main gap described by practitioners and stakeholders was the need to address 'food literacy', a term that had not existed five years earlier when the document was written (Queensland Public Health Forum 2009). The original document, instead, referred to 'cooking skills', 'nutrition knowledge', and 'food skills' (Queensland Public Health Forum 2002).

As governments do, the next step was to find an existing food literacy pro-gramme used in another jurisdiction, and roll it out on a state-wide basis. The programme that was in their sights focused on budgeting, shopping and cooking for low income groups. Other practitioners looked to programmes focused on local food production, growing your own food, food labelling and providence. And celebrity chefs were knocking on the door of government for sponsorship. The food literacy agenda seemed very much influenced by one's personal experience with food and opinion of what were the significant antecedents to their self-defined 'healthy' relationship with food. As the only nutritionist in the team with both a home economics and dietetics background, I was concerned that we had missed out a few steps – most importantly, some process in determining what is food literacy? And then how does it influence what we eat?

With this in mind, I left the health department and began my PhD investi-gating precisely this. Part of my work was funded by my former employer, which meant practitioners and policy makers were involved in interpreting and contributing to my research. As intended, research links you with people around the world studying and working in related fields. The contributors to this book are these people. They come from a range of different countries where their work is applied both locally and further afield. They work in varying sectors such as health, education, consumer behaviour, food security, sustainable food ways and food policy. It is hoped that these varying perspec-tives will give the reader an introduction to the emerging concept of food literacy. This book aims to gather current insights and provide a platform for discussion to further understanding and application in this field. I hope this book stimulates you to conceptualize what food literacy means in your practice and critically review its potential contribution to a range of outcomes.

References

Queensland Public Health Forum 2002, *Eat Well Queensland 2002–2012: Smart Eating for a Healthier State*, Brisbane, viewed 22 September 2010, <http://www.health.qld.gov.au/qphf/documents/30434.pdf>.

Queensland Public Health Forum 2009, *Eat Well Queensland: Are We Half Way There Yet?* Midpoint Implementation Review, Queensland Public Health Forum, Brisbane, viewed 22 September 2010, <http://www.health.qld.gov.au/qphf/>.

1 Introduction

Food literacy for contemporary food and eating

Helen Vidgen

Globally, the food system, and the relationship of the individual to that system, continues to change and grow in complexity. Food is a basic human need in that it is essential for healthy growth and development. It has an important role to play in enhancing wellbeing and quality of life. In their definition of food ahead of the second International Congress on Nutrition, the Public Interest Civil Society Organizations acknowledge the broad contribution of food and nutrition in our lives by stating:

> It is our common understanding that food is the expression of values, cultures, social relations and people's self-determination, and that the act of feeding oneself and others embodies our sovereignty, ownership and empowerment. When nourishing oneself and eating with one's family, friends, and community, we reaffirm our cultural identities, our ownership over our life course and our human dignity. Nutrition is foundational for personal development and essential for overall wellbeing.
>
> (Public Interest Civil Society Organizations 2014: 2)

This definition recognizes the multiple dimensions of food and eating and the roles that it plays in the lives of individuals, households, communities, nations and globally.

Eating is an everyday event that is part of everyone's lives. While this seems a fairly unremarkable statement to make, it is important to ponder because it means that what we eat constantly changes in response to the changes in the world around us. These changes can be at the individual (e.g. changes in work status), household (e.g. changes in relationships and who is in the household), community (e.g. changes in the proximity of food retail outlets), national (e.g. changes in competition laws regarding supermarkets) and global levels (e.g. free trade agreements that open up markets to global multinational food companies). There is also a reciprocity in our response to these changes, in that they too change the world around us. As eating is a daily activity, our actions change the nature of food gradually, but constantly. For example, the increase in women's participation in the workforce has influenced the nature of domestic food work, urbanization has influenced the increase in food consumed outside the home and exposure to other foods and cultures through travel and the internet has influenced a greater diversity of food tastes and ingredients beyond traditional local cuisines.

There are many commentaries on the nature of these changes and their socio-cultural, environmental, educational, economic and health consequences. Authors describe a 'gastronomic revolution' (Bifulco & Caruso 2007: 2058), a 'culinary skills transition' (Lang & Caraher 2001: 2), the 'industrial eater' (Berry 1990), and the 'passive consumer, unwilling or unable to make informed decisions about the food they eat' (Begley & Gallegos 2010b: 26).

Irrespective of their paradigm, these commentaries all describe a period of rapid change in the past century. They assert that these changes have impacted on food intake, food preparation and rituals of eating. The commentaries differ in viewing these changes as a loss, a trend, a transition or an evolution; something that must be halted or something that must be adapted to. While it is true that there have been significant changes in how, what, when and with whom we eat, it is important to acknowledge that individuals, households, communities, nations and global factors have all had a part in shaping that.

Among this discussion, the term 'food literacy' has emerged. Its use in the literature, policy and practice implies that the term is an attempt to encapsulate the knowledge, skills and behaviours needed for everyday eating. This is echoed in contemporary public food and nutrition policies and plans through-out the world that have begun to recognize that these documents need to connect with the everyday practicalities of eating. The term is most often applied to the outcome of nutrition but is also applied to other food related outcomes, particularly environmental sustainability, informed consumerism, active citizenship and food security. This chapter will first review the use of the term in policy and practice, and then go on to review what is known about contemporary food and eating and its influence on the emergence of this term.

The use of the term in policy and practice

Food literacy in policy

Recent local, national and international nutrition policies and plans echo the sentiments of the practitioners they guide in calling for a renewed emphasis on the practical food aspects of nutrition and connecting nutrition messages with food solutions. The International Union of Nutrition Science's Giessen Declaration calls for a 'new nutrition science' that extends beyond a 'biological science' to include a comprehensive understanding of 'how food is grown, processed, distributed, sold, prepared, cooked and consumed' (International Union of Nutrition Sciences 2005). The Rome Declaration affirms the need for nutrition action to engage with all elements of the food system and for individuals, communities, governments and nations to have the knowledge and skills for informed action (Food and Agriculture Organization and World Health Organization 2014). The Public Interest Civil Society Organizations' definition of food described previously further supports this by recognizing the cultural and social position of nutrition within everyday food and eating.

This points to a broad set of knowledge, skills and behaviours that come into play when feeding individuals, communities and nations. The United Kingdom's *Foresight Report on Obesity*, the European Union's *Discussion Paper on Sustainable Food Consumption*, the Conference Board of Canada's *What's to Eat?* report and the United States Institute of Medicine's Committee on *Accelerating Progress in Obesity Prevention* report all use the term 'food literacy'; however, its meaning varies from its application to sustainable food to instruction on dietary guidelines in schools (Conference Board of Canada 2013; Glickman et al. 2012; Reisch, Lorek & Bietz 2011; Vandenbroeck, Goossens & Clemens 2007).

The Australian example demonstrates how food literacy is implicitly and explicitly expressed in food and nutrition policy. The *Australian Dietary Guidelines* identify 'low levels of food literacy' (National Health and Medical Research Council 2013: 8) as a possible barrier to compliance with these recommendations and as one of the significant social and environmental changes that have led to the increasing prevalence of overweight and obesity (National Health and Medical Research Council 2013). The Australian *National Food Plan* identified 'a food literate community accessing safe, affordable and nutritious food' as a key goal (Department of Agriculture, Fisheries and Forestries 2012). Consultation papers for the Australian Health and Physical Education Curriculum and National Food Policy attracted several submissions calling for a recognition of the practical skills aspects of healthy eating (Australian Curriculum and Assessment Reporting Authority 2012; Department of Agriculture, Fisheries and Forestries 2012). The *National Aboriginal and Torres Strait Islander Nutrition Strategy and Action Plan* identifies skills in cooking, budgeting and food selection, food preparation areas, storage facilities for food, cooking equipment and other health hardware as key issues to progress in order to improve nutritional status (Strategic Intergovernmental Nutrition Alliance 2001).

The practitioner context

Governments and practitioners are currently investing in strategies to address components of food literacy which they intuitively believe to be useful. Evaluation, if conducted, is often limited to process, such as use of recipes, and impact level, such as confidence in cooking and changes in awareness of nutrition recommendations (Herbert et al. 2014; Rees et al. 2012; Reicks et al. 2014). Food literacy is inconsistently defined and measured. The practical dimensions of everyday eating do not form part of any national monitoring or surveillance systems against which progress can be benchmarked.

In the health sector, food literacy work is undertaken by a range of practitioners, particularly nutritionists. However, what their role is in this space, what behaviours they can hope to modify and what outcome they are aiming to influence by addressing food literacy are unclear. As a result, nutritionists and their managers may not consider this very practical nutrition work legitimate

(Begley & Gallegos 2010a). This is despite the recognized need to support clients in the practicalities of following nutrition recommendations.

Addressing food literacy is likely to have benefits well beyond physical health both at an individual and community level. Outside the nutrition paradigm, food is used by a range of health, education and welfare service practitioners to build rapport, self-confidence, self-efficacy, empowerment and social inclusion. In the welfare sector food literacy is being addressed in the context of life skills for those experiencing multiple levels of disadvantage. Food literacy is likely to be both a risk factor and an asset for food security, but this relationship is unknown and unexplored. In the agriculture and food production sectors, food literacy is linked to the origins of food, including the environmental, ethical and ecological implications of food choice (Bellotti 2010; Farnworth, Thomas & Jiggins 2008). Gastronomes and governments in nations with more famous food cultures talk about maintaining or enhancing a food culture where food literacy includes an appreciation and understanding of flavour and quality, the pleasure and artistry of food production and convivial eating (Ministry of Agriculture and Fisheries n.d.; UNESCO 2010, 2013).

The public context

High profile advocates have weighed into the debate regarding optimal govern-ment investment in nutrition, most notably celebrity chef Jamie Oliver (Oliver 2010) and several other local examples (Alexander 2010). These programmes tend to extend the knowledge and skills of an already engaged client rather than shift the non-engaged (Flego et al. 2014). The effectiveness and sustainability of these substantial investments are yet to be established. It is particularly unclear if these programmes serve to contribute to the celebrity's brand rather than the health issue. What remains salient, however, is that interventions should not further marginalize and stigmatize disadvantaged groups but rather support the generation of a common healthy food culture of empowerment, sustainability and informed food citizenship. Food literacy needs to be framed as an essential life skill, irrespective of social class, which empowers an individual to take control over what they eat (Caraher & Lang 1999). This should reflect the different lives people live.

Beyond the nutrition paradigm

Acknowledging that nutrition is only one of the many outcomes of eating, it is interesting to consider the positioning of food literacy in public health nutrition strategies. Caraher warns against the linking of food literacy to only one agenda, such as obesity, as this diminishes its importance in the broader context and threatens to cut short investment in the area (Caraher & Seeley 2010). It may be that a nutrition outcome is not the most appropriate measurable end-point of food literacy. Nutrition may be better positioned as a consequential by-product on the way to meeting other more highly prioritized needs such as social connectedness, financial management, ecological sustainability or food security. The concept of sustainable diets may be a more useful outcome for food literacy (Burlingame & Dernini 2010).

Contemporary food and eating

Public policies, plans and practice aim to improve the lives of the people they serve. If food literacy is considered a resource for everyday life, then it is useful to reflect on what is known about contemporary food and eating. This following section reviews the evidence to support key themes that are reflected in the published use of the term food literacy.

Food and physical health

There is irrefutable evidence that the prevalence of overweight and obesity is high and has increased over time (Cook, Rutishauser & Seeling 2001; World Health Organization 2010). Increased food intake and decreased physical activity are established risk factors for overweight and obesity (World Health Organization 2010). Additionally, poor food choice impacts on non-communicable disease and overall wellbeing, independent of its contribution to body weight (National Health and Medical Research Council 2003). Non-communicable disease has now overtaken communicable disease with respect to global deaths (World Health Organization 2014). This is related to the poor nutritional quality of food rather than insufficient calories as had occurred previously. In low and middle income countries, this has been described as a 'nutrition transition' in which starvation is occurring alongside rapidly increasing rates of obesity. Globally, diets are consistently shifting away from these recommendations as core foods are replaced by high sugar, high fat, high salt, ready to eat processed foods (World Health Organization 2014).

Despite calls to consider social, cultural, economic and environmental systems, nutrition recommendations predominantly continue to remain within a biological frame (National Health and Medical Research Council 2011, 2013). In doing so, recommendations fail to acknowledge the 'day-to-dayness' of healthy eating. Diet-related disease typically develops over a lifetime of poor eating habits, and prevention, therefore, involves maintaining healthy habits over the long term (World Health Organization 2004). Consistency in diet quality over a lifetime is a critical element to the relationship between diet and health. It is implied in recommendations and practice, but not specifically and typically addressed. Food literacy may be a useful construct to describe the knowledge, skills and behaviours required to consistently meet food needs through change and over time.

Domestic food preparation

Nutritionists' interest in meal preparation, food skills and cooking is underpinned by the assumption that they will be associated with a higher intake of core foods, increased dietary variety and a greater control over the nutritional quality of foods eaten. Evidence to support the link between preparing food and diet quality comes predominantly from cross-sectional studies which aim to demonstrate an association between the two, and evaluation of cooking programmes. Both have their methodological problems which weaken the strength of this evidence. Most significant is the ability to consistently define what is meant by food preparation, and identify and measure the aspects which may influence diet quality.

Despite this, there is some evidence of the link between food preparation and healthy eating. Studies suggest a positive association between diet quality and food preparation, but this does not appear to extend to an association with healthy body weight. This is most often an increase in the self-reported number of fruit and vegetables and a decrease in the consumption of take-away foods (Crawford et al. 2007; Larson, Perry, et al. 2006).

Time spent preparing food has decreased in some but not all countries and still takes up more time than any other domestic task (Australian Bureau of Statistics 2008). The US *Time Use* survey reports that time spent preparing food has dropped. The greatest drop occurred between 1965 and 1992, with the time levelling from the mid-1990s to 2007. Interestingly, just over 50% of people were involved in any food preparation, despite all registering that they spent time eating (Bureau of Labor Statistics 2015). Food preparation continued to be predominantly done by women although this differential has reduced substantially.

The decision of who prepares meals tends to be based on expertise, enjoyment and fairness, rather than gender (Lupton 2000). The meal preparer tended to be the individual in the household who was better at it, liked it more, was more often home around meal times or was the main household manager (Lupton 2000). However, due to social and economic systems, women tend to more often meet these criteria (Blake et al. 2009; Schubert 2008).

Gender highlights the importance of context and broader social, cultural and economic systems. It also helps to describe the diversity of potential food literacy components, particularly beyond cooking. The dilution of gender roles in the provisioning of food may be a contributor to the emergence of the term food literacy. The knowledge, skills and behaviours used to meet food needs may not have been considered essential when this work was fundamentally only done by women.

The value and meaning of preparing food

Food preparation can be viewed as less about the end-product of the food or meal produced and more about the meaning of the process (Caraher & Lang 1999; Charles & Kerr 1988; DeVault 1991; Lang & Caraher 2001; Murcott 1982). Caraher identified that informal everyday meals were associated with convenience foods and fast foods, but special occasion meals involved some element of cooking, particularly from basic ingredients (Caraher, Baker & Burns 2004). Blake observed 'scripts' for evening meals which were dependent upon the specific eating context (Blake et al. 2008). The values which inform these scripts, such as nutrition, socialization and convenience, were also contextually driven. These findings reinforce the seminal work of Douglas and Murcott in describing the hierarchy of meals (Douglas 1972; Murcott 1982). These are important points to ponder when one is considering the various outcomes of enhanced food literacy. From a nutrition and environmental sustainability perspective, it is the day-to-day food intake that is of greater interest than special occasion eating. When one considers, however, the broader role of food in social wellbeing, this may also be an important part of food literacy. This differentiation in the value of meals and its relationship to their preparation is important to note when determining how confidence and ability to prepare food correspond with the frequency of actually performing these tasks.

The imperative to prepare food also has meaning for those who have experienced disadvantage. In a study of Bulgarian food habits as they transitioned from a communist economy to a free market economy, it was noted that despite tripling in food prices, employed people tended to spend less time preparing meals at home and were less likely to grow vegetables at home (Florkowski et al. 2000). The authors note that similar trends were observed in the former East Germany, Czech Republic and Hungary. While at the time of the study, food service and food processing industries in Bulgaria were minimal, it was anticipated that they would proliferate. Studies of the proliferation of street foods in Asia in the past century have linked it with growing informal economies and changes in family structures which saw women with less time to prepare traditional meals with multiple dishes and men going away from home for work (Dixon, Hinde & Banwell 2006). These changes could also be a result of greater autonomy and empowerment following economic freedom with its expression happening through food.

Commentators have noted the emergence of cooking as a 'leisure' activity rather than a daily task to explain the popularity of cooking shows and books. There is, however, no evidence to support that their increase in popularity has translated into an increase in everyday cooking. British data showed people spent less time in the kitchen on a day-to-day basis but did view cooking as 'enjoyable' and 'de-stressing' (Caraher & Lang 1999). In the Australian *Time Use* survey, Australians spent slightly more time preparing food on the weekend than on weekdays; this was particularly true for men (Australian Bureau of Statistics 2008). This indicates that weekend meals are determined for pleasure with greater preparation time allowed for, and weekday meals are determined by convenience with minimal preparation time. Convenience and pleasure also imply the presence of choice. Disadvantage is defined by the limitations of choice. The value and meaning of preparing food, and its relationship to diet quality, for these populations, therefore are likely to be influenced by their disadvantage.

Food preparation hardware

Access to the facilities and equipment, including fuel, will also influence the ability to prepare food (Bailie et al. 2010; Strategic Intergovernmental Nutrition Alliance 2001). Access to and use of food preparation equipment has been contrasted with other common food security strategies in a cross-sectional study of low income Indian households. This examined the relationship between food insecurity and foods grown for own use, use of soya (a locally available crop) and pressure cooker ownership (van Elsland et al. 2012). Of these three factors, pressure cooker ownership was most strongly protective against very low food security (compared with low food security) with this association remaining strong and statistically significant even after controlling for socio-economic status. The authors conclude that access to adequate equipment is a largely unexplored and under-utilized strategy in addressing food and nutrition security. Inadequate access to equipment or facilities is also likely to be of significance for those with unstable housing. Access to appropriate facilities and equipment may be an important policy issue for key housing and welfare agencies. Emergency accommodation, for example, is typically in hotels where equipment is limited to a kettle and possibly a small microwave oven which significantly limits the range of foods that can be prepared and their nutritional quality. For couch surfers, they often feed themselves in secret to keep themselves hidden from other household members and so cannot store food beyond a single eating occasion. In low and middle income countries the impact of facilities to prepare food is likely to be even more significant, particularly in the context of emergency and relief feeding (personal communication, World Food Programme and Red Cross).

Food supply

Globally there have been significant changes in the food supply and the extent to which dietary intake is made up of food prepared completely or partly outside the home. This is a reflection of shifts in both the food retail and food service sector. Data from the United States and Australia indicate that the majority of food consumed is still prepared in the home; however, the proportion of food consumed outside the home is growing (Smith, Ng & Popkin 2013).

Household Expenditure Survey data show expenditure on meals prepared outside the home is the single item that takes the biggest part of the Australian fortnightly food budget and that this has gone up significantly in the past twenty years (Australian Bureau of Statistics 2006a). The amount and proportion of household income spent on food consumed outside the home differ according to income. Households in the highest household income quintile spent around a third of their total food budget on foods eaten outside the home; this was double the proportion spent by those in the lowest quintile (Australian Bureau of Statistics 2006b). This could reflect the frequency of meals consumed outside the home or the cost of those meals.

There has also been an exponential increase in where food is available and the number of foods available to choose from. Supermarkets grew in high income countries in the 1950s, with this growth reaching low and middle income countries in South America in 1990s, Asia in the 2000s and more recently in Africa (Reardon & Berdegué 2006). This growth has been described as being driven by improved incomes, urbanization, female workforce participation, global media and time-poor consumers (Kelly et al. 2015). Free trade agreements and decreased regulation of foreign investment have further supported this growth, particularly in low and middle income countries (Hawkes 2005).

In Australia, between 1990 and 2008, the number of food and beverages products in a typical full service supermarket increased by 67% from 11,700 products to 19,540 (National Heart Foundation 2010). Supermarkets and hypermarkets are most competitive when they stock processed and packaged foods (Reardon & Berdegué 2006). Fresh foods, such as fruit and vegetables, are less profitable for this type of retailer (Kelly et al. 2015). Given that fresh foods are also those promoted for good health, it is likely that this dominance by supermarkets has created a dominance of processed and packaged foods in the everyday food supply. In low and middle income countries where the growth has been especially rapid, the health consequences are significant and alarming (Hawkes 2005; Kelly et al. 2014; Popkin 2004).

Clearly the increased consumption of foods prepared outside the home is real rather than perceived. The knowledge, skills and behaviours needed to meet nutrition recommendations, clearly, must interface with food prepared outside the home, as a reflection of contemporary food and eating. Food literacy as a term has evolved to reflect that this knowledge and skills must extend beyond food preparation.

The rituals of eating

Food intake is profoundly influenced by social and cultural meanings attached to food and eating. These include when, where and with whom certain foods and combinations of foods are eaten. This might broadly be described as the rituals of eating. Social commentators observing a 'gastronomic revolution' and the 'industrial eater' are as concerned with the changes in these aspects as they are with what is eaten (Berry 1990; Bifulco & Caruso 2007). Some authors cite the proliferation of the fast food and convenience food industries as applying new standards and expectations on eating; these include preparation speed, individual likes and dislikes being catered for within one sitting, consistency of end-product and the pace and environment of eating (Dixon, Hinde & Banwell 2006). Others describe an anomie or individualization of eating rituals resulting from an overabundance of rules about food, eating and nutrition (Fischler 1979; Kristensen & Holm 2006; Poulain 2002; Sobal 2006).

The relationship between these rituals and nutritional status is complex as their relative importance and value are culturally and socially constructed. Most studies which examine the relationship between the rituals of eating and nutrition focus on two aspects: daily eating structures, particularly meals and meal-times, and commensal eating. These aspects are related as the conceptualization and definition of meals often include people eating together.

Meals

How a meal is defined and what constitutes a meal have been the subject of much research. Meals in themselves have been defined by the rituals that surround them regarding what, when, how and with whom they are eaten (Douglas 1972; Murcott 1982).

Keeping to a conventional meal pattern is associated with taking care of your body (Kristensen & Holm 2006; Poulain 2002). Nutrition studies often assume that following a meal pattern means meals are planned for and are more likely to be healthy. It is proposed that people develop a script or flow chart of what procedures to follow in a particular context when preparing meals or making food choices (Bisogni et al. 2007); for example, the evening meal is surrounded by values of a time to connect with family and friends, a time for relaxation and separating from the working day (Blake et al. 2008). It is also proposed that having a consistent structure around eating such as planned eating occasions will result in a more conscious eater who can better monitor their intake.

Commensality

For many, thoughts of a 'proper meal' include not eating alone. The importance of sharing meals has been formally recognized in Japan's Shokuiku Food Law (Ministry of Agriculture and Fisheries n.d.), the Brazilian *Dietary Guidelines* (Primary Health Care Department 2014) and the UNESCO Heritage listings of the Mediterranean and French diets (UNESCO 2010, 2013).

Nutrition studies which examine commensality assume a relationship with healthy eating (Abbott et al. 2007; Demory-Luce et al. 2004; Larson et al. 2006). Findings of a US study are likely to be consistent in many countries in that most ate alone for breakfast, alone or with co-workers for lunch and the large majority ate dinner with others, usually co-habiting family. Around a quarter of people ate breakfast, lunch and dinner with others, around one seventh ate all of these meals alone (Sobal & Nelson 2003). A Danish study found that those who ate alone were less likely to plan their eating, more likely to control the amount of food they ate and more likely to eat high energy, low nutrient snack foods frequently throughout the day when compared to those who planned to eat together (Kristensen & Holm 2006). It should be noted that eating together does not always mean the food is prepared at home (Blake et al. 2009) and family meals might not mean all family members are present always (Gallegos et al. 2011). Sharing food is important in establishing and developing relationships. It can engage those who may otherwise be socially excluded or exclude and privilege groups and individuals (Sobal & Nelson 2003).

Conclusions

This chapter has introduced the use of the term food literacy in policy and practice. It has described key elements of contemporary food and eating that warrant particular consideration when conceptualizing food literacy. This book has been written at a time when this term is in its infancy. As editor, I have gathered researchers and practitioners, each working in different areas of food literacy, to present their thoughts on this emerging area.

This book begins with an overview of the use of the term in the literature, the history of its use in diverse paradigms and nations. Other terms used to describe the everyday practicalities of feeding yourself are also reviewed in considering what the term food literacy might add. Chapters 3 and 4 define the term and its components, and model its relationship to food intake and health status. These chapters are based on empirical research I conducted in two separate studies with food experts and then young people experiencing disadvantage. This definition and conceptualization is then further interrogated by examining its parallels with health literacy and its links with food choice in Chapters 5 and 6 respectively.

Food literacy is highly contextual and, as this chapter has explored, our contemporary food system is complex and not equally available to all people. In describing food literacy as the knowledge, skills and behaviours to meet food needs, the influence of broader social, economic, cultural and geographic factors must be acknowledged. In Chapter 7, food literacy is deconstructed to consider the development of personal knowledge, skills and behaviours from the perspective of both victim blaming and capacity building. Chapter 8 further explores the tensions between agency and systems by focusing on food literacy and food security.

The book then explores the development of food literacy. Three key settings of health, schools and food production are examined in more detail. Chapter 13 discusses the measurement of food literacy. In particular, what are the key considerations in developing a measure and what already exists that might be useful? We conclude with a conversation about what all the ideas presented in this book mean for practice and policy in food literacy. What are the key concepts to take away and what are the bits that still need wrestling with?

I hope this book is of use to both new and experienced practitioners. My aim was to gather key thinkers in this field to document their ideas in one spot, not in an effort to provide a definitive guide on food literacy but rather to create a starting point for further work in this area. Food literacy emerged as a term to acknowledge the broad role food and eating play in our lives and the empowerment that comes from meeting food needs well. The pioneers of this term used 'literacy' to convey that food and eating is at the centre of everyone's lives. It certainly is for the authors of this book! I hope you enjoy their contributions.

References

Abbott, R., Macdonald, D., Mackinnon, L., Stubbs, C., Lee, A., Harper, C. & Davies, P. 2007, *Healthy Kids Queensland Survey 2006 – Summary Report*, Queensland Health, Brisbane.

Alexander, S. 2010, *Stephanie Alexander Kitchen Garden Foundation*, viewed 22 September 2010, <http://www.kitchengardenfoundation.org.au/>.

Australian Bureau of Statistics 2006a, *6530.0 Household Expenditure Survey Australia 2003–4*, Commonwealth Government of Australia, viewed 30 September 2010, <http://www.abs.gov.au/AUSSTATS/abs@.nsf/DetailsPage/6535.0.55.0012003-04%20(Reissue)?OpenDocument>.

Australian Bureau of Statistics 2006b, *6535.0.55.001 Household Expenditure Survey Australia: Detailed Expenditure Items, 2003–04 (Reissue)*, Commonwealth Government of Australia, viewed 30 September 2010, <http://www.abs.gov.au/>.

Australian Bureau of Statistics 2008, *4153.0 How Australians Use their Time, 2006*, Australian Bureau of Statistics, viewed 30 September 2010, <http://www.abs.gov.au/AUSSTATS/abs@.nsf/Latestproducts/4153.0Main%20Features12006?opendocumentandtabname=Summaryandprodno=4153.0andissue=2006andnum=andview=>.

Australian Curriculum and Assessment Reporting Authority 2012, *Draft Shape of the Australian Curriculum: Health and Physical Education*, Commonwealth Government of Australia, Sydney, viewed 12 December 2012, <http://www.acara.edu.au/verve/_resources/DRAFT_Shape_of_the_Australian_Curriculum-HPE-FINAL.pdf>.

Bailie, R., Stevens, M., McDonald, E., Brewster, D. & Guthridge, S. 2010, 'Exploring cross-sectional associations between common childhood illness, housing and social conditions in remote Australian Aboriginal communities', *BMC Public Health*, vol. 10.

Begley, A. & Gallegos, D. 2010a, 'Should cooking be a dietetic competency?', *Nutrition and Dietetics*, vol. 67, no. 1, pp. 41–46.

Begley, A. & Gallegos, D. 2010b, 'What's cooking for dietetics? A review of the literature', *Nutrition and Dietetics*, vol. 67, no. 1, pp. 26–30.

Bellotti, B. 2010, 'Food literacy: reconnecting the city with the country', *Agricultural Science*, vol. 22, no. 3, pp. 29–34.

Berry, W. 1990, 'The pleasure of eating', Center for Ecoliteracy, viewed 10 December 2015, <http://www.ecoliteracy.org/essays/pleasures-eating>.

Bifulco, M. & Caruso, M.G. 2007, 'From the gastronomic revolution to the new globesity epidemic', *Journal of the American Dietetic Association*, vol. 107, no. 12, pp. 2058–2060.

Bisogni, C.A., Falk, L.W., Madore, E., Blake, C.E., Jastran, M., Sobal, J. & Devine, C.M. 2007, 'Dimensions of everyday eating and drinking episodes', *Appetite*, vol. 48, no. 2, pp. 218–231.

Blake, C.E., Bisogni, C.A., Sobal, J., Jastran, M. & Devine, C.M. 2008, 'How adults construct evening meals. Scripts for food choice', *Appetite*, vol. 51, no. 3, pp. 654–662.

Blake, C.E., Devine, C.M., Wethington, E., Jastran, M., Farrell, T.J. & Bisogni, C.A. 2009, 'Employed parents' satisfaction with food-choice coping strategies. Influence of gender and structure', *Appetite*, vol. 52, no. 3, pp. 711–719.

Bureau of Labor Statistics 2015, 'Time spent in primary activities and percent of the civilian population engaging in each activity, averages per day by sex, 2014 annual averages', United States Department of Labor, viewed 8 July 2015, <http://www.bls.gov/news.release/atus.t01.htm>.

Burlingame, B.A. & Dernini, S. 2010, 'Sustainable diets and biodiversity', in *International Scientific Symposium Biodiversity and Sustainable Diets United Against Hunger*, Rome, Italy.

Caraher, M., Baker, H. & Burns, M. 2004, 'Children's views of cooking and food preparation', *British Food Journal*, vol. 106, no. 4, p. 255.

Caraher, M. & Lang, T. 1999, 'Can't cook, won't cook: a review of cooking skills and their relevance to health promotion', *International Journal of Health Promotion and Education*, vol. 37, no. 3, pp. 89–100.

Caraher, M. & Seeley, A. 2010, 'Cooking in schools: lessons from the UK', *Journal of the Home Economics Institute of Australia*, vol. 17, no. 1, pp. 2–9.

Charles, N. & Kerr, M. 1988, *Women, Food and Families*, Manchester University Press, Manchester.

Conference Board of Canada 2013, *What's to Eat?: Improving Food Literacy in Canada*, viewed 8 July 2015, <https://appetite4change.files.wordpress.com/2013/12/cbofc-food-literacy.pdf>.

Cook, T., Rutishauser, I. & Seeling, M. 2001, 'Comparable data on food and nutrient intake and physical measurements from the 1983, 1985 and 1995 national nutrition surveys', Australian Food and Nutrition Monitoring Unit, Canberra, viewed 16 February 2016, <http://www.health.gov.au/internet/main/publishing.nsf/Content/health-pubhlth-strateg-food-pdf- comp-data-cnt>.

Crawford, D., Ball, K., Mishra, G.D., Salmon, J. & Timperio, A. 2007, 'Which food-related behaviours are associated with healthier intakes of fruits and vegetables among women?', *Public Health Nutrition*, vol. 10, no. 3, pp. 256–265.

Demory-Luce, D., Morales, M., Nicklas, T., Baranowski, T., Zakeri, I. & Berenson, G. 2004, 'Changes in food group consumption patterns from childhood to young adulthood: The Bogalusa Heart Study', *Journal of the American Dietetic Association*, vol. 104, no. 11, pp. 1684–1691.

Department of Agriculture Fisheries and Forestries 2012, *National Food Plan: Green Paper*, Department of Agriculture, Fisheries and Forestries, Canberra, viewed 19 December 2012, <http://www.daff.gov.au/__data/assets/pdf_file/0009/2175156/national-food- plan-green-paper-072012.pdf>.

Department of Agriculture Fisheries and Forestries 2013, *National Food Plan*, Department of Agriculture, Fisheries and Forestries, Canberra, viewed 23 June 2013, <http://www.daff.gov.au/__data/assets/pdf_file/0011/2293328/national-food-plan-white-paper.pdf>.

DeVault, M.L. 1991, *Feeding the Family*, University of Chicago Press, Chicago.

Dixon, J., Hinde, S. & Banwell, C. 2006, 'Obesity, convenience and "phood"', *British Food Journal*, vol. 108, no. 8, p. 634.

Douglas, M. 1972, 'Deciphering a meal', *Daedalus*, Winter.

Farnworth, C., Thomas, E. & Jiggins, J. 2008, 'Towards a new agenda', in C. Farnworth, J. Jiggins & E. Thomas (eds), *Creating Food Futures: Trade, Ethics and the Environment*, Gower Publishing Company, Aldershot, Hampshire.

Fischler, C. 1979, 'Gastro-nomie et gastro-anomie', *Communications*, vol. 31, pp. 189–210.

Flego, A., Herbert, J., Gibbs, L., Waters, E., Swinburn, B. & Moodie, M. 2014, *The Evaluation of Jamie's Ministry of Food, Ipswich: Final Evaluation Report*, Melbourne, <http://www.thegoodfoundation.com.au/wp-content/uploads/2010/08/Deakin-Study-2014-Jamies-Ministry-of-Food-Australia1.pdf>.

Florkowski, W.J., Moon, W., Resurreccion, A.V.A., Jordanov, J., Paraskova, P., Beuchat, L.R., Murgov, K. & Chinnan, M.S. 2000, 'Allocation of time for meal preparation in a transition economy', *Agricultural Economics*, vol. 22, no. 2, pp. 173–183.

Food and Agriculture Organization and World Health Organization 2014, *The Rome Declaration on Nutrition*, viewed 8 February 2015, <http://www.fao.org/3/a-ml542e.pdf>.

Gallegos, D., Dziurawiec, S., Fozdar, F. & Abernethie, L. 2011, 'Adolescent experiences of "family meals" in Australia', *Journal of Sociology*, vol. 47, no. 3, pp. 243–260.

Glickman, D., Parker, L., Sim, L.J., Del Valle Cook, H. & Miller, E.A. (eds) 2012, *Accelerating Progress in Obesity Prevention: Solving the Weight of the Nation*, National Academies Press Washington, viewed 10 December 2015, <http://www.nap.edu/op enbook.php?record_id=13275>.

Hawkes, C. 2005, 'The role of foreign direct investment in the nutrition transition', *Public Health Nutrition*, vol. 8, no. 04, pp. 357–365.

Herbert, J., Flego, A., Gibbs, L., Waters, E., Swinburn, B., Reynolds, J. & Moodie, M. 2014, 'Wider impacts of a 10-week community cooking skills program – Jamie's Ministry of Food, Australia', *BMC Public Health*, vol. 14.

International Union of Nutritional Sciences 2005, *The Giessen Declaration*, viewed 22 September 2010, <http://www.iuns.org/features/05-09%20NNS%20Declaration. pdf>.

Kelly, M., Seubsman, S., Banwell, C., Dixon, J. & Sleigh, A. 2015, 'Traditional, modern or mixed? Perspectives on social, economic, and health impacts of evolving food retail in Thailand', *Agriculture and Human Values*, vol. 32, no. 3, pp. 445–460.

Kristensen, S.T. & Holm, L. 2006, 'Modern meal patterns: tensions between bodily needs and the organization of time and space', *Food and Foodways: Explorations in the History and Culture of Human Nourishment*, vol. 14, no. 3, pp. 151–173.

Lang, T. & Caraher, M. 2001, 'Is there a culinary skills transition? Data and debate from the UK about changes in cooking culture', *Journal of the Home Economics Institute of Australia*, vol. 8, no. 2, pp. 2–14.

Larson, N.I., Perry, C.L., Story, M. & Neumark-Sztainer, D. 2006, 'Food preparation by young adults is associated with better diet quality', *Journal of the American Dietetic Association*, vol. 106, no. 12, pp. 2001–2007.

Larson, N.I., Story, M., Eisenberg, M.E. & Neumark-Sztainer, D. 2006, 'Food preparation and purchasing roles among adolescents: associations with sociodemographic characteristics and diet quality', *Journal of the American Dietetic Association*, vol. 106, no. 2, pp. 211–218.

Lupton, D. 2000, 'Where's me dinner? Food preparation arrangements in rural Australian families', *Journal of Sociology*, vol. 36, no. 2, pp. 172–186.

Ministry of Agriculture and Fisheries (n.d.) *What is 'Shokuiku (Food Education)'?*, Ministry of Agriculture and Fisheries, Tokyo, viewed 7 July 2015, <http://www.maff.go.jp/ e/pdf/shokuiku.pdf>.

Murcott, A. 1982, 'On the social significance of the "cooked dinner" in South Wales', *Social Science Information*, vol. 21, no. 4–5, pp. 677–696.

National Health and Medical Research Council 2003, *Dietary Guidelines for Australian Adults*, Commonwealth Department of Health and Ageing, Canberra, viewed 10 December 2015, <http://www.nhmrc.gov.au/_files_nhmrc/file/publications/synopses/ n33.pdf>.

National Health and Medical Research Council 2011, *A Review of the Evidence to Address Targeted Questions to Inform the Revision of the Australian Dietary Guidelines*, Commonwealth of Australia, Canberra, viewed 10 December 2015, <http://www.eatforhealth.gov.au/ sites/default/files/files/the_guidelines/n55d_dietary_guidelines_evidence_report.pdf>.

National Health and Medical Research Council 2013, *Australian Dietary Guidelines*, Commonwealth Department of Health and Ageing, Canberra, viewed 15 March 2013, <http://www.nhmrc.gov.au/_files_nhmrc/publications/attachments/n55_australian_ dietary_guidelines_0.pdf>.

National Heart Foundation 2010, *Consumer Behaviour Change*, National Heart Foundation of Australia, Canberra, viewed 24 March 2011, <http://www.heartfoundation.org.au/SITES/TICK/HEALTH_PROFESSIONALS/TICKPUBLICHEALTHIMPACT/Pages/ConsumerBehaviourChange.aspx>.

Oliver, J. 2010, *Jamie's Ministry of Food*, viewed 22 September 2010, <http://www.jamieoliver.com/jamies-ministry-of-food/>.

Popkin, B.M. 2004, 'The nutrition transition: an overview of world patterns of change', *Nutrition Reviews*, vol. 62, no. 7, pp. 140–143.

Poulain, J.P. 2002, 'The contemporary diet in France: "de-structuration" or from commensalism to "vagabond feeding"', *Appetite*, vol. 39, no. 1, pp. 43–55.

Primary Health Care Department 2014, *Dietary Guidelines for the Brazilian Population*, Brazil.

Public Interest Civil Society Organizations 2014, *Vision Statement for Nutrition*, viewed 8 February 2015, <http://www.fao.org/fileadmin/user_upload/faoweb/ICN2/documents/CSO_Vision_Statement_-_Final.pdf>.

Reardon, T. & Berdegué, J.A. 2006, *The Retail-led Transformation of Agrifood Systems and its Implications for Development Policies*, November 2006 edn, Rimisp-Latin American Center for Rural Development, viewed 13 July 2015, <https://openknowledge.worldbank.com/bitstream/handle/10986/9233/WDR2008_0033.pdf?sequence=1>.

Rees, R., Hinds, K., Dickson, K., O'Mara-Eves, A. & Thomas, J. 2012, *Communities that Cook: A Systematic Review of the Effectiveness and Appropriateness of Interventions to Introduce Adults to Home Cooking*, EPPI-Centre, Social Science Research Unit, Institute of Education, University of London.

Reicks, M., Trofholz, A.C., Stang, J.S. & Laska, M.N. 2014, 'Impact of cooking and home food preparation interventions among adults: outcomes and implications for future programs', *Journal of Nutrition Education and Behavior*, vol. 46, no. 4, pp. 259–276.

Reisch, L.A., Lorek, S. & Bietz, S. 2011, *CORPUS Discussion Paper 2 on Policy Instruments for Sustainable Food Consumption*, Brussels, European Commission, viewed 12 December 2012, <http://www.scp-knowledge.eu/sites/default/files/Food_Policy_Paper.pdf>.

Schubert, L. 2008, 'Household food strategies and the reframing of ways of understanding dietary practices', *Ecology of Food and Nutrition*, vol. 47, pp. 254–279.

Smith, L.P., Ng, S.W. & Popkin, B.M. 2013, 'Trends in US home food preparation and consumption: analysis of national nutrition surveys and time use studies from 1965–1966 to 2007–2008', *Nutrition Journal*, vol. 12, p. 45.

Sobal, J. 2006, 'Individualization of eating', *Appetite*, vol. 47, no. 3, p. 400.

Sobal, J. & Nelson, M.K. 2003, 'Commensal eating patterns: a community study', *Appetite*, vol. 41, no. 2, pp. 181–190.

Strategic Intergovernmental Nutrition Alliance 2001, *National Aboriginal and Torres Strait Islander Nutrition Strategy and Action Plan*, National Public Health Partnership, Canberra.

UNESCO 2010, *The Gastronomic Meal of the French*, United Nations, viewed 10 December 2015, <http://www.unesco.org/culture/ich/en/RL/gastronomic-meal-of-the-french-00437>.

UNESCO 2013, *Mediterranean Diet*, United Nations, viewed 7 July 2015, <http://www.unesco.org/culture/ich/RL/00884>.

van Elsland, S.L., van der Hoeven, M., Joshi, S., Doak, C.M. & Ponce, M.C. 2012, 'Pressure cooker ownership and food security in Aurangabad, India', *Public Health Nutrition*, vol. 15, no. 05, pp. 818–826.

Vandenbroeck, P., Goossens, J. & Clemens, M. 2007, *Foresight: Tackling Obesities: Future Choices – Obesity System Atlas*, Government Office for Science, London, viewed 12 December 2012, <http://www.bis.gov.uk/assets/foresight/docs/obesity/11.pdf>.

World Health Organization 2004, *Global Strategy on Diet, Physical Activity and Health*, World Health Organization, Geneva, viewed 14 June 2012, <http://www.who.int/dietphysicalactivity/strategy/eb11344/strategy_english_web.pdf>.

World Health Organization 2010, *Overweight and Obesity Facts Sheet*, World Health Organization, Geneva, viewed 29 September 2010, <http://www.who.int/media centre/factsheets/fs311/en/index.html>.

World Health Organization 2014, *Global Status Report on Noncommunicable Diseases 2014*, World Health Organization, Geneva, viewed 8 July 2015, <http://apps.who.int/iris/bitstream/10665/148114/1/9789241564854_eng.pdf?ua=1>.

2 An overview of the use of the term food literacy

Andrea Begley and Helen Vidgen

Introduction

The use of the term food literacy has emerged in an attempt to encapsulate the range of activities associated with eating food. Eating as a daily activity requires numerous thought and skill based applications to achieve and given its utility extends across many disciplines. Eating and its associated activities such as cooking are generally described as a mundane, ordinary activity in people's everyday lives and it is exactly this everydayness that makes it difficult to study, as people are not always aware of how they use knowledge and skills. Interest in food literacy has been most recently driven by evidence of poor dietary intakes and impact on health which has resulted in heightened anxiety about how people are feeding themselves.

Taking a health or biomedical focus is not that useful to describe collectively this knowledge and skills as they are innately associated with everyday life. A biomedical approach on its own may be counterproductive to attaining further health achievements, particularly with the way health practitioners communicate nutrition knowledge and skills (Bisogni et al. 2012). Food literacy has emerged as one of a range of literacies required for functioning in everyday life (Renwick 2013; Vidgen & Gallegos 2014). This focus places an emphasis on food not nutrition. While nutrition education focuses on food intake and how the body utilizes nutrients for growth, development, and health, food literacy has a wider scope that ranges across food management, planning, production, selection, preparation, and processing to food choice and eating.

The concept of food literacy has been proposed to have emerged from the conceptualization of the term health literacy. Nutbeam (2000) identified various stages of health literacy, ranging from basic everyday function to the application of social, personal and cognitive skills that enable individual empowerment over one's health (Nutbeam 2000). Nutbeam (2008) conceptualized health literacy as a key component of health promotion focused on the development of skills and capacities that enable people to exert greater control over their health and the range of personal, social and environmental determinants of health (Nutbeam 2008). The meaning of health literacy has been broadened to indicate both a skill and an enabler. These concepts and their application to food literacy are examined in more detail in Chapter 5.

Food, however, has greater benefits than just health. Food needs to be considered for the social and cultural connections it brings. It is largely agreed by researchers interested in the other roles that food plays in everyday life that food in general has been under-researched in the field of sociology and that the use of different paradigms will enable a broader view (Germov & Williams 2008; Mennell, Murcott & van Otterloo 1992).

This chapter aims to describe the various terms used in the academic literature that are conflated with the broad intent of the term food literacy. In the past five years, the use of the term has increased significantly in both the literature and in practice. We begin this chapter with a history of the use of the term and a review of its published use currently. We will describe the use of other terms and justify why these are not sufficient in their own right.

Published use of the term food literacy

The first locatable published use of the term food literacy is from 1990 in an American Dietetic Association (Committee on Labor and Human Resources 1990) response to a Senate enquiry into food labelling. The term is not defined and is used in the following manner:

> ADA believes that nutrition information on food labels, as addressed in S 1425, and in food advertising, government by the FTC, can improve the food literacy of Americans.
>
> (Committee on Labor and Human Resources 1990: 107)

It does not appear as though the term was widely used at the time. Perhaps the representative before the Senate made it up on the spot! There are few examples of its use in the 1990s (Demas 1998; Solin & Dalton 1997).

The first paper that defined the term appeared in 2001 (Kolasa et al. 2001). It defined food literacy as:

> The capacity of an individual to obtain, interpret and understand basic food and nutrition information and services as well as the competence to use that information and services in ways that are health enhancing.
>
> (Kolasa et al. 2001: 2)

The paper was written by dietitians and describes a programme developed as part of a range of responses by the local health area to overweight and obesity in adults. The programme involved community volunteers working with food stamp recipients. The definition extends a health literacy definition developed by the local area's Joint Committee on National Health Education Standards replacing the word 'health' with 'food and nutrition'. Throughout the paper, the term is used interchangeably with 'nutrition education'. This narrow, individualistic use of the term, which implies that a lack of knowledge is responsible for high rates of obesity, has evolved over time.

The term is now used throughout the world. In English speaking countries it is particularly used in Canada (Colatruglio 2015; Department of Health and Wellness 2012; Desjardins & Azevedo 2013; Howard & Brichta 2013), Australia (Department of Agriculture, Fisheries and Forestries 2013; National Health and Medical Research Council 2013; Public Health Association of Australia 2009), the United States (Glickman et al. 2012; Joshi et al. 2014) and to a lesser extent in the United Kingdom (European Union Committee 2011; Macdiarmid et al. 2011). It is difficult to accurately determine its use in non-English speaking countries, but publications containing the term have been written by authors from Korea (Kim & Lee 2014), Malaysia (Ibrahim & Ahmad 2014), China (Lai-Yeung 2015), India (Pailoor 2012), Mexico (Acevedo-Rojas 2015), Germany (Dreas & Hassel 2010), Italy (Bifulco & Caruso 2007; Vezzosi, Carruci & Picciolli 2014), Spain (España, Cabello Garrido & Blanco López 2014), Austria (Sedlacko, Reisch & Scholl 2013), Sweden (Anderson 2014; Brunosson et al. 2014), Denmark (Benn 2014; Coff & Kemp 2014), Belgium (Prové 2013), Finland (Närvänen, Saarijärvi & Simanainen 2013), Hungary (Baumbach 2012), Malta (Piscopo 2015), Nigeria (Onyene & Bakare 2011) and in documentation by the European Union (BEST Institut für berufsbezogene Weiterbildung und Personal Training 2006) and World Bank (Shrimpton & Rokx 2013).

Table 2.1 shows the use of the term in academic publications, specifically journal articles, academic books and theses, over time. This results from a search for the term 'food literacy' in Google Scholar, Quick Find, Eric, PubMed and CINAHL. No date restrictions were applied and included the term in any part of the publication. References were checked, and duplicates and grey literature such as reports, magazines and news articles were excluded. From 2011 to 2013, several publications offer definitions of the term, but this is less common in more recent years where publications are more likely to cite one of these definitions or assume a common understanding of the term.

The term food literacy has been used in publications across a range of sectors, particularly health, education, life skills and sustainability. It is perhaps an attempt by these sectors to describe the totality of food and eating rather than focus on just one purpose, e.g. health. Table 2.1 lists published definitions of the term from 1999 to 2014. Despite the increased use of the term, it continues to be inconsistently applied and understood. Definitions vary considerably in the range of knowledge, skills and behaviours they consider food literacy to include. They are common in describing food literacy at an individual level. The danger of food literacy being considered only as a function of the individual, resulting in victim blaming and drawing attention away from well-established political, social and economic determinants of health, is discussed in more detail in Chapters 7 and 8. Despite the increased use of the term, the definition developed by Vidgen and Gallegos remains the only one based on empirical data. This data and how it contributed to the definition is detailed in Chapter 3.

Table 2.1 Published definitions of the term food literacy

Source	Definition
(Kolasa et al. 2001: 2)	'the capacity of an individual to obtain, interpret and understand basic food and nutrition information and services as well as the competence to use that information and services in ways that are health enhancing.'
(Probst 2006: xxiii)	'The level of understanding of foods and their nutrient interactions.'
(Drummond & Caraher 2007: eprint)	'Food literacy comprises knowledge, skills and capacities to grow, select, store, prepare, cook and serve food.'
(Von Sehlen 2007: 51)	'means educating all people about the food system, making apparent and meaningful the role they play within the system, and the effect the food system has on their lives, in an effort to encourage wide-spread, informed participation as a "food citizen" in a "food democracy".'
(Vandenbroeck, Goossens & Clemens 2007: 40)	'Degree to which people are able to assess nutritional quality and provenance.'
(Farnworth, Thomas & Jiggins 2008: 231)	'food literacy is not just about the physical origin of food but also about the social context and quality of life aspirations of those who produce it. If consumers have not grasped this then they will not have achieved food literacy ... food literacy is not just a matter of factual knowledge about the origin of food. Food literacy involves an enmeshment of one's life with the process of growth. This instils a deep sense in "things", a sense that has been largely lost in the modern world.'
(Bellotti 2010: 29, 34)	'"Food Literacy" is described as a concept involving three main domains: food, nutrition and health; agriculture, environment and ecology; and social development and equity.' 'Food literacy provides a framework for rediscovering our relationship with food, learning how our food choices impact on our health, our environment, and on the businesses and communities that provide our food.'
(Schlegel et al. 2010: 187)	'the understanding and motivation to act on the interrelated social, economic, and ecological dimensions of food production, distribution, preparation, consumption, and waste management, recognising the roles of individuals, communities, and societies at local to global scales.'
(Stinson 2010: 2)	'a deeper understanding of the complex environmental and social components of food in our lives.'

Source	Definition
(Block et al. 2011: 7, 8)	'Food literacy entails both understanding nutrition information and action on that knowledge in ways consistent with promoting nutrition goals and food wellbeing.... The conceptual or declarative component of food literacy involves reading and acquiring knowledge about food, food sources, nutrition facts and other knowledge acquisition and apprehension activities involving food and nutrition. In contrast, procedural knowledge involves applying such knowledge to food decision making, including food shopping and preparation skills. Procedural knowledge involves the development of food scripts. ... The development of food literacy involves the ability, opportunity, and motivation to identify, understand, interpret, communicate and use information about food in various contexts.'
(Bublitz et al. 2011: 3)	'Food literacy expands traditional measures of nutrition knowledge to include not only what people know about food but also their ability to use that information to facilitate higher levels of food wellbeing. Food literacy ranges from declarative knowledge (e.g. knowing what asparagus is and what types of nutrients asparagus might provide) to procedural knowledge (e.g. how to cook this vegetable).'
(Fordyce-Voorham 2011: 119)	'Food literacy was seen mainly as an individual's ability to read, understand, and act upon labels on fresh, frozen, canned, frozen, processed, and takeout food.'
(Pendergast, Garvis & Kanasa 2011: 418)	'More recently, the term "food literacy" as a component of health literacy has emerged, adopting the three levels generally used in the health schema. That is, an amalgamation of functional, interactive, and critical dimensions of food and nutrition that collectively can be described as food literacy.'
(Thomas & Irwin 2011: 2)	'the ability to make healthy food choices by having the skills and knowledge necessary to buy, grow and cook food with implications for improving health.'
(Vaughan 2011: 191)	'Food literacy refers to the participants' engagement with food including its preparation; knowledge about where food is sourced from, and familiarity with traditional foods as well as new foods experienced in the UK.'
(Chambers 2012: 4)	'food literacy encompasses using basic food preparation knowledge that has been learned, understood, and practiced to make better food decisions.'
(Vrhovnik 2012: 12)	'the ability to read and understand food information.'

Table 2.1 (continued)

Source	Definition
(Slater 2013: 623)	'Functional *food literacy*: basic communication of credible, evidence-based food and nutrition information, involving accessing, understanding and evaluating information. Interactive *food literacy*: development of personal skills regarding food and nutrition issues, involving decision making, goal setting and practices to enhance nutritional health and well-being. Critical *food literacy*: respecting different cultural, family and religious beliefs in respect to food and nutrition (including nutritional health), understanding the wider context of food production and nutritional health, and advocating for personal, family and community changes that enhance nutritional health.'
(Moe 2014: 62)	'*Food literacy* refers to food knowledge, including the food system, nutrition, and food preparation.'
(Vidgen & Gallegos 2014: 54)	'*Food literacy* is the scaffolding that empowers individuals, households, communities or nations to protect diet quality through change and strengthen dietary resilience over time. It is composed of a collection of inter-related knowledge, skills and behaviours required to plan, manage, select, prepare and eat food to meet needs and determine intake.'

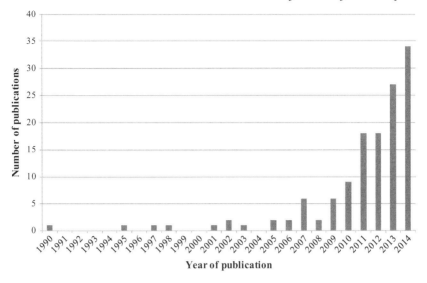

Figure 2.1 Use of the term food literacy in academic literature from 1990 to 2014

Other terms used to describe food knowledge, skills and behaviours

This section will expand on a range of terms used to indicate the knowledge and skills required for eating that have been used in the academic literature but have limitations for describing the scope of the intent that using food literacy entails. In many instances these terms are used without much problematizing as to their meanings. The terms to be explored are cooking, cooking skills, food skills, food provisioning, foodwork, food wellbeing, nutrition literacy and other constructs.

Cooking

Eating is associated with the term cooking and this term is often used to reflect the basic activities undertaken for people to feed themselves. Traditional dictionary definitions of cooking refer to the conversion of raw material into cooked food with the use of fire or heat. The *Macquarie Dictionary* defines the verb 'to cook' as to prepare (food) by the action of heat, as by boiling, baking, roasting, etc. Used as a noun, the word means someone who cooks, someone whose occupation is the preparation of food for the table. Cookery is seen as the art or practice of cooking (*Macquarie Dictionary* 2008). These definitions in themselves are limiting for research into the conceptualization of cooking skills for health; for example, when trying to promote the increased consumption of vegetables, this would appear to exclude salads.

It may be that given the pervasive nature of cooking, many authors and researchers overlook the possible meanings of cooking as an everyday practice.

A review of definitions used in the literature uncovers diverse descriptions of cooking. For example, Symons (2002) has considered cooking as a method that enhances nutritional properties and pleasure of food but has more broadly proposed that 'cooking is the organization and provision – that is, the production – of meals, and the essence of this is food distribution' (Symons 2002: 435).

Symons poses the question 'what's cooking?' in an attempt to provide a specific definition. This definition focuses on the process of cooking and the technical skills required. Others allude to the need to consider a broader view than just the traditional ideal of cooking from scratch, which usually is described as taking raw, basic or unprocessed foods and transforming these into a meal or snack as opposed to opening packages and reheating meals/snacks, which is seen as meal assemblage (Stead et al. 2004). A more recent description of cooking emphasizes a broad perspective and suggests that cooking should be considered as 'any process that involves some level of transformation of foodstuffs' (Meah & Watson 2011: 1). Other authors take a more sociological view of cooking as 'the making of food' (Furst 1997: 442), for example: 'Cooking … is a process – a source of pleasure, a means of exercising skill – not simply a collection of ingredients or taste' (Duruz 2000: 289).

This view of cooking as a source of 'pleasure' implies a privileging of those with time and resources to enjoy cooking. There is an assumption that cooking is satisfying and rewarding (Bittman 2011). Short (2006) concludes from her research with several middle income households in the United Kingdom that cooking has ambiguous meanings. Short's research demonstrates that some people see cooking as the verb form, for example, the preparation of food, and others see cooking as the adjectival form, describing a domestic task.

In conclusion, the use of the term 'cooking' to encapsulate the range of activities associated with eating food is likely to be misinterpreted and narrowed to specific activities that are unlikely to represent the broad intention of food literacy. What is clear from research on this topic is that cooking is an important part of a food literacy approach.

Cooking skills

The interest in cooking from a variety of sectors is related to the concern that practices are changing due to a decline and/or devaluing of skills resulting in a loss of skills and potentially a changing set of skills driven by the food supply. Skills are described as 'embodied' activities: they are not visible until put into practice and they take time to develop. Much of human activity is constituted by skills and the way people incorporate knowledge (Sun, Merrill & Peterson 2001). Education theory defines various stages that people progress through to develop skills in an area. In the acquisition of declarative knowledge, the first step is acquiring the explicit knowledge of how to perform the task, and once a skill is practised, then people are reliant on procedural or implicit knowledge, whereby they can extend their skills into other areas like problem solving. Through continual engagement with food, some people build an internal consciousness related to the knack or feel of food that is combined with senses of taste, smell and sounds of cooking (Jaffe & Gertler 2006). This type of consciousness is evident in people who may not learn to cook at home but develop cooking skills through other means. This is what Giard refers to as a sense of culinary consciousness in 'doing cooking' in research on everyday life (Giard 1998: 153). Over time, it would be expected that cooking skills would be reconfigured as part of ongoing skill development.

Skills develop through formal learning such as home economics, and informal learning such as observing in the home. They enable people to experiment and try new foods and develop confidence related to food. Cooking skills, although an important set of skills required to feed oneself, are not sufficient on their own. There are many other skills needed, particularly for contemporary food and eating which includes many eating occasions and foods prepared outside the home. It is therefore important that cooking is not conflated with food literacy.

Food skills

The focus on skills has led some researchers and programme developers to refer to a collective set of skills as food skills or food. Conceptualizing the skills related to food recognizes a range of practical activities that need to be undertaken to eat.

Used in a home economics sense to break down the mechanics for teaching purposes or what are referred to as microskills (Fordyce-Voorham 2009, 2011), food skills in this sense are defined as 'the process of purchasing, preparing and cooking food materials (ingredients) using available resources to produce well-balanced and tasty meals appropriate to the age and needs of the individuals consuming them' (Fordyce-Voorham 2009).

Research with food experts in Australia documented food skills as a collection of aspects of knowledge, information, skills and resources. The focus on microskills is important from a home economics perspective in teaching cooking and other food skills but does not capture the macro level influences on eating.

Foodwork

Sociological discourses on food skills substitute this term as 'food work' (Beagan et al. 2008; Bove & Sobal 2006; Foley 2010; Sydner et al. 2007; Szabo 2013). Foodwork is a reference to the domestic set of chores associated with feeding households and families and therefore is seen as women's work (Wright, Maher & Tanner 2015) or feminized labour (Beagan et al. 2008). Foodwork is one such complex of practices, here understood as referring to all the tasks associated with planning, purchasing, storing, cooking and preparing food, as well as related tasks such as washing up and clearing away (Meah 2014). Szabo (2013) distinguishes between foodwork and foodplay as a gender divide, reflecting how men may engage with cooking. Given the gender implications of this term it is less useful in trying to encapsulate the knowledge and skills required for feeding oneself. There is also no explicit relationship of this term to the knowledge and skills required to choose healthy foods by considering nutrition.

Food provisioning

There are several references to the concept of food provisioning as a way of recognizing the work required to feed individuals and households (Bava, Jaeger & Park 2008; Slater et al. 2011). The term was first used by DeVault in her seminal work and defined as the broad scope of activities entailed in feeding the self and others, including shopping, gardening, farming, bartering, cooking and serving, and providing an essential link between markets and home (DeVault, 1991). Specifically, other authors use the term food provisioning to refer to the 'life cycle of food' outlined by Goody (1982) and which captures the process from food acquisition through to cleaning up (see also Table 2.2).

Neysmith and Reitsma-Street also use the term food provisioning to capture this domestic work representing 'the work of securing resources and providing the necessities of life to those for whom one has relationships of responsibility' (Neysmith and Reitsma-Street 2004: 383). The limitation of this use of the term to encapsulate the knowledge and skills required is that food provisioning strategies are seen as different for working and non-working people, particularly mothers. Time use surveys described in Chapter 1 demonstrate that whilst there are changes, domestic chores are still primarily done by women in traditional households. Food provisioning is a gender specific term as it is seen as the role of women and applied at a household level. These are valid applications of the term but limit its usefulness in describing an array of knowledge and skills for all the population. The use of this term has been criticized for focusing on individual responsibility, unpaid work, the potential to place guilt on women, or over-emphasize the emotional labour of food provisioning (Koch 2015). It also focuses on the eating within a household, and not on the knowledge and skills to choose foods outside the home, prepared by others including the food industry.

Food wellbeing

Wellbeing is a broad concept which lacks a single definition; however, it is important to consider how people perceive wellbeing in relation to food decisions. Wellbeing as a notion has only recently found its way into public policy. Block et al. (2011) document food literacy as one of five constructs

Table 2.2 Steps in food provisioning process

Step	Activity
Acquisition	Going to supermarket, purchasing grocery items
Preparation	Peeling, chopping, blanching, etc. of meal components
Cooking	Boiling, baking, roasting, etc. of meal components
Eating	Meal consumption
Disposal	Cleaning up, freezing and storing leftovers, etc.

Marshall (1995)

including food availability, policy, socialization and marketing but describe this as being built from the concept of health literacy. The authors propose a restructuring of the 'food as health' paradigm to 'food as well-being'. This requires shifting from an emphasis on restraint and restrictions to a more positive, holistic understanding of the role of food in overall wellbeing. Food wellbeing is defined as a positive psychological, physical, emotional and social relationship with food at both individual and societal levels (Block et al. 2011); however, it is most strongly associated with physical wellbeing (Ares et al. 2014).

Drawing principally from the capabilities approach as described by Fleuret and Atkinson (2007), wellbeing can be considered to arise through the utilization of competencies and skills that enable a positive engagement with the social and cultural aspects of everyday life. This means that an association between food and wellbeing arises when the person develops a food involvement that enhances their sense of having a flourishing, pleasurable engagement with and through the social and cultural context of their everyday life (Hooper, Ivory & Fougere 2015). Other research has also emphasized that important elements in the use of this term are the positive emotions and pleasure and emotional aspects related to food (Ares et al. 2015). A feature of some of the conceptualization of food literacy is the emphasis on the enjoyment or pleasures around cooking, eating and experiencing food as an aspect (Schnögl et al. 2006) which highlights the importance of the cultural, social and emotional factors that need to be considered.

There is a clear need to consider how food literacy might contribute to wellbeing (Deer et al. 2014), but the use of food wellbeing as a term has been to capture five primary domains: food socialization, food literacy, food marketing, food availability, and food policy (Block et al. 2011). This conceptualization highlights the need for research that bridges other disciplines and paradigms outside and within health.

Nutrition literacy

There are only a few papers in the literature that refer to nutrition literacy (Cornish & Morres 2015; Guttersrud et al. 2014; Harley et al. 2013; Silk et al. 2008). It is described as the capacity to obtain, process and understand nutrition information and the materials needed to make appropriate decisions regarding one's health and nutrition decisions (Guttersrud et al. 2014). Nutrition literacy can be defined similarly to health literacy. The focus on the term nutrition literacy is an acknowledgement that deciphering nutrition information is clearly challenging (Murimi 2013). Some form of nutrition literacy is likely to be one part of the overall food literacy required in everyday life.

Other constructs

In attempts to label or define the required knowledge and skills for everyday eating, the importance of considering psychological constructs is also important.

Primary constructs such as confidence, self-efficacy and resilience are associated with the ability to select, prepare and eat a healthy and acceptable meal. Self-efficacy has long recognized importance in public health nutrition as the belief in one's capabilities under action to succeed in selecting and eating a healthy diet. Bandura recognized that high self-efficacy enables people to attempt complex behaviour change and be willing to potentially try behaviour change several times before success (Bandura 1977). Dietary resilience focuses on the development and use of adaptive strategies to maintain diet quality through change. This may include prioritizing eating well, doing whatever it takes to keep eating well, being able to do it yourself, and getting help when you need it.

Conclusions

The use of the term food literacy has increased exponentially but at the same time there is a lack of empirical research on what food literacy actually is and how it relates to health outcomes and other aspects of everyday life. The search for a term to encapsulate the knowledge and skills required to eat has uncovered no single reality or truth about these activities. What is evident is that there is richness to the activities constructed from multiple realities in a wide variety of disciplines. Much of the other terminology used applies to aspects of food literacy, for example cooking.

Given the changing food environment and the economic power of the food industry, it would seem that improved food literacy empowers individuals to make informed food choices (Lang et al. 1999). Caraher and Lang refer to food literacy as necessarily life or citizenship skills (Lang & Caraher 2001). Without food literacy, the consumer becomes reliant on the food industry to define their eating options. Food literacy may be a key 'protective factor' that supports an individual or a community in making healthy food choices (Vidgen & Gallegos 2010). However, food literacy is often trivialized or assumed, as it can be missing from conceptual food and nutrition systems (Heywood & Lund-Adams 1991), strategic plans and population nutrition monitoring and surveillance systems. To improve health and a number of other outcomes, it is clear that a common term and meaning would assist research, practice and policy initiatives. Research into food literacy may also help to re-orientate practice and policy initiatives.

References

Acevedo-Rojas, N.I., Dávalos-Flores, J.L.Torres-Torres, F. 2015, 'Importance of certified quality of bovine milk for consumer of the metropolitan area of México city', *Agrociencia*, vol. 49, no. 1, pp. 101–112.

Anderson, M. 2014, 'Building community capacity through urban agriculture', Master of Science in Environmental Management and Policy thesis, Lund University, viewed 20 February 2015, <http://lup,lub.lu.se/uur/download?func=downloadFile&recordOId= 4697730>.

Ares, G., De Saldamando, L., Giménez, A., Claret, A., Cunha, M., Guerrero, L., Pinto De Moura, A., Oliveira, D., Symoneaux, R. & Deliza, R. 2015, 'Consumers' associations with wellbeing in a food-related context: a cross cultural study', *Food Quality and Preference*, 40.

Ares, G., De Saldamando, L., Gimenez, A. & Deliza, R. 2014, 'Food and wellbeing. Towards a consumer-based approach', *Appetite*, vol. 74, no. 1, pp. 61–69.

Bandura, A. 1977, 'Self-efficacy: toward a unifying theory of behavioral change', *Psychological Review*, vol. 84, pp. 191–215.

Baumbach, L.K. 2012, 'Urban food production: A contribution to urban food resilience in Berlin?', Master of Science thesis, Central European University, Budapest, viewed 12 December 2012, <http://www.etd.ceu.hu/2012/baumbach_lea.pdf>.

Bava, C.M., Jaeger, S.R. & Park, J. 2008, 'Constraints upon food provisioning practices in "busy" women's lives: trade-offs which demand convenience', *Appetite*, vol. 50, no. 2–3, pp. 486–498.

Beagan, B., Chapman, G., D'sylva, A. & Bassett, B. 2008, '"It's just easier for me to do it': Rationalising the family division of foodwork', *Sociology*, vol. 42, pp. 653–671.

Bellotti, B. 2010, 'Food literacy: reconnecting the city with the country', *Agricultural Science*, vol. 22, no. 3, pp. 29–34.

Benn, J. 2014, 'Food, nutrition or cooking literacy: a review of concepts and competencies regarding food education', *International Journal of Home Economics*, vol. 7, no. 1, pp. 13–35.

BEST Institut für berufsbezogene Weiterbildung und Personal Training 2006, *Savoury Dishes for Adult Education and Counselling: Food Literacy Guidelines and Toolbox*, European Commission, Vienna.

Bifulco, M. & Caruso, M.G. 2007, 'From the gastronomic revolution to the new globesity epidemic', *Journal of the American Dietetic Association*, vol. 107, no. 12, pp. 2058–2060.

Bisogni, C., Jastran, M., Seligson, M. & Thompson, A. 2012, 'How people interpret healthy eating: contributions of qualitative research', *Journal of Nutrition Education and Behavior*, vol. 44, no. 4, pp. 282–301.

Bittman, M. 2011, *Cooking Solves Everything: How Time in the Kitchen Can Save Your Health, Your Budget, and Even the Planet*, itunes edn, Bytliner, San Francisco.

Block, L.G., Grier, S.A., Childers, T.L., Davis, B., Ebert, J.E.J., Kumanyika, S., Laczniak, R.N., Machin, J.E., Motley, C.M., Peracchio, L., Pettigrew, S., Scott, M. & van Ginkel Bieshaar, M.N.G. 2011, 'From nutrients to nurturance: a conceptual introduction to food well-being', *Journal of Public Policy & Marketing*, vol. 30, no. 1, pp. 5–13.

Bove, C. & Sobal, J. 2006, 'Foodwork in newly married couples', *Food Culture & Society*, vol. 9, pp. 69–89.

Brunosson, A., Brante, E., Sepp, H. & Mattsson Sydner, Y. 2014, 'To use a recipe – not a piece of cake. Students with mild intellectual disabilities' use of recipes in home economics', *International Journal of Consumer Studies*, vol. 38, no. 4, pp 412–18.

Bublitz, M.G., Peracchio, L.A., Andreasen, A.R., Kees, J., Kidwell, B., Miller, E.G., Motley, C.M., Peter, P.C., Rajagopal, P., Scott, M.L. & Vallen, B. 2011, 'The quest for eating right: advancing food well-being', *Journal of Research for Consumers*, no. 19, pp. 1–12.

Chambers, C. 2012, 'A pilot study: the use of a survey to assess the food knowledge of nutrition students at various levels of nutrition education', Master of Science thesis, University of Nebraska, Lincoln, viewed 12 December 2012, <http://digitalcommons.unl.edu/cehsdiss/151/>.

Coff, C. & Kemp, P. 2014, 'Food Ethics and Policies', in P.B. Thompson & D.M. Kaplan (eds), *Encyclopedia of Food and Agricultural Ethics*, Springer, Netherlands, pp. 1–8, viewed 16 February 2016, <http://dx.doi.org/10.1007/978-94-007-6167-4_149-1>.

Colatruglio, S. 2015, 'Understanding food literacy from perceptions of young Canadian adults: a qualitative study', Master of Science thesis, University of Manitoba, Winnipeg, viewed 10 December 2015, <http://mspace.lib.umanitoba.ca/bitstream/1993/30169/1/Colatruglio_Sarah.pdf>.

Committee on Labor and Human Resources 1990, *Nutrition Labeling and Education Act of 1989: Hearing before the Committee on Labor and Human Resources, United States Senate*, by Committee on Labor and Human Resources, First Session edn, U.S. Government Printing Office, Washington DC, viewed 10 December 2015, <http://hdl.handle.net/2027/mdp.39015042569072>.

Cornish, L. & Moraes, C. 2015, 'The impact of consumer confusion on nutrition literacy and subsequent dietary behaviour', *Psychology & Marketing*, vol. 32, no. 5, pp. 558–574.

Deer, F., Falkenberg, T., McMillan, B. & Sims, L. 2014, *Sustainable Well-Being Concepts, Issues and Educational Practices*, ESWB Press, Manitoba, Canada.

Demas, A. 1998, 'Low-fat school lunch programs: achieving acceptance', *American Journal of Cardiology*, vol. 82, no. 10, supplement 2, pp. 80–82.

Department of Agriculture, Fisheries and Forestries 2013, *National Food Plan*, Canberra, viewed 23 June 2013, <http://www.daff.gov.au/__data/assets/pdf_file/0011/2293328/national-food-plan-white-paper.pdf>.

Department of Health and Wellness 2012, *Thrive: A Plan for a Healthier Nova Scotia*, Province of Nova Scotia, viewed 10 December 2015, <https://thrive.novascotia.ca/sites/default/files/Thrive-Strategy-Document.pdf>.

Desjardins, E. & Azevedo, E. 2013, *Food Literacy for Life*, The Locally Driven Collaborative Project, Ontario, viewed 13 June 2014, <http://www.osnpph.on.ca/resources/Food%20Literacy%20Study.LDCPOntario.Final.Dec2013.pdf>.

DeVault, M. 1991, *Feeding the Family: The Social Organisation of Caring as Gendered Work*, Chicago University Press, Chicago.

Dreas, J.A. & Hassel, H. 2010, 'What accounts for good practice? Assessment of obesity prevention projects for kindergarten children in Germany', *Journal of Public Health*, vol. 18, no. 2, pp. 145–152.

Drummond, C.E. & Caraher, M. 2007, 'The imperative for consultation and involvement in child nutrition research: adding perspectives from qualitative research', in L. Carter (ed.), *Child Nutrition Research Advances*, Nova Science Publications, Hauppauge, NY, viewed 10 December 2015, <http://openaccess.city.ac.uk/474/4/caraher-drummond_chap_NOVA.pdf>.

Duruz, J. 2000, 'A nice baked dinner…or two roast ducks from Chinatown? Identify grazing', *Continuum*, vol. 14, no. 3, pp. 289–301.

España, E., Cabello Garrido, A. & Blanco López, Á. 2014, 'A framework for developing food competence in compulsory education', *Enseñanza de las ciencias*, vol. 32, pp. 611–629.

Farnworth, C., Thomas, E. & Jiggins, J. 2008, 'Towards a new agenda', in C. Farnworth, J. Jiggins & E. Thomas (eds), *Creating Food Futures: Trade, Ethics and the Environment*, Gower Publishing Company, Aldershot, Hampshire.

Fleuret, S. & Atkinson, S. 2007, 'Wellbeing, health and geography: a critical review and research agenda', *New Zealand Geographer*, vol. 63, pp. 106–118.

Foley, W. 2010, 'Family food work: lessons learned from urban Aboriginal women about nutrition promotion', *Australian Journal of Primary Health*, vol. 16, pp. 268–274.

Fordyce-Voorham, S. 2009, 'Essential food skills required in a skill-based healthy eating program', *Journal of the Home Economics Institute of Australia*, vol. 16, no. 2, pp. 16–20.

Fordyce-Voorham, S. 2011, 'Identification of essential food skills for skill-based healthful eating programs in secondary schools', *Journal of Nutrition Education and Behavior*, vol. 43, no. 2, pp. 116–122.

Furst, E. 1997, 'Cooking and femininity', *Women's Studies International*, vol. 20, no. 3, pp. 441–449.

Germov, J. & Williams, L. 2008, 'Introducing the social appetite: towards a sociology of food and nutrition', in J. Germov & L. Williams (eds), *A Sociology of Food and Nutrition: The Social Appetite*, 3rd edn, Oxford University Press, South Melbourne.

Giard, L. 1998, 'Doing-Cooking', in M. de Certeau, L. Giard & P. Mayol (eds), *The Practice of Everyday Life*, University of Minnesota Press, Minnesota.

Glickman, D., Parker, L., Sim, L.J., Del Valle Cook, H. & Miller, E.A. (eds) 2012, *Accelerating Progress in Obesity Prevention: Solving the Weight of the Nation*, National Academies Press, Washington, viewed 10 December 2015, <http://www.nap.edu/openbook.php?record_id=13275>.

Goody, J. 1982, *Cooking, Cuisine and Class: A Study in Comparative Sociology*, Cambridge University Press, Cambridge.

Guttersrud, O., Dalane, J.O. & Pettersen, S. 2014, 'Improving measurement in nutrition literacy research using Rasch modelling: examining construct validity of stage-specific "critical nutrition literacy" scales', *Public Health Nutrition*, vol. 17, no. 4, pp. 877–883.

Harley, A., Zilber, J., Lemke, M. & Kingery, L. 2013, 'Youth chef academy: results from a cooking and nutrition literacy program for middle-school students piloted in an urban, public school system', American Public Health Association, 141st Annual General Meeting, Boston.

Heywood, P. & Lund-Adams, M. 1991, 'The Australian Food and Nutrition System: a basis for policy formulation and analysis', *Australian Journal of Public Health*, vol. 14, no. 4, pp. 258–270.

Hooper, C., Ivory, V. & Fougere, G. 2015, '"Dinner's ready!": a qualitative exploration of the food domain across the lifecycle', *Appetite*, vol. 92, pp. 133–142.

House of Lords 2011, *Innovation in EU Agriculture: 19th Report of Session 2010–12*, European Union Committee, vol. 171, Stationery Office, viewed 12 December 2012, <http://www.publications.parliament.uk/pa/ld201012/ldselect/ldeucom/171/171.pdf>.

Howard, A. & Brichta, J. 2013, *What's to Eat? Improving Food Literacy in Canada*, The Conference Board of Canada, Canada, viewed 16 February 2016, <https://appetite4change.files.wordpress.com/2013/12/cbofc-food-literacy.pdf>.

Ibrahim, M.B. & Ahmad, N.B. 2014, 'Review of peri-urban agricultural concept and its place in solving food crisis of developing countries: a community development approach', *Africa Development and Resources Research Institute Journal*, vol. 5, no. 2, pp. 1–19.

Jaffe, J. & Gertler, M. 2006, 'Victual vicissitudes: consumer deskilling and the (gendered) transformation of food systems', *Agriculture & Human Values*, vol. 23, no. 2, 143–162.

Joshi, A., Henderson, T., Ratcliffe, M. & Feenstra, G. 2014, *Evaluation for Transformation: A Cross-Sectoral Evaluation Framework for Farm to School*. National Farm to School Network, Chicago, viewed 10 December 2015, <http://www.farmtoschool.org/Resources/Evaluation_Transformation_FINAL-Web.pdf>

Kim, J.-W.. and Lee, E.-J. 2014, 'Evaluation of dietary habits and dietary life competency of elementary school students', *Journal of Korean Practical Arts Education*, vol. 27, no. 4, pp. 17–37.

Koch, S. 2015, 'Leave a bowl of fruit on the kitchen table': the missing work of food provisioning in food and nutrition policy in the United States, *Social Currents*, vol. 2, pp. 231–238.

Kolasa, K., Peery, A., Harris, N. & Shovelin, K. 2001, 'Food literacy partners program: a strategy to increase community food literacy', *Topics in Clinical Nutrition*, vol. 16, no. 4, pp. 1–10.

Lai-Yeung, T. 2015, 'Hong Kong parents' perceptions of the transference of food preparation skills', *International Journal of Consumer Studies*, vol. 39, no. 2, pp. 117–124.

Lang, T. & Caraher, M. 2001, 'Is there a culinary skills transition? Data and debate from the UK about changes in cooking culture', *Journal of the Home Economics Institute of Australia*, vol. 8, no. 2, pp. 2–14.

Lang, T., Caraher, M., Dixon, P. & Carr-Hill, R. 1999, *Cooking Skills and Health*, Health Education Authority, London.

Macdiarmid, J.I., Loe, J., Douglas, F., Ludbrook, A., Comerford, C. & McNeill, G. 2011, 'Developing a timeline for evaluating public health nutrition policy interventions. What are the outcomes and when should we expect to see them?', *Public Health Nutrition*, vol. 14, no. 4, pp. 729–739.

Macquarie Dictionary 2008, *The Macquarie Dictionary Online* Macquarie Dictionary Publishers Pty Ltd., Sydney, viewed 29 August 2008, <http://www.macquariedictionary.com.au/begley@9191788078647/-/p/thes/index.html>.

Marshall, D.W. 1995, 'Introduction: Food choice, the food consumer and food provisioning', in D.W. Marshall (ed.), *Food Choice and the Consumer* (pp. 1–17). Blackie Academic & Professional, London.

Meah, A. 2014, 'Reconceptualising power and gendered subjectivities in domestic cooking spaces', *Progress in Human Geography*, vol. 38, no. 5, pp. 671–690.

Meah, A. & Watson, M. 2011, 'Saints and slackers: challenging discourses about the decline of domestic cooking', *Sociological Research Online*, vol. 16 no. 2.

Mennell, S.J., Murcott, A. & van Otterloo, A. 1992, *The Sociology of Food: Eating, Diet and Culture*, Sage Publications, London.

Moe, J.L. 2014, 'Hard to stomach: food insecurity and inequitable access to nutritious food in Vancouver', Master of Public Policy thesis, Simon Fraser University, British Columbia.

Murimi, M. 2013, 'Healthy literacy, nutrition education, and food literacy', *Journal of Nutrition Education and Behavior*, vol. 45, no. 3, p. 195.

Närvänen, E., Saarijärvi, H. & Simanainen, O. 2013, 'Understanding consumers' online conversation practices in the context of convenience food', *International Journal of Consumer Studies*, vol. 37, no. 5, pp. 569–576.

National Health and Medical Research Council 2013, *Australian Dietary Guidelines*, Commonwealth Department of Health and Ageing, Canberra, viewed 15 March 2013, <http://www.nhmrc.gov.au/_files_nhmrc/publications/attachments/n55_australian_dietary_guidelines_0.pdf>.

Neysmith, S., Reitsma-Street, M. 2005, '"Provisioning": conceptualizing the work of women for 21st century social policy', *Women's Studies International Forum*, vol. 28, no. 5, pp. 381–391.

Neysmith, S., Reitsma-Street, M., Collins, S. & Porter, E. 2004, 'Provisioning. Thinking about all of women's work', *Canadian Women Studies*, vol. 23, pp. 192–198.

Nutbeam, D. 2000, 'Health literacy as a public health goal: a challenge for contemporary health education and communication strategies into the 21st century', *Health Promotion International*, vol. 15, no. 3, pp. 259–267.

Nutbeam, D. 2008, 'The evolving concept of health literacy', *Social Science and Medicine*, vol. 67, no. 12, pp. 2072–2078.

Onyene, V. & Bakare, T.V. 2011, 'Women in post harvest management of food production in Nigeria', *Journal of Stored Products and Postharvest Research*, vol. 2, no. 16, pp. 292–300.

Pailoor, A. 2012, 'Magic of millets', *Appropriate Technology*, vol. 39, no. 1, pp. 18–20.

Pendergast, D., Garvis, S. & Kanasa, H. 2011, 'Insight from the public on home economics and formal food literacy', *Family and Consumer Sciences Research Journal*, vol. 39, no. 4, pp. 415–430.

Piscopo, S. 2015, 'Are food convenience and sustainable consumption mutually exclusive?', in V.W. Thoresen, D. Doyle, J. Klein and R.J. Didham (eds), *Responsible Living: Concepts, Education and Future Perspectives*, Springer International Publishing, New York, pp. 197–215.

Probst, Y.C. 2006, *An Evaluation of Automated Dietary Assessment: A Case Study into the Development, Implementation and Evaluation of Computer-Assisted Survey Technology as an Adjunct to Professional Dietary Consultation*, Doctor of Philosophy thesis, University of Wollongong.

Prové, C. 2013, 'Did you Say Urban Agriculture in Ghent? An Exploratory Case-study', Master of Science in Nutrition and Rural Development thesis, University of Ghent, viewed 20 December 2015, <http://lib.ugent.be/fulltxt/RUG01/002/063/690/RUG01-002063690_2013_0001_AC.pdf>.

Public Health Association of Australia 2009, *A Future for Food: Addressing Public Health, Sustainability and Equity from Paddock to Plate*, Public Health Association of Australia, Deakin.

Renwick, K. 2013, 'Food literacy as a form of critical pedagogy: implications for curriculum development and pedagogical engagement for Australia's diverse student population', *Victoria Journal of Home Economics*, vol. 52, no. 2, pp. 6–17.

Schlegel, W., Reynolds, H.L., Getty, V.M., Henshel, D. & Reidhaar, J.W. 2010, 'Food for thought: a multidisciplinary faculty grassroots initiative for sustainability and service-learning', in H. Reynolds, E. Brondizio & J. Robinson (eds) *Teaching Environmental Literacy: Across Campus and Across the Curriculum*, Scholarship of Teaching and Learning Series, Indiana University Press, Bloomington, IN.

Schnögl, S., Zehetgruber, R., Danninger, S., Setzwein, M., Wenk, R., Freudenberg, M., Muller, C. & Groeneveld, M. 2006, *Savoury Dishes for Adult Education and Counselling: Food Literacy Guidelines and Toolbox*, BEST Institut, Vienna.

Sedlacko, M., Reisch, L. & Scholl, G. 2013, 'Sustainable food consumption: When evidence-based policy making meets policy-minded research. Introduction to the special issue', *Sustainability: Science, Practice, & Policy*, vol. 8, pp. 1–6.

Short, F. 2006, *Kitchen Secrets. The Meaning of Cooking in Everyday Life*, Berg Publishers, New York.

Shrimpton, R. & Rokx, C. 2013, *Double Burden of Malnutrition: A Review of Global Evidence*, The International Bank for Reconstruction and Development/The World Bank, Washington DC, viewed 20 December 2015, <http://www-wds.worldbank.org/external/default/WDSContentServer/WDSP/IB/2013/07/15/000445729_20130715150604/Rendered/PDF/795250WP0Doubl00Box037737900PUBLIC0.pdf>.

Silk, K.J., Sherry, J., Winn, B., Keesecker, N., Horodynski, M.A. & Sayir, A. 2008, 'Increasing nutrition literacy: testing the effectiveness of print, web site, and game modalities', *Journal of Nutrition Education and Behavior*, vol. 40, no. 1, pp. 3–10.

Slater, J. 2013, 'Is cooking dead? The state of Home Economics Food and Nutrition education in a Canadian province', *International Journal of Consumer Studies*, vol. 37, no. 6, pp. 617–624.

Slater, J., Sevenhusen, G., Edginton, B. & O'Neil, J. 2011, '"Trying to make it all come together"; structuration and employed mothers' experience of family food provisioning in Canada', *Health Promotion International*, vol. 27, no. 3, pp. 405–415.

Solin, M.S. & Dalton, S. 1997, 'Knowledge of food identification, food preparation techniques, and attitudes toward the professional need for food skills of registered dietitians and dietetic students', *Journal of the American Dietetic Association*, vol. 97, no. 9, supplement 1, pp. A104-A.

Stead, M., Caraher, M., Wrieden, W., Longbottom, P., Valentine, K. & Anderson, A. 2004, 'Confident, fearful and hopeless cooks. Findings from the development of a food-skills initiative', *British Food Journal*, vol. 106, no. 4, pp. 274–287.

Stinson, E. 2010, 'Eating the world: food literacy and its place in secondary school classrooms', Master of Education thesis, University of Victoria, Canada.

Sun, R., Merrill, E. & Peterson, T. 2001, 'From implicit skills to explicit knowledge: a bottom-up model of skill learning', *Cognitive Science*, vol. 25, pp. 203–244.

Sydner, Y.M., Sidenvall, B., Fjellström, C., Raats, M. & Lumbers, M. 2007, 'Food habits and foodwork: the life course perspective of senior Europeans', *Food, Culture and Society: An International Journal of Multidisciplinary Research*, vol. 10, pp. 367–387.

Symons, M. 2002, 'Cutting up cultures', *Journal of Historical Sociology*, vol. 15, no. 4, pp. 431–448.

Szabo, M. 2013, '"I'm a real catch": the blurring of alternative and hegemonic masculinities in men's talk about home cooking', *Women's Studies International Forum*, vol. 44, pp. 228–235.

Thomas, H.M.C. & Irwin, J.D. 2011, 'Cook It Up! A community-based cooking program for at-risk youth: overview of a food literacy intervention', *BMC Research Notes*, vol. 4, no. 495, pp. 1–7.

Vandenbroeck, P., Goossens, J. & Clemens, M. 2007, *Foresight: Tackling Obesities: Future Choices – Obesity System Atlas,*, Government Office for Science, London, viewed 12 December 2012, <http://www.bis.gov.uk/assets/foresight/docs/obesity/11.pdf>.

Vaughan, L.T. 2011, 'A socio-cultural study investigating the influences on food and lifestyle choices, and the cultural transition, of British Bangladeshis living in Tower Hamlets East London', PhD in Food Policy thesis, City University, viewed 20 December 2015, <http://openaccess.city.ac.uk/1158/1/Vaughan%2C_Lisa.pdf>.

Vesnaver, E., Keller, H.H., Payette, H. & Shatenstein, B. 2012, 'Dietary resilience as described by older community-dwelling adults from the NuAge study "if there is a will there is a way!"', *Appetite*, vol. 58, no. 2, pp. 730–738.

Vezzosi, S., Carruci, M. & Picciolli, P. 2014, 'Traditional food systems. Harmony in Tuscany', *World Nutrition*, vol. 5, no. 10, pp. 870–883.

Vidgen, H. & Gallegos, D. 2010, 'Food literacy: time for a new term or just another buzzword?', *Journal of the HEIA*, vol. 17, no. 2, pp. 2–8.

Vidgen, H.A. & Gallegos, D. 2014, 'Defining food literacy and its components', *Appetite*, vol. 76, pp. 50–59.

Von Sehlen, J.A. 2007, 'Beyond organic: defining alternatives to USDA certified organic', University of Montana, Missoula, viewed 20 December 2015, <http://scholarworks.umt.edu/cgi/viewcontent.cgi?article=1113&context=etd>.

Vrhovnik, L. 2012, 'A pilot study for the development of a food skills survey tool', Master of Science thesis, Queen's University, Ontario, viewed 20 December 2012, <https://catspaw.its.queensu.ca/handle/1974/7323>.

Wright, J., Maher, J. & Tanner, C. 2015, 'Social class, anxieties and mothers' foodwork', *Sociology of Health and Illness*, vol. 37, no. 3, 422–436.

3 A definition of food literacy and its components

Helen Vidgen

Introduction

This chapter and the next report the findings of two qualitative research studies undertaken to define food literacy, including its components, and model its relationship to nutrition. The two studies were undertaken in 2010 and 2011 as part of my PhD thesis. The first was a Delphi study of Australian food experts (n=43) and the second was a study of young adults across a spectrum of disadvantage (n=37). This chapter expands on data reported in Vidgen & Gallegos (2014).

Defining food literacy and identifying its components was an iterative process. Grounded theory was used to code themes that emerged from the data. The results of both studies were considered separately and then compared to each other. In this way, each study informed the other. At various points throughout the research, interim findings were also 'tested' and discussed with practitioners to see if they were useful in informing their work in food literacy. Vidgen (2014) describes the methodology in more detail. This chapter instead will focus on the results and describe the components of food literacy, the data used to identify them and how they combined to produce a definition of food literacy.

The identification of food literacy components by food experts

Participants in the Food Experts Delphi Study came from nutrition, food industry, agriculture, retail, gastronomy, welfare and education sectors. They were practitioners, policy makers, advocates and academics. The study was made up of three rounds, starting with individual telephone interviews, the results of which were then used to develop surveys that went out to participants in the subsequent two rounds to measure their level of agreement with key food literacy concepts. During individual semi-structured interviews, food experts were asked what they needed to know and understand about food to use it to meet their needs, and whether this differed from the set of knowledge, skills and behaviours needed to meet nutrition needs. They were asked about the relative importance of cooking, their use and understanding of the term 'food literacy', the application of health literacy constructs of 'functional, interactive and critical literacy', and programmes and practitioners that they considered were addressing food literacy.

A broad range of eighty potential components of food literacy were described by food experts in their individual interviews (see Table 3.1). These were grouped into eight domains of access, planning and management, selection, knowing where food comes from, preparation, eating, nutrition and language. The words used by food experts to describe these components were retained so as to keep their meaning as much as possible. These eighty components were then collectively presented to the same food experts in a survey where they were asked to rate each of these components as either 'irrelevant', 'core' (need to know) or 'desirable' (nice to know). At least 75% of the experts agreeing was considered to represent consensus. There was very little agreement on potential components in the second round survey. Frequencies are reported in Table 3.1. Of the eighty possible components of food literacy presented, only six achieved consensus. They are highlighted in the table. Participants were then given a third chance to rate the remaining statements in another survey when one more statement achieved consensus. The breadth of views from food experts on what food literacy includes reinforces the need for an empirically generated and agreed definition.

Experts found it difficult to identify core components without a particular context applied. Few items of knowledge, skills and behaviours were considered critical in all contexts. Components were also considered to be interdependent. That is, the absence of one component may require the strengthening of another. For example, if food preparation skills were poor and the individual relied on food prepared by others, understanding food origins may become more important.

After this study, published food literacy interventions were reviewed by a nutritionist external to the research to test the face validity of findings, that is, to see if they were useful in describing the sorts of work that practitioners typically consider to be 'food literacy' (Cullerton, Vidgen & Gallegos 2012). The reviewer categorized the elements of each intervention into the food literacy component domains identified in the Expert Study. The results demonstrated that food literacy domains identified in the Expert Study were consistent with what practitioners more broadly considered to be part of food literacy. This review revealed that interventions rarely address all domains of food literacy. Furthermore, addressing all domains within the one intervention did not appear to be necessary. Individuals are likely to be at different levels of ability within each domain. It may be more effective for practitioners to work with clients to explore which domains require greater focus as determined by the individual and their context. These findings all contributed to an overall conceptualization and definition of food literacy which is described later in this chapter.

Table 3.1 Identification of food literacy components and percentage agreement by food experts (consensus defined as at least 75% agreement)

Domain	Food literacy components identified in round one (n=43) (Components that experts agreed were 'core' are highlighted. Those receiving the highest 'irrelevant' scores are bolded)	Round two % agreement (n=34)			Round three % agreement (n=24)
		Irrelevant	Core	Desirable	Core
1. Access	1.1. Being able to find food anywhere, that you can eat.	23.5	50.0	26.5	50.0
	1.2. Being able to access food through some source on a regular basis with very limited resources.	14.7	**79.4**	5.9	
	1.3. Knowing that some places are cheaper than others.	23.5	17.7	58.8	
	1.4. Knowing how to access the shop, how to access the funds to purchase what you require and the knowledge in regards to if it's not coming from a shop for example, bush foods, aid agencies.	5.9	64.7	29.4	62.5
	1.5. Getting out in the garden and growing food, even if it's herbs in a pot.	**50.0**	2.9	47.1	
	1.6. Being critical of the food supply system and being able to advocate for improvements.	**50.0**	11.8	38.2	

Table 3.1 (continued)

Domain	Food literacy components identified in round one (n=43) (Components that experts agreed were 'core' are highlighted. Those receiving the highest 'irrelevant' scores are bolded)	Round two % agreement (n=34)			Round three % agreement (n=24)
		Irrelevant	Core	Desirable	Core
2. Planning and management	2.1. Looking forward about what you are going to be eating and how to access that.	11.8	61.8	26.5	37.5
	2.2. Planning ahead to make sure you meet your nutrition requirements.	14.7	52.9	32.4	37.5
	2.3. Knowing quantities of food to buy so that nothing's wasted.	5.9	41.2	52.9	
	2.4. The ability to handle and manage money.	14.7	58.8	26.5	50.0
	2.5. Knowing which foods fill your belly so that everyone has got something to eat. What food goes the furthest and costs the least.	11.8	44.1	44.1	
	2.6. Being able to plan in terms of how long something's going to take to prepare.	14.7	47.1	38.2	
	2.7. Being able to choose foods that are within your skill set and available time.	8.8	**76.5**	14.7	
	2.8. Consuming food in the context of the total responsibilities placed on individuals and also within families.	17.7	52.9	29.4	37.5
	2.9. Parenting skills; some sort of ability to talk to their family and say 'no' and be able to moderate their intake.	20.6	50.0	29.4	29.2

Domain	Food literacy components identified in round one (n=43) (Components that experts agreed were 'core' are highlighted. Those receiving the highest 'irrelevant' scores are bolded)	Round two % agreement (n=34)			Round three % agreement (n=24)
		Irrelevant	Core	Desirable	Core
3. Selection	3.1. Understanding how the foods that are grown influence the environment and how our food choices influence the environment and also the other way around. How climate change is going to influence what we eat.	20.6	29.4	50.0	
	3.2. Knowing the environmental, social and ethical consequences of the ways in which foods are produced, packaged and distributed.	23.5	35.3	41.2	
	3.3. Knowing how to choose culturally and socially acceptable food. So I'm not going to be stigmatized because I've chosen a particular food and not others.	29.4	32.4	38.2	
	3.4. Being able to critically judge advertisements, promotions, marketing and everything that's coming your way.	2.9	67.7	29.4	70.8
	3.5. Having the critical skills so that when a new food comes onto the market you're able to make an informed decision about it.	2.9	73.5	23.5	54.2
	3.6. Being able to judge the quality of raw and processed food which might include freshness and how does the price compare to other times in the year.	5.9	58.8	35.3	58.3

Table 3.1 (continued)

Domain	Food literacy components identified in round one (n=43) (Components that experts agreed were 'core' are highlighted. Those receiving the highest 'irrelevant' scores are bolded)	Round two % agreement (n=34)			Round three % agreement (n=24)
		Irrelevant	Core	Desirable	Core
	3.7. Choosing native and seasonal foods in keeping with where you live.	17.7	29.4	52.9	
	3.8. Knowing how to read the labels but also being able to read what's not on the label.	8.8	58.8	32.4	50.0
	3.9. Being able to read the nutrition information panel and how to use the per 100g versus the per serve column and compare.	8.8	47.1	44.1	
	3.10. Being able to understand what the ingredient list means.	5.9	58.8	35.3	37.5
	3.11. Having enough English language literacy skills to understand what the food is.	5.9	61.8	32.4	41.7
	3.12. Being able to understand what's in the product and how to store and use it.	0.0	73.5	26.5	**79.2**
	3.13. Being able to read the label and understand that information in context.	0.0	58.8	41.2	54.2

Domain	Food literacy components identified in round one (n=43) (Components that experts agreed were 'core' are highlighted. Those receiving the highest 'irrelevant' scores are bolded)	Round two % agreement (n=34)			Round three % agreement (n=24)
		Irrelevant	Core	Desirable	Core
4. Knowing where food comes from	**4.1. Getting down and dirty, experience food, plant it, grow it, harvest it, prepare it, eat it.**	**35.3**	11.8	52.9	
	4.2. Just being able to look at a processed food and know what's in it so you might be able to categorize what it is. Being able to recognize what would have been the primary form of that food.	14.7	44.1	41.2	
	4.3. Some knowledge of where the food came from and what resources were required for its production. Was this healthy, sustainable or ethical?	23.5	32.4	44.1	
	4.4. Trusting your food supply.	23.5	35.3	41.2	
	4.5. Knowing where your food was farmed.	**35.3**	14.7	50.0	
	4.6. Being aware of the broader political, ecological and social contexts in which the food is grown.	32.4	17.7	50.0	
	4.7. Having enough food preparation experience to know what might have gone into a food or dish.	11.8	44.1	44.1	

Table 3.1 (continued)

Domain	Food literacy components identified in round one (n=43) (Components that experts agreed were 'core' are highlighted. Those receiving the highest 'irrelevant' scores are bolded)	Round two % agreement (n=34)			Round three % agreement (n=24)
		Irrelevant	Core	Desirable	Core
5. Preparation	5.1. Knowing how to prepare foods in a way that's attractive and edible.	8.8	70.6	20.6	70.8
	5.2. Knowing what tastes and flavours go together.	8.8	38.2	52.9	
	5.3. Knowing how to follow a recipe.	5.9	55.9	38.2	37.5
	5.4. Being able to make four to six meals by yourself that you can repeat week in week out.	20.6	41.2	38.2	
	5.5. Knowledge of some basic commodities and how to prepare them.	0.0	**82.4**	17.7	
	5.6. Knowing how to prepare some foods from all of the food groups, for example, how to prepare meat, how to cook pasta, how to prepare vegetables and then there are spin-offs from there.	2.9	**79.4**	17.7	
	5.7. Knowing how to prepare the same foods that you have access to in different ways so that they're interesting.	5.9	35.3	58.8	
	5.8. Having a whole repertoire of skills so you can try more adventurous recipes, make up your own recipe or cooking style, adapt things to suit your preferences and equipment.	20.6	20.6	58.8	

Domain	Food literacy components identified in round one (n=43) *(Components that experts agreed were 'core' are highlighted. Those receiving the highest 'irrelevant' scores are bolded)*	Round two % agreement (n=34)			Round three % agreement (n=24)
		Irrelevant	*Core*	*Desirable*	*Core*
	5.9. Being able to pull a meal together that might consist of four or five different parts, for example a baked dinner.	23.5	38.2	38.2	
	5.10. Being able to prepare foods in the most efficient manner.	17.7	32.4	50.0	
	5.11. Being able to prepare a meal for two to six people without any difficulty.	14.7	41.2	44.1	
	5.12. Knowing how to stretch food if more people come over or are staying at your house.	11.8	38.2	50.0	
	5.13. Being able to conceptualize what you want to put together.	11.8	44.1	44.1	
	5.14. Having knife skills.	23.5	26.5	50.0	
	5.15. Being able to confidently use common pieces of kitchen equipment such as a stove top, oven, microwave, can opener and saucepans.	2.9	**76.5**	20.6	
	5.16. Knowing a few little short cuts so you can prepare food without it taking much time.	11.8	35.3	52.9	
	5.17. Being able to substitute with alternatives if what you want is unavailable.	0.0	52.9	47.1	62.5
	5.18. Enough food hygiene and food safety so that you don't poison anyone.	0.0	**85.3**	14.7	

Table 3.1 (continued)

Domain	Food literacy components identified in round one (n=43) (Components that experts agreed were 'core' are highlighted. Those receiving the highest 'irrelevant' scores are bolded)	Round two % agreement (n=34)			Round three % agreement (n=24)
		Irrelevant	Core	Desirable	Core
	5.19. Knowing how to store food to optimize its value and quality.	0.0	70.6	29.4	70.8
	5.20. How to dispose of waste in an environmentally considerate manner.	14.7	38.2	47.1	
6. Eating	6.1. Being able to join in, sit down and eat in a social way.	11.8	55.9	32.4	50.0
	6.2. Interacting with food and being able to eat in a way that doesn't restrict you being able to be part of a group.	17.7	52.9	29.4	37.5
	6.3. Knowing what food transports well and how to pack it so it still looks appetising when you're going to eat it.	20.6	32.4	47.1	
	6.4. Being willing to try an unfamiliar food.	11.8	23.5	64.7	
	6.5. Knowing principles for everyday eating: only eat when you're hungry, try and get some routine, slow down, eat consciously and reflectively, and be more contemplative about what you're doing and how you're relating to the world.	5.9	44.1	50.0	

Domain	Food literacy components identified in round one (n=43) (Components that experts agreed were 'core' are highlighted. Those receiving the highest 'irrelevant' scores are bolded)	Round two % agreement (n=34)			Round three % agreement (n=24)
		Irrelevant	Core	Desirable	Core
7. Nutrition	7.1. Just what's healthy and what's not.	14.7	58.8	26.5	33.3
	7.2. Understand the overall message of a food selection guide such as the dietary pyramid or plate.	8.8	61.8	29.4	50.0
	7.3. Knowing that all foods are good. It's just the amounts you eat them in. So you need to know about portions and frequency.	14.7	58.8	26.5	33.3
	7.4. Knowing how to categorize foods into the food groups, that you need generally some of each every day and what sort of proportions to eat them in.	11.8	52.9	35.3	37.5
	7.5. Knowing the composition of food groups, for example, meats give you iron and protein.	29.4	32.4	38.2	
	7.6. I don't want to be locked into saying food groups, but knowing what are the components for a healthy basic diet.	5.9	73.5	20.6	50.0
	7.7. Understanding the Australian Dietary Guidelines.	26.5	26.5	47.1	
	7.8. Understanding of what a diverse diet looks like and why it is important from a health and ecological perspective. It doesn't make sense to get our foods from a limited number of agricultural sources or limited number of corporate actors.	20.6	38.2	41.2	

Table 3.1 (continued)

Domain	Food literacy components identified in round one (n=43) (Components that experts agreed were 'core' are highlighted. Those receiving the highest 'irrelevant' scores are bolded)	Round two % agreement (n=34)			Round three % agreement (n=24)
		Irrelevant	Core	Desirable	Core
	7.9. Understanding how to translate the Australian Dietary Guidelines into food and food habits.	29.4	38.2	32.4	
	7.10. Being aware of the role of fats, proteins, carbohydrates and so on.	26.5	38.2	35.3	
	7.11. Knowing what your food is made up of in terms of nutrients and how they all interact.	32.4	23.5	44.1	
	7.12. Knowing that you need vitamins and minerals in certain quantities and what foods they are in.	32.4	26.5	41.2	
	7.13. Knowing about different requirements for different stages of life.	11.8	47.1	41.2	
	7.14. Knowing the specifics of nutrition recommendations, for example, how much fat is too much fat, what does low salt mean on a label.	14.7	55.9	29.4	29.2
	7.15. Understanding the interaction between food and physical activity, and monitoring that by looking at body composition.	23.5	47.1	29.4	
	7.16. Being aware that you have unique individual requirements and understanding how food affects your body when you look at your blood results, etc.	**38.2**	26.5	35.3	

Domain	Food literacy components identified in round one (n=43) (Components that experts agreed were 'core' are highlighted. Those receiving the highest 'irrelevant' scores are bolded)	Round two % agreement (n=34)			Round three % agreement (n=24)
		Irrelevant	*Core*	*Desirable*	*Core*
	7.17. Understanding how your body functions so you can understand how to fuel it or feed it. Not just nutrition but satiety, sensory factors, things like that.	17.7	35.3	47.1	
	7.18. Understanding how a particular food might interact with your physiology and what the implications might be if you have a diet-related disease.	17.7	32.4	50.0	
8. Language	8.1. Being able to communicate around food, be able to articulate and explain things about it.	14.7	47.1	38.2	
	8.2. Knowledge of terminology, so that you can, for example, follow recipes, read labels, make consumer choices. Read stuff in popular magazines and know that you can follow the terminology.	11.8	52.9	35.3	62.5

Components that experts agreed were 'core' are highlighted. Those receiving the highest 'irrelevant' scores appear in bold type.

Knowledge, skills and behaviours used by young people to meet food needs: identifying a final set of food literacy components

In the second study, young people (16–25 year olds) who were responsible for feeding themselves were asked how they went about it. They were asked if they thought they were 'good with food' and, if they knew anyone who was, what they did. They were asked if they thought 'being good with food' was related to healthy eating and how. They were also asked about their usual dietary intake and this was then analysed against nutrition recommendations.

The study involved face to face qualitative interviews with people across a spectrum of disadvantage. Disadvantage was described in terms of source of income, education, housing, social exclusion and employment. Participants were recruited from the Australian Red Cross Night Café for homeless young people; Edmund Rice Flexible Learning Centres for young people who have experienced homelessness, juvenile detention, expulsion from mainstream schooling or some other significant life event which has meant their participation in the mainstream education system has been difficult; people classified as disadvantaged by where they live (i.e. a geographically defined area derived from census data); and university business graduates and their friends. The study took a strengths based approach in that it looked for and privileged the responses of those individuals who used food well to look for enablers rather than barriers.

Data was then compared to the results of the Expert Study using constant comparison techniques until a final set of eleven components of food literacy were determined. They are grouped into four domains of planning and management, selection, preparation and eating (see Table 3.2). This section uses the voices of young people to describe each component and their relationship to food intake across the spectrum of disadvantage and in different contexts. Determinants of this context are many and include the social determinants of health. While it is unlikely that an individual will demonstrate all components of food literacy all of the time, these descriptors help practitioners to identify where to focus their efforts. Components may not always be present in every individual but each is an important piece of scaffolding to strengthen our relationship with food. Conversely, in the absence of one or more components, diet quality will be more vulnerable.

1 Planning and management

The components within this domain describe making time for food in your life, having a plan to make sure it happens but also having the skills to make sure the plan is feasible and likely to deliver the expected outcome. The planning and management components give some predictability or certainty to food intake. These components also help the individual minimize the impact of restricted resources or other changes in circumstance on food choice.

Table 3.2 The domains and components of food literacy

	Food literacy is the ability to …	
Domain	**Components**	
1. Planning and management	1.1	Prioritize time and money for food.
	1.2	Plan food intake (formally and informally) so that food can be regularly accessed through some sources, irrespective of changes in circumstances or environment.
	1.3	Make feasible food decisions which balance food needs (e.g. nutrition, taste, hunger) with available resources (e.g. time, money, skills, equipment).
2. Selection	2.1	Access food through multiple sources and know the advantages and disadvantages of these sources.
	2.2	Determine what is in a food product, where it came from, how to store it and use it.
	2.3	Judge the quality of food.
3. Preparation	3.1	Make a good tasting meal from whatever food is available. This includes being able to prepare commonly available foods, efficiently use common pieces of cooking equipment and having a sufficient repertoire of skills to adapt recipes (written or unwritten) to experiment with food and ingredients.
	3.2	Apply basic principles of safe food hygiene and handling.
4. Eating	4.1	Understand food has an impact on personal wellbeing.
	4.2	Demonstrate self-awareness of the need to personally balance food intake. This includes knowing foods to include for good health, foods to restrict for good health, and appropriate portion size and frequency.
	4.3	Join in and eat in a social way.

Planning and management emerged as strong themes when young people reflected on unsatisfying food arrangements in households where they had lived over their life-course, particularly when reflecting on the key skills they had acquired since living independently. Similarly, participants in the Expert Study discussed the fundamental nature of this domain, particularly when negotiating the complex food supply to routinely select and consume healthy foods.

1.1 Prioritize money and time for food

Prioritizing food was a strong theme that emerged in young people's conceptualizations of someone who was 'good with food'. This differed from having adequate money for food. This component referred to a person who, with limited resources, be it money or time, will consider food and eating above other needs. This differs from someone who is a 'foodie' and will spend time and money on food predominantly for pleasure. This component refers to routinely prioritizing food. For those with limited income, this usually refers to prioritizing money for food, for others, it may refer to prioritizing time. While it is unlikely that prioritizing money and time for food will automatically result in healthier choices, it is clear that in order to make healthy choices, food needs to be prioritized.

Angelica, 20, reflects on when she first left her parental home as a pregnant 15 year old:

> I had to try and feed myself for $30 a week. I was just 'I really want chocolate. Do I want chocolate, or do I want food?' And it was the first time I'd ever lived in my own house, as well. It was different money-wise, I was used to always going into shops and just putting whatever I wanted into the trolleys, and now it's sort of like – it's – yeah. I think money's a big factor.
>
> Angelica

This can be contrasted with Vince, 23, a father of two, who was chronically unemployed, and couch surfing:

> I was in a relationship and I had a little girl and so I had to take off, that's when I did time and went down a very bad path for three months, hit drugs real hard and stuff like that. Yeah, I wasn't in a very good state back then. So, yeah, I never had money for food.
>
> *So what would you do?*
>
> Nothing, just not eat 'til I get paid. You know, there was like 13 of us in the house so just wait for someone to get paid and get some food. It'd all be gone by that afternoon. Yeah, I never ate at all. I'd eat probably maybe once, maybe twice a fortnight if I'm lucky.
>
> Vince

1.2 Plan food intake (formally and informally) so that food can be regularly accessed through some source irrespective of changes in circumstances or environment

This component describes the ability to adapt to changes in the macro and micro environment. Themes of resilience were strong throughout interviews with young people. They described the types of skills they use to adapt to change. From a nutrition perspective, resilience and adaptability to change is an important component of maintaining a healthy diet over time. Planning was a key aspect of this component. It involved consciously considering eating ahead of time and determining how this would happen. In the examples that follow, this typically involved planning to meet a range of needs. This component particularly highlights that food literacy needs to extend beyond food preparation.

Ann had been homeless for three months. Here she describes her typical eating pattern and demonstrates her ability to think ahead about her food intake and where it might come from:

> Usually for breakfast, we go to Coles® and steal some pies for breakfast. But that's usually our dinner and our breakfast, but during the day, we go to YOS, the Youth Outreach Service. We go there, have a feed for lunch and then when that closes at 12, so we're there from nine to 12, and then from one to four, we go to BYS, Brisbane Youth Service, and we have another feed there. So we – we're always well fed during the day, it's just the morning when you wake up and you're hungry, that's all you can do is steal like something to eat, or for dinner.
>
> Ann

Some people described quite formalized planning while others tended to start with what food was available and then planned their food intake from there. This appeared to be a personal preference, rather than related to income or disadvantage. It may be that when first being responsible for feeding yourself, formalized planning is helpful, with this process becoming more automatic with experience.

Here, Amy, 17, who had recently returned to her parental home, describes how she plans her weekly food expenditure:

> I will write down – I will sit down – Monday, Tuesday, Wednesday, Thursday, Friday, Saturday, Sunday, and plan it out every day what I'm going to eat and only buy that amount, so I'm not going over what I need. I'm not buying chocolates and lollies and crap, unless I have the money for it.
>
> Amy

Tina, 24, had been responsible for feeding herself and her son for the past six years. Here she describes her approach to planning her food intake:

> I tend to buy whatever's on special, like in the meat section and stuff, and then plan meals from that. I do the meat section first, because it is first in my grocery store. So if I get mince, then I'm going to have spaghetti bolognaise or rissoles, if I buy sausages then I'm going to have a casserole or sausage and veggies, steaks, or steak and veggies. So I just work it out from whatever meat's on special.
>
> Tina

1.3 Make feasible food decisions which balance food needs (for example, nutrition, taste, hunger) with available resources (for example, time, money, skills, equipment)

People who described this behaviour spoke of the need to consider a range of resource limitations and to be able to compromise between the range of needs food can fulfil. This rarely meant deciding between a simple set of factors. The relative importance of needs and restriction of resources varied regularly and this meant food decisions would also. This component tended to require an element of self-awareness which typically came from self-reflection, particularly of prior unsatisfactory food decisions.

Julia, 16, had been living under a bridge for the past four months and had been homeless on and off for the past two years. She describes how she used extremely limited resources to meet a diverse range of identified food needs. Here she talks about how she decides how to spend a food voucher when she happens to receive one.

> *It must be hard to work out what to do when you know you're not getting it all the time.*
>
> Yeah. I try to get things like – I get some bread because you know that it will last at least – tonight's meal and then maybe tomorrow, toast for breakfast. Some sausages, just sausages for everyone. I try to get things that – will last or feed people. We have a kitchen and stuff at our place. Last night we go to like to Roma Street or to Southbank, they have barbecues and stuff like that … I try to get meat, more meat than anything, meat, and bread, because they'll eat it. Yeah. I like seafood salad, I'll get myself seafood salad. Ham sandwiches, try and get some tomatoes or something like that just to mix it up a bit … I make sure I have enough because there's a – there's a lot of us, oh well not – a lot of us, but a lot of people live under the bridge, easy 20 sometimes and we all kind of care about each other, so I always make sure everyone is fed.
>
> Julia

Angelica, 20, who left her parental home for the first time as a pregnant 15 year old, used self-reflection to evaluate her previous food decisions to improve future ones:

> I guess it took me a while to figure it out. You, sort of, have to get yourself in a routine sort of thing. Because when I first used to go to the shops, I used to just get things – 'I'm going to make this, I'm going to make that'. And half the time, I never made it. You have to really think about if you're actually going to be able to make a roast on Wednesday at 5 o'clock in the afternoon to have for dinner. Do you know what I mean? Because I used to do that; and I'd get home at six and try and make a really nice dinner. And I would be trying to keep Ruby awake and everyone's hungry. Now I cook really basic and easy meals that take 10 minutes. Like pasta or even Chicken Tonight®. I guess a lot of my meals are pretty similar in the way they always have rice or pasta and meat in them. Or if they're not like a dish like that, I'll have lamb chops with potatoes and – yeah. So I always have the same things in my cupboard; I've always got veggies and potatoes and pasta packets and stuff like that.

All the sides that I can put with something or the jars for the flavours of something that I want to make. I guess for me it's organization. Because when I'm not organized a big thing doesn't go well. And I end up eating noodles at 8 o'clock.

Angelica

2 Selection

This domain refers to the skills needed to choose individual food items. It refers to both grocery (for example, choosing a cut of meat) and food service items (for example, choosing from a range of options in a food court). The selection of food was referred to much more often in the Expert Study (see Table 3.1). Although even for food experts an awareness of the provenance of foods was often indentified in the first round interviews, but not seen as a core component of food literacy in the subsequent two rounds of the Delphi process. 'Knowing where food comes from' was of interest to very few young people. Participants tended to refer to previous experiences when determining their criteria for food selection. This came from both their own behaviour and those of others, typically the person they mainly learnt about food from.

'Being willing to try new foods' is often considered an important attribute by practitioners; however, young people rarely mentioned adding new foods to their day-to-day eating, rather food routines were commonly referred to in interviews with young people. This is consistent with the findings of other studies (Blake et al. 2008; Jastran et al. 2009; Meat and Livestock Australia 2009).

2.1 Access food through multiple sources and know the advantages and disadvantages of these sources

This component refers to knowledge of the local food supply and the ability to make an informed decision about where to access food to best meet needs. This component is highly contextual. This can mean understanding options to access food without an income, understanding the options in a new geographical location or when income is secure, having a more critical understanding of the food supply to make a more empowered choice.

Todd, a second-year university student, describes how he has organized feeding himself since leaving his parental home for the first time:

Well, when I was at home Mum cooked most of my dinners, and generally there was food in the pantry for breakfast. ... Now, I grocery shop, like, semi regularly. 'Cause I, kind of, need to be fairly frugal when I buy food, so I obviously go to shopping centres to save money. When I go shopping I usually buy single serve microwave or oven meals, which are a big one – pizzas particularly. I have, like, lasagnes and pastas that you can just microwave and eat. So yeah – and I always go to the Coles® down the road from my house because it's the closest, and I don't have a car. I know Coles® is too expensive though, if I had a choice I would shop elsewhere, and probably go to markets and stuff if I could, but without the transport possibility I have to go to Coles®.

Todd

2.2 Determine what is in a food product, where it came from, how to store it and use it

This component refers to a broad range of information about the food itself. In the Expert Study it was referred to as 'Being able to understand what's in a product and how to store and use it'. The level of knowledge required to make a good food selection is highly contextual and was influenced by needs and values. Young people more often referred to the lack of food knowledge of others rather than consciously reflecting on their own food knowledge. Many young people used their experience in preparing food to help them select foods prepared outside the home, be they bought in a grocery or food service outlet. An understanding of what was in the food tended to come from having some experience preparing it. From a nutrition perspective, this component is particularly important as it helps consumers make a choice when confronted with foods outside their standard repertoire and to reassess the foods they currently consume.

The importance of this component differed between experts and young people. Experts talked a lot more about the importance of the 'conscious consumer' and a greater knowledge of food, particularly its components and origins, contributing to this. This did not appear to be a strong theme in the Young People Study. The composition and origins of food were of little interest. It remains unclear, therefore, what level of consumer knowledge is useful in supporting healthy eating as few participants sought this information even when it was available. The interview excerpts for this component demonstrate the limited extent of participants' knowledge and interest in food in comparison to the expectations of experts as expressed in the earlier study. In keeping with an assets-based approach, these interview excerpts are taken from those participants who actively discussed the origins of foods; for the majority, it simply was not a consideration.

Kelli, a 24 year old university graduate, left her parental home at 20. Kelli, her separated parents and two sisters were all morbidly obese during her adolescence. Kelli had lost 85kg over the past three years with the help of a personal trainer. When reflecting on learning about food at home, Kelli did not consider her weight was related to her parental home environment. To lose weight, Kelli followed a very rigid meal regime for a fortnight at a time and complemented this with home delivered diet meal packs. Kelli relied heavily on her personal trainer to help her select food:

I think I have a lot to thank her, because I could text her, and it would be 'I'm out – my options are like McDonald's® or Red Rooster®, what's the best?' and she would text me back and say 'you want the skin free chicken from Red Rooster® and salad'.

Kelli

Todd, a 19 year old university student, describes the tension between knowing where food comes from and the feasibility of selection decisions:

> I research a fair bit about global warming and stuff, I understand that food gets transported a lot, and if it were my choice I would eat locally to avoid that. But I can't really do that with my transport issues. Also with noodles, like mi goreng and stuff, it's alarming to me because I have no idea what's in it, and it comes from a foreign country, but I, kind of, sacrifice those for the ease of use. Yeah.

Todd

Todd was the only participant to discuss the ethics and origins of food, although as Todd states, this has little influence on his food intake decisions. In the 24 hours prior to the interview, Todd had eaten pizza. Every Tuesday Todd buys two for one take-away pizza, then eats only this for the next 1–2 days. He indicated that part of the appeal of this food choice is the lack of washing up which was also why he chooses noodles.

2.3 Judge the quality of food

This component involves using the information about the food, where it came from and how to store it and use it to judge the quality of an available food and make a selection that will meet their food needs. This can contribute to the predictability and pleasure of eating.

3 Preparation

Almost all young people agreed that the ability to prepare food was an essential life skill. This is consistent with findings of the Expert Study. Most described the level of ability needed as 'basic', but ideas of 'basic' differed. This is also consistent with the findings of the Expert Study. Young people also had an expectation or desire that everyday food and eating should 'taste good' and that the level of skill needed to produce food that 'tasted good' was beyond 'basic'.

3.1 Make a good tasting meal from whatever food is available. This includes being able to prepare commonly available foods, efficiently use common pieces of kitchen equipment and having a sufficient repertoire of skills to adapt recipes (written or unwritten) to experiment with food and ingredients

In the Expert Study, the ability to prepare commonly available foods was described as 'knowledge of some basic commodities and how to prepare them' and 'knowing how to prepare some foods from all of the food groups, for example, how to prepare meat, how to cook pasta, how to prepare vegetables and then spin-offs from there' (see Table 3.1). Consistent with the findings of the Expert Study, participants in the Young People Study discussed the use of 'basic' commodities. The food groups, were, however, rarely used to categorize these commodities. It was more appropriate to refer to 'commonly available' foods rather than 'basic' foods, as the need to be able to prepare these was defined more by what was typically available in their food environment rather than what society as a whole used. Additionally, for people not born in Australia, there were foods that may have been 'basic commodities' in their home country but were now unavailable and so the skill included adapting to this new environment.

The main motivation to prepare foods was taste. Being able to make a good tasting meal from whatever food is available was very strongly identified across all participant groups in their conceptualization of someone who was 'good with food'. This requires being familiar enough with a range of foods and techniques to be able to deliver a predictable result. The extent of one's repertoire, or the number of foods participants considered one needed to know how to prepare, was highly variable. The following interview excerpts demonstrate this and the variation in conceptualizations of 'taste'.

This component includes several ambiguous terms: 'meal', 'taste' and 'common'. The meaning of each can be largely contextual and broadly inter-preted, so their use has been criticized in the literature. However, as this research was committed to capturing the insights of young people, a range of meanings, as defined by the participant, were documented. This is an important finding to highlight in the planning of interventions.

Tina was a 24 year old mother of a six year old living in a disadvantaged area. She had been responsible for feeding herself and others since she was 16. Throughout her interview she describes a very routine approach to eating. In this series of excerpts she describes preparing food:

> I can cook good, I'm a good cook. I've got five basic meals that I do really well … I think by the time you leave home you need to know how to make a roast, a good stir fry and the basic pasta – then if you can know how to cook meat without making it chewy, vegetables, the basic pasta and roast, you're pretty much set. I think you're right with that … My partner, he made really, really good, you know that pasta you get in the packet, you add the milk and the butter? He made that really good.
>
> Tina

Aiden, a university graduate who lived in an advantaged area, reflects on former housemates and describes what he considers the skills needed by the time you leave your parental home:

> Just the basics, you know, how to prepare food; how to handle it; how to store it, like, those sort of really basic things that you should know about

food. And it doesn't have to be like, you don't have to cook a three course meal. But just to be able to sustain and be somewhat interesting rather than putting a bowl, you know, a can of baked beans in the microwave and with a slice of toast for dinner, you know. Be able to cook yourself a balanced, nutritious meal for yourself. I think that's a key essential that you need to know before leaving.

Aiden

Meg had been homeless since she was 12 and could not recall ever having a meal prepared in her parental home. Here she reflects on her own ability to prepare commonly available foods:

> I do know how to make some things. I can make a stir fry 'cause like when you stay in youth shelters they make you cook, and you have to cook a new recipe every week. So I can make stir fry and I can make potato bake and I can make spaghetti, but like really dero spaghetti like bogan spaghetti, not like the Italian one.
> *So what's bogan spaghetti?*
> Bogan spaghetti is like frozen vegetables and pasta sauce. You know how like Australians take everything that's really nice and cultured from overseas and then they just simplify it and make it bogan, yeah like.
> *So could you cook pasta?*
> Yeah I can cook pasta, but it's always either too soft or too hard, but it's edible.

Meg

Young people across all groups described needing to know how to use common pieces of kitchen equipment. This included those experiencing homelessness who typically transitioned in and out of a range of different living arrangements and whose eating on the street sometimes involved the use of equipment, for example, microwaves in convenience stores and barbeques in parks.

Unlike food ingredients, kitchen equipment was less culturally and socially defined and so 'common pieces' were consistent across participant groups. When asked if they could use common pieces of cooking equipment, all participants indicated they could. When asked what equipment that included, they tended to list off ovens, stoves, and microwaves. It was difficult to determine their ability to use other pieces of equipment, for example, knives, in the most efficient way. Efficient use of equipment can influence the time spent preparing food and the satisfaction with the end result; for example, using a large knife to chop a small ingredient is cumbersome and slow; using a low temperature to seal meat will result in it being chewy rather than juicy. In this way, being able to efficiently use common pieces of kitchen equipment is a sub-component of being able to 'make a good tasting meal from whatever food is available' (Component 3.1 in Table 3.2). In describing what they considered fundamental knowledge, participants were more likely to describe people they had lived with who could not use equipment. Here Sharni reflects on her time living in shared youth accommodation where typically residents take turns preparing food:

> This girl she was trying to make vegetables one day and she was steaming them. And she was steaming cucumber and capsicum with peas and carrot and I'm like, 'Oh, my God'. And she didn't put any water in the bottom of the pan and it was burning. And so she put some water in, it was like this much, and they just tasted burnt at the end.
>
> Sharni

Having a sufficient repertoire of skills to adapt recipes (written or unwritten) to experiment with food and ingredients refers to having enough experience with food preparation to adapt to a range of environments and circumstances. Participants often referred to recipes, but not in the formal sense of a written recipe in a book, rather a procedure they followed in order to get a predictable result. If used, written recipes more often served as inspiration rather than being followed per se. This component was highly linked to taste. It implies the individual has sufficient food experiences to draw on to produce a meal that is palatable despite unfamiliar circumstances. It is unclear what a 'sufficient' repertoire would be. This is likely to depend upon the individual. The repertoire would need to include commonly available foods and be adequate to meet nutrition needs. Beyond this, it may depend upon the individual's requirements. This component also requires self-efficacy, which is influenced by experience and mastery.

Experimentation was often referred to by participants, but more typically for the purposes of being resourceful and adaptable rather than being inquisitive and innovative in a foodie sense. Here Tyler, 16, is asked to think of someone whom he considers is 'good with food'. He describes his friend's mum with whom he was currently living. She was feeding three young people in her home using her welfare payment.

> She'll cook up some spaghetti chops and get the cans of spaghetti, heat that – there up, and mix it all in together and it tastes really mad. She can work with anything and make a really mad meal.
>
> Tyler

Bella, a university graduate who moved out of her parental home for the first time in the last twelve months, gives her description of someone who is 'good with food':

> I have a good friend and he is very good with cooking meat, I guess, maybe that's the thing – like he'll be very specific and then he'll take a photo and send it to me, and it always looks amazing and he's always got

like ten different ingredients going on. And I've been over to his house for dinner a few times and he never seems to be stressed when he's cooking, and he comes out and it's like this amazing meal and it's like often like some Moroccan tagine thing, and I'm like, 'How did you do that? Awesome.'

Bella

3.2 Apply basic principles of safe food hygiene and handling

In the Expert Study the component which achieved the highest level of consensus was 'enough food hygiene and food safety so that you don't poison anyone'. Similarly, in the Young People Study it was primarily described in relation to higher risk foods, for example:

If you eat meat, you should probably know how to cook meat, so that you don't die of food poisoning or something.

Dan

These excerpts describe a 'broad brush', 'general principles' level of safe food handling knowledge.

4 Eating

This component includes both the act of eating and the consequences of eating, including nutritional status. In both studies, conceptualizations of being 'good with food' or 'what you need to know and understand about food to be able to use it to meet your needs' included nutrition. In both the studies, participants considered there were two main elements to nutrition knowledge: (i) an understanding of the effects of healthy eating and (ii) an understanding of what healthy eating means. Commensal eating is the other key component of this domain. The combination of these components emphasizes the importance of balancing a range of food needs which is further highlighted in the planning and management domain. Those that valued eating with others tended to prioritize food and plan their eating and food intake.

4.1 Understand that food has an impact on personal wellbeing

This component refers to an understanding that food intake and health, which extend beyond obesity prevention, are related. These interview excerpts demonstrate the individualized nature of this.

Laura was 20. She suffered from a mental illness which she described as currently being managed well. Throughout the interview she reflected on when she had not managed as well, including a seven month period when she was homeless and lived in a tent. In this interview excerpt Laura describes the relationship between her food intake and her wellbeing.

I've always been very organized with food and eating and stuff like that because I know it affects the way that I think. 'Cause I've some mental health issues and I know if I don't eat or if I don't eat properly or regularly then it can affect the way that I think. So I've always been pretty good with that … So a lot of people that I speak to don't really – I think that kids get told like – it's sort of like the anti-smoking campaigns, where junk food is bad for you and all this other kind of stuff. But I know they're not really educated on how it sort of affects the way that you think, like it can affect you mentally and no, I don't think they really realize that.

Laura

Hamish, a university student, talked about going through phases of healthy eating. Here he describes what prompts him to enter a healthy phase:

It gets to a point where I just realize that I'm just, like, I'm feeling – I don't want to sound, like, weird, but, like, I feel, like, I feel heavy, I feel gross, like, up until about a week or two ago, I constantly felt – although I was hungry, I constantly felt, like, full and bloated. And so since then – I think that was 'cause I was eating not fantastically, but I've started to, like, smaller down my intake, eat more meals, and that sort of stuff.

Hamish

Tyler, 17, from a highly disadvantaged area, describes his motivation for eating healthy foods. This domain includes several quotes from Tyler who demonstrates a deep understanding of food, nutrition and health.

I'm just Aboriginal-Australian. I think that because most Aboriginals have fairly bad health, it's sort of encouraged me to sort of look at what I eat and try to stay a bit healthier.

Tyler

4.2 Demonstrate self-awareness of the need to personally balance food intake. This includes knowing foods to include for good health, foods to restrict for good health and appropriate portion size and frequency

Restriction and balance were two concepts which were strongly associated with healthy eating. Across all participant groups, valuing self and self-efficacy were key themes that emerged among those young people who were more likely to restrict and balance their food intake. Young people needed to consider that they were worth looking after and needed to believe that they were able to make healthy changes. This was not to say that young people considered their dietary intake to be completely self-determined. Participants that proactively considered nutrition in their food selection were able to identify a range of other factors that made healthy choices more difficult. These included the cost of healthy food in comparison to unhealthy food, the disproportionate marketing of unhealthy foods, the importance of introducing healthy foods early in life and a range of lifestyle factors and changes that impacted on the ability to maintain a healthy diet, for example, relationship breakdowns.

In examining foods to include and restrict for good health, participants were asked if they could name the five core food groups to get a sense of their knowledge of common nutrition messages. The interviewer stressed that exact names of groups were not important, rather knowledge of the general categories of foods recommended for good health. Participants tended to recite them as something that had been learnt at school but they were not used as a guide to healthy eating. Several of the quotes below demonstrate that while this basic nutrition tool was not used, many still understood the concepts of healthy eating. It is interesting to note, however, that healthy eating was conceptualized as that which prevents overweight and obesity, rather than that which nourishes. In this excerpt we again hear from Tyler who had spent his whole life living in disadvantage, including interrupted and delayed schooling.

> *So with nutrition, would you know the food groups?*
> Nope.
> *Could you sort of guess? If you had to guess what the general groups of food are?*
> I wouldn't have a clue.
> *Okay. Okay. So do you think of nutrition at all when deciding what to eat?*
> I try to eat healthier things on a regular basis.
> *So what things do you think of – the healthy?*
> Fruit, vegetables, meat and stuff like that. Dairy products, milk and bread and eggs. Other than that I don't know.
>
> Tyler

Jewel had been homeless for several years. Here he describes his decision-making regarding foods to steal. He does not identify these as nutritious food choices; in fact, later in the interview he actively distances himself from nutrition and health. However, his decision is based on foods that will nourish and sustain him.

> *And when you've got no money, what do you do?*
> Me and my brother normally go to Coles® and grab a few things.
> *So what sort of stuff do you normally take?*
> Oh, the same thing every time; chicken, mayonnaise, bread, butter. I've been on and off streets for five years of my life. And I've always learnt one major rule. When you steal, steal for what you need, not for what you want. Something that you really, really, need, then yeah, I'll steal. But if it's something small it's like I'm hungry I want some chips or I want some chocolate, no. I have rules to breaking the law. I mean like, if I'm busking for a whole day and not made any money and it's raining, so no one's out, I'll go steal that one day, yeah. Because I know I'm not going to make any money …

Do you ever think about nutrition when you - - -
No.
Do you think there'd ever be a time where you'd think that that was important?
No.
Okay.
I'm the total opposite of healthy. I know what's healthy, I know how to eat healthy; I choose not to.
So if you had to sort of name the food groups, what would the food groups be?
What do you mean by food groups? Triangle of food group thingy?
Yeah, that stuff.
Everything I eat is on the bottom two. That goes with ice-cream, chocolates, fatty foods, fried foods, I can keep going.

Jewel

Dietary recommendations typically include appropriate portion size and frequency. However, participants did not reference these recommendations when discussing these concepts.

4.3 Join in and eat in a social way

Commensal eating was a very strong theme in interviews, with all participant groups acknowledging that being 'good with food' included being able to socialize with food. This was strongly linked with pleasure. Sharing meals was an important part of building a sense of belonging and social inclusion. Participants tended to share meals with people they could identify with. Young people who did not typically eat commensally in their parental home sometimes found it difficult to do so now with others which impacted on their ability to make social connections. Participants who enjoyed sharing meals also tended to prioritize food in their lives (Component 1.1 in Table 3.2). For financial reasons, few young people prepared food to feed groups of people outside their household. More often they took turns in supplying or preparing food and identified times and places where they could eat together regularly. The fragmentation of time meant that this did not necessarily occur on a daily basis but was highly valued when it did occur. For individuals and families experiencing disadvantage, the ability to prepare and share food was described by service providers in the Expert Study as being associated with a feeling of being in control of their lives and their capacity to care for others.

Evidence in the literature of the importance of commensal eating on diet quality is unclear (Demory-Luce et al. 2004; Kristensen & Holm 2006; Larsen et al. 2006, 2009). Some propose that shared meals are more often planned and so more likely to be nutrient dense. Others consider that shared meals may mean more conscious and therefore measured consumption. Here James and Angelica talk about their experiences of living alone and its impact on their eating.

I hate cooking for myself 'cause you cook for yourself, you eat by yourself, you clean up by yourself. It's the most depressing thing in the world, and I see food as a social thing. Food to me is really social and I hated living by myself for that reason.

James

When I have people that live with me, I eat a lot better, because you know, I cook. And it's more the atmosphere, I like it. But when I'm on my own, I sort of just don't.

Angelica

This study focused on young people experiencing disadvantage. For young people at the extremes of social exclusion, traditional images of family meals and familial handing down of food knowledge were not representative of their lived experience. However, the value of sharing eating occasions with others, having meal times and learning about food from the people you are living with were all strongly represented in the data collected from this group. Several young people in our study went to extraordinary lengths to sustain shared meal times. There were several stories of the parent no longer preparing food and the children instead taking on this role, despite the parent not participating in the meal. Young mothers saw shared meal times as part of defining their role as a mother and establishing a family. Our study would suggest that while the structure of families and provisioning of food within them may be more het-erogeneous, young people still seek to share eating occasions in a planned and social way.

A definition of food literacy

The components are descriptors of a food literate person. This inter-related set of components, and the results of both studies more broadly, were used to develop the following definition of food literacy:

> Food literacy is a collection of inter-related knowledge, skills and behaviours required to plan, manage, select, prepare and eat foods to meet needs and determine food intake.
>
> Food literacy is the scaffolding that empowers individuals, households, communities or nations to protect diet quality through change, and support dietary resilience over time.

The definition has three elements: (i) what food literacy includes, that is, its components; (ii) its purpose; and (iii) its action. Food literacy can be thought of as a basket of knowledge, skills and behaviours whose specific contents will vary over the life-course in response to changes. Change may be at the individual level, for example, feeding dependants for the first time, or at the environ-mental level, for example, changes in the local food supply. While this study focused on individuals, it was clear from the data that food literacy could be used at multiple levels, that is, to describe households, communities and nations.

Conclusions

Many terms and tools have been used to measure the everyday practicalities of food and eating. In each of these constructs and the tools that measure them, the 'expert', be it the researcher, practitioner or policy maker, has determined what the knowledge, skills and behaviours to meet food needs are. These parameters are then measured alongside food intake to look for correlations to determine their importance. This research, however, considered this phenomenon from multiple perspectives, privileging that of the eater.

The four domains of planning and management, selection, preparation and eating reflect a social, environmental and functional understanding of food systems consistent with contemporary public health nutrition policy and practice. The conceptualization of food literacy existing at individual, household, community and national levels reflects an understanding of these systems and their reciprocal relationship to food intake and nutritional status. Unlike other literacies, food literacy has no end-point of competence. Within each domain, there may be a continuum of knowledge, skills or behaviours, but the optimal position will be context dependant. Additionally, the individual may slide up and down these continua over their life-course, and simultaneously sit at different levels of competency across different components. Food literacy has also been conceptualized as supporting resilience. Broader conceptualizations of resilience acknowledge that it too is dynamic, rather than being a fixed attribute that is shaped by social context.

This definition of food literacy and its components describes a way of considering the temporal and dynamic nature of everyday eating. It emphasizes that healthy eating is about more than meeting nutrition recommendations; it's about how to do this on a day to day basis over a lifetime.

References

Blake, C.E., Bisogni, C.A., Sobal, J., Jastran, M. & Devine, C.M. 2008, 'How adults construct evening meals. Scripts for food choice', *Appetite*, vol. 51, no. 3, pp. 654–662.

Cullerton, K., Vidgen, H. & Gallegos, D. 2012, *A Review of Food Literacy Interventions Targeting Disadvantaged Young People*, Queensland University of Technology, Brisbane, Queensland, viewed 10 December 2015, <http://eprints.qut.edu.au/53753/>.

Demory-Luce, D., Morales, M., Nicklas, T., Baranowski, T., Zakeri, I. & Berenson, G. 2004, 'Changes in food group consumption patterns from childhood to young adulthood: the Bogalusa Heart Study', *Journal of the American Dietetic Association*, vol. 104, no. 11, pp. 1684–1691.

Jastran, M.M., Bisogni, C.A., Sobal, J., Blake, C. & Devine, C.M. 2009, 'Eating routines. Embedded, value based, modifiable, and reflective', *Appetite*, vol. 52, no. 1, pp. 127–136.

Kristensen, S.T. & Holm, L. 2006, 'Modern meal patterns: tensions between bodily needs and the organization of time and space', *Food and Foodways: Explorations in the History and Culture of Human Nourishment*, vol. 14, no. 3, pp. 151–173.

Larson, N.I., Nelson, M.C., Neumark-Sztainer, D., Story, M. & Hannan, P.J. 2009, 'Making time for meals: meal structure and associations with dietary intake in young adults', *Journal of the American Dietetic Association*, vol. 109, no. 1, pp. 72–79.

Larson, N.I., Perry, C.L., Story, M. & Neumark-Sztainer, D. 2006, 'Food preparation by young adults is associated with better diet quality', *Journal of the American Dietetic Association*, vol. 106, no. 12, pp. 2001–2007.

Meat and Livestock Australia 2009, *Last Night's Dinner*, Meat and Livestock Australia, Sydney, viewed 5 November 2010, <http://www.redmeatandnutrition.com.au/NR/rdonlyres/37C22E0A-83F6-408B-BD79-45DC620F3AA4/0/LastnightsdinnerFINAL.pdf>.

Vidgen, H. 2014, *Food Literacy: What is it and Does it Influence what we Eat?* PhD dissertation, Queensland University of Technology, Brisbane, viewed 10 December 2015, <http://eprints.qut.edu.au/66720/>.

Vidgen, H. & Gallegos, D. 2014, 'Defining food literacy and its components', *Appetite*, vol. 76, pp. 50–59.

4 Relating food literacy to nutrition and health

Helen Vidgen

Introduction

This chapter describes the evolution of a model to propose the relationship between food literacy and nutrition. As described in the previous chapter, this is based on the results of two studies, the first being a three round Delphi study of Australian food experts and the second being a qualitative study of young people across a spectrum of disadvantage. Both studies contributed to the development of this model. This chapter sequentially presents the results of each study to describe how and why the model developed and the contribution of each to this process.

The first iteration of the model of the relationship between food literacy and nutrition was developed following the Expert Study. Its application and face validity were then tested with practitioners using it to describe and evaluate existing interventions. Data from the Young People Study was analysed to look for intersecting themes when participants described feeding themselves. These were then compared with concepts described in the Expert Study model. In addition, throughout the research process, the model was presented to peers in a range of forums to test the clarity of the representation of concepts. This resulted in a final 'Conceptual model of the relationship between food literacy and nutrition' which is the subject of this chapter. This model is not only useful in describing the relationship between food literacy and nutrition, it can also be used as a framework for programme planning, implementation and evaluation. It helps to identify outcomes, impacts, strategies and partners. This is discussed in more detail in the latter part of this chapter.

Both studies also reinforce that practitioners and policy makers invest in food literacy with outcome expectations beyond diet quality. For this reason, a second model was developed to conceptualize the role of food literacy with respect to food security, body weight and chronic disease risk. This model is less developed as this research was designed to explore the relationship between food literacy and nutrition. This second model, however, is useful in positioning food literacy within multi-strategic public health nutrition and chronic disease plans.

Food experts' conceptualization of the relationship between food literacy and nutrition

This section describes how data from the Expert Study was used to develop a model of the relationship between food literacy and nutrition. The profile of participants (described in the previous chapter) allowed for a deep exploration and discussion of this relationship with them that was not possible with the Young People Study. Expert Study participants were selected as a result of their extensive and diverse experience and expertise in food. As such, they had very considered views of the potential relationship between food literacy and nutrition. This section describes supporting data for each of the constructs presented in the model. These were used to develop an initial model shown in Figure 4.1.

Experts considered the relationship between food literacy and nutrition to be indirect. In discussing possible mechanisms for this relationship, the three themes of providing security and certainty, improving choice, and making eating more pleasurable emerged. Experts discussed that the strength of this relationship was likely to be mediated by the food supply and the individual's values. Experts talked about the relative importance of components of food literacy being dependent upon these mechanisms and mediators. Food literacy interventions targeting individuals living in a remote town with limited fresh fruit and vegetables, for example, may focus more on selection components. The level of nutrition outcome being sought may also impact on the relative importance of proposed components. For example, a client needing to avoid a particular food ingredient, such as gluten, may need to focus more on knowing where food comes from.

Mechanisms

The mechanisms by which food literacy improved nutrition were by:

- providing more *choice* and consequently being less restricted by the local food environment and resources;
- making healthy foods more *pleasurable* and so more likely to be eaten; and
- improving food *security* by providing greater certainty in the availability, accessibility and acceptability of food.

These three mechanisms were all considered in the context of empowering the individual, giving more control over food and eating, and consequently, greater resilience to protect diet quality through change.

Choice was conceptualized in two ways by food experts. The first related to individualism: the right to exercise choice and establish one's own goals and needs. The second related to the proliferation of food choices and the need to make sense of these. This second interpretation is linked with food security and certainty. These constructs presented a paradox. Several participants talked about the emergence of a focus on food literacy being related to the increase in

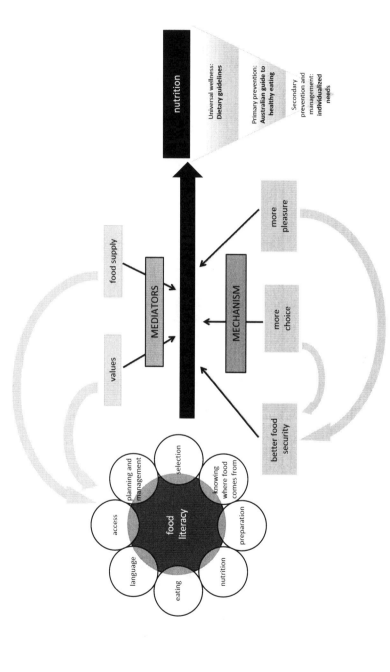

Figure 4.1 A preliminary model of the relationship between food literacy and nutrition resulting from a study of Australian food experts

the number and diversity of foods in our contemporary food supply and the complexity of skills and knowledge needed to navigate through it. In contrast, others discussed the limited number of healthy choices.

> It was much easier before we were so sophisticated with the food products that are out there in the supermarket, because the majority of people still shop in a supermarket and are faced with a barrage of, as you know, breakfast cereals and dairy and yoghurts and ice-creams. And because everything's fortified and we're taught nutrients, it's difficult for kids to think, 'Oh, I can get my calcium from orange juice, or I can get my ...' It's not easy to teach. It's much harder to teach. So I think we've got the challenges. It's more challenging for us now, I think, than ever before, from a nutrition point of view, to help people get through the myriad of information.
>
> Industry practitioner 3

Pleasure was conceptualized broadly. It ranged from taste, flavour and content-ment to satisfaction and accomplishment. It included pleasure in healthy eating.

> Food that you genuinely like and that you're genuinely happy with. If that is just a simple lamb chop and some steamed vegetables, that's fine. That's a fabulous meal.
>
> Gastronomy practitioner 1

It was noted that often, however, nutrition is not associated with pleasure and that other sectors perform much better in this domain.

Both choice and pleasure are relevant to both the food secure and the food insecure. This mechanism predominantly examined the construct of certainty, which was more significant for those who were food insecure but could also be interpreted more broadly.

> I guess around the issue of choice I could comment, you know, and I would agree that much of the definition, if you like, crudely of what constitutes poverty is around the levels of choice that people are able to exercise.
>
> Welfare researcher 1

In the context of food security, food literacy was conceptualized as providing greater resilience and resistance to changing economic and social changes. It was seen as helping to protect diet quality. This could also be interpreted as giving a greater degree of certainty around food, particularly its availability and quality.

Mediators

Food experts considered the extent to which food literacy might influence nutrition being mediated by values and the local food supply. Some respondents discussed these in terms of 'pre-requisites' or 'facilitators'. These factors were also described as influencing the relative importance of food literacy components. For example, for a food insecure young mother, knowing how to stretch food further might be more important than understanding the provenance of a food product. A chef who values taste and appearance over health may have high food literacy but this will have little impact on their nutrition. This link with values and food supply may indicate where food literacy could be positioned within broader food and nutrition systems.

Food experts identified food supply as the key determinant of nutrition and the irrelevance of food literacy when food supply was inadequate. Others discussed the increased need for food literacy given the complexity of the food supply and how its relative importance depended on this complexity.

> I think if you're a poor person, or you're a person living in an area where you can't get easy access to cheap, good, fresh products, which is actually a lot of people, then it's going to be really hard.
>
> Welfare researcher 2

> You had to get people 'housing ready' was the terminology [used] and one of the critical parts of that` around what they call 'living skills' was learning how to cook. But often, in my interviews and research with people experiencing homelessness, the majority of them found it very insulting and unnecessary. And, in fact, their nutritional capacity among most of them was quite good and in effect on par with the general community, their food literacy levels. But again, it's simply a question, as I said at the outset of the interview, that it's their capacity to exercise their food literacy is diminished by their financial poverty. Yeah, that was the governing factor, it wasn't a lack of nutrition knowledge, it was a lack of money to execute that knowledge.
>
> Welfare researcher 1

> We've been doing some research about what one would call the Depression era Australians and what they ate, and this was prior to Dietary Guidelines, and they would describe their meat and three veg meals. They'd describe a highly routinized diet without much going out to eat and very little use of convenience foods. That generation, because of the local food environment that they inhabited with far less choice, they didn't need to consciously have nutritional knowledge to eat well.
>
> Gastronomy researcher 1

In public health nutrition plans, food literacy is most often categorized as a component of food supply (Prime Minister's Science Engineering and Innovation Council 2010; Queensland Public Health Forum 2009). Its relationship, however, is more likely to be multidirectional. Improved food literacy improves individual food supply; however, concurrently, the extent to which food literacy can influence nutrition is limited by the food available. The relative importance of components of food literacy will also be influenced by the food supply; for example, in a remote community with one store and typically poor quality fruits and vegetables, preparation or growing food may be more important.

Nutrition

When experts were asked specifically about the relationship between food literacy and nutrition, three main nutrition themes emerged. They were the mutual exclusivity of food literacy and nutrition; the variability in interpretation of healthy eating and its influence on food literacy; and nutritionism.

For most experts, it was acknowledged that nutrition was a specific component of food literacy and that it would not naturally follow if other components were met. Views varied as to why and to what extent this was important. Some considered this to be a function of our contemporary food environments, that is, in years past or in nations where the local food environment is predominantly made up of core foods, food literacy is more likely to result in a healthy diet. Some considered nutrition knowledge to be a subset of food literacy. Others considered it to be a different set of knowledge, skills, attitudes and beliefs. Participants discussed the need to explicitly focus on nutrition. The depth of this focus was a function of the nutrition end-point being sought.

> Thais don't need nutrition science to tell them what is a healthy diet. They, until very recently, have done it, because the traditional diet for them has been a healthy diet. I think the same pertains to Italy and to Greece where there have been their traditional diets, perhaps haven't had the diversity that nutritionists would want. But, the reliance on fruit and vegetables and complex carbohydrate, I mean it's fantastic. So, there are many places in the world where the traditional diet is so lined up with now what nutrition science is saying, that you actually didn't need the knowledge to eat healthily. But, I think things have changed in all those countries and in Australia, with the rise of food offerings and the local – our local food environments have changed so dramatically, so that there's food on every corner.
>
> Gastronomy researcher 1

> I think back to the messages that we give out in nutrition, like, two serves of fruit a day, five serves of veg, no more than three or four meat meals per week, ideally two sorts of fish meals. That really goes back to the planning and the access for people, that it's not a matter of just selecting what's on special, or perhaps what a family preference is, or people's own preferences, but that you'd have to specifically be undertaking some sort of plan, really, to make sure that you've met those requirements.
>
> Nutrition researcher 1

This study sought the views of a diverse group of experts with interest and experience in healthy eating. Non-nutritionists in particular expressed strong views on nutrition promotion and its impact on people's relationship with food. These views were often in conflict with how nutritionist participants described their role.

> Rather than constantly bombarding people with the latest nutrition science as X, Y and Z, because I think that that adds to this under confidence, this fear of food, this, 'look I don't know what to do'. (non-nutritionist)
>
> Gastronomy researcher 1

> I've got a very strong view, because for me, if you're, let's use the term 'good with food' – if you grow your own vegetables, or buy from farmer's markets, you go with the seasons, you cook just simply and beautifully, nutrition is just a by line for it. (non-nutritionist)
>
> Gastronomy practitioner

> We're so confused, we're so frightened. That sends us into the embrace of commercial food providers and other food providers, because we say, 'Oh, we can't do it.' And, for me, unless we reclaim that mastery over food, that ease with it, then we're in deep trouble. And that's far more than ease and mastery over nutrients. (non-nutritionist)
>
> Gastronomy researcher 2

> Well, I live in a world where the amount of nutrition information, misinformation overwhelms the nutritional information and it's me just trying to get a few people to get their heads above all the crap. (nutritionist)
>
> Industry practitioner 1

> I think that there has been distortion of quantities and people I think have lost their way in terms of what is reasonable to eat, how often to eat certain foods. (nutritionist)
>
> Industry advocate 3

> I'm not at all in favour of professionalism but it strikes me that we actually are not able to effectively communicate to our colleagues what this nutrition stuff is about. Them appreciating that we're not being exclusive or precious but that to sort of eat well and appropriately is complex. But on the other hand I guess I don't, I think that it's complex largely because of all the, the messiness around eating in society at the moment. (nutritionist)
>
> Nutrition policy 1

Food experts differed in what they thought was an important level of nutrition knowledge. The nutrition end-point sought appeared to differ depending upon the setting and context. Many discussed overall broad nutrition goals, perhaps best described as universal population-wide wellbeing. This included knowing the general proportions in which to eat foods and broad principles regarding foods to include and avoid for general good health. These sorts of broad goals are probably best articulated in dietary guidelines although most participants had limited familiarity with these nutrition tools and measures and so did not mention them specifically. Food literacy was also considered with respect to its relationship to meeting food group serve recommendations and further to individualized nutrition needs, for example when following a special diet.

The relative importance of food literacy components also seemed to differ depending upon the nutrition end-point being sought, as did the mechanism through which nutrition would be improved. It may be that the importance of each of these components is relative to each other. For example, if you do not prepare food from raw ingredients then the labelling aspects from the selection domain may be more important. Components of food literacy that a dietitian focuses on with an individual client following a restricted renal diet, for example, may be motivated by increasing the choice of foods within the client's usual food environment.

Summary

Experts described that food literacy was made up of multiple, inter-related dynamic components. These all had an influence on diet quality by making nutrition recommendations more certain, more pleasurable or that gave more choice. The extent to which this could occur would be mediated by the individual's values, particularly for health, and the food supply which was accessible to them. The specificity of the nutrition end-point would determine the nature of each component of food literacy and the aspects the practitioner would need to focus on. This model was used to review interventions and was then subsequently modified using the results of the Young People Study (Cullerton, Vidgen & Gallegos 2012). The latter process, which led to the development of a final model, is discussed in the next section.

Results of the Young People Study: a final model of the relationship between food literacy and nutrition

Data from the Young People Study was examined for new themes and then re-examined against the results of the Expert Study to look for areas of intersection. This led to the development of a final model. Unlike the Expert Study, participants in the Young People Study were not asked about the relationship between food literacy and nutrition; rather they were asked about how they go about feeding themselves, and what they considered meeting food needs 'well' meant – that is, their conceptualizations of 'being good with food'. This data was considered alongside information on dietary intake, and attitudes towards nutrition and healthy eating. From this, the Expert Study model was re-examined and modified to better communicate the relationship between food literacy and nutrition. This section describes each of the constructs presented in the final model. Many of the constructs as described in the results of the Expert Study model were retained; however, the understanding of their meaning and contribution to the overall model deepened following the Young People Study and tests of its application with practitioners.

The construction of the model involved both the development of a theory of the relationship between constructs and the clarity of their representation graphically. The latter process was informed by peer debriefing. Various model options were first presented and discussed with a project reference group composed of practitioners and researchers from health, community and education sectors. The final model is presented in Figure 4.2.

In the final model, the inner circle describes the core relationship between food literacy and nutrition. It illustrates that food literacy improves diet quality by contributing to the certainty, choice and/or pleasure of food intake. Diet quality can be described at varying levels of specificity. Food literacy may also result in other outcomes such as social connectedness and food security. The outer circle illustrates the importance of context. The extent to which food literacy can influence nutrition will be influenced by the food supply and early childhood experiences with food, shown in the first circle. These in turn will be influenced by the social determinants of health, particularly poverty, geography, social exclusion and social support. The overarching influence of these contextual factors on all of these relationships, that is, the nature of food literacy components, their contribution to certainty, choice and pleasure, and the extent to which they will contribute to improving diet quality, is depicted by the circle shapes. The following section describes the model and each of these constructs in detail.

Food literacy

Food literacy has been defined in the previous chapter as:

> A collection of inter-related knowledge, skills and behaviours required to plan, manage, select, prepare and eat foods to meet needs and determine food intake. It is the scaffolding that empowers individuals, households, communities or nations to protect diet quality through change and support dietary resilience over time.

The diagrammatic representation of food literacy aims to reflect the key themes in this definition. The final model shows that food literacy is made up of several components. In the revised model they are grouped into four domains. All four domains are essential parts of food literacy. Domains are also related in that competence within a domain may influence the level of competence needed in another. For example, if one has limited food preparation skills and relies on pre-made foods, a higher level of competence in food selection may be needed to maintain diet quality. Circles are linked to represent this relationship and food literacy as a whole concept, rather than separate parts.

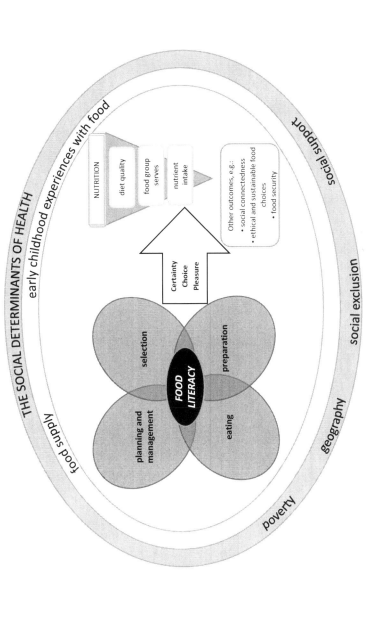

Figure 4.2 A model of the relationship between food literacy and nutrition

Data from both studies revealed that food literacy is contextually driven and changes over time. The relative importance of domains to improving or maintaining diet quality will constantly vary. For example, within the same individual, the level of food preparation skills needed to feed themselves will differ from that needed to feed dependants. Similarly, the planning and management knowledge would differ between when an individual is in stable housing and when they are not. As a consequence, the degree to which a set of knowledge, skills and behaviours can influence diet quality will also vary.

Mechanisms

As with the Expert Study model, this model shows that the relationship between food literacy and nutrition is not direct; rather, it improves nutrition by making food intake more certain (or predictable), more pleasurable and gives more choice (or helps to inform choice in our complex food environment). These mechanisms aligned well with the main themes identified in young people's conceptualizations of being good with food. For example, Component 3.1 (Table 3.2) of food literacy is the ability to:

> Make a good tasting meal from whatever food is available. This includes being able to prepare commonly available foods, efficiently use common pieces of kitchen equipment and having a sufficient repertoire of skills to adapt recipes (written or unwritten) to experiment with food and ingredients.

The mechanisms of certainty, choice and pleasure all contribute to this component.

In the final model these mechanisms have been given greater emphasis than in the Expert Study model. This reinforces that they are the mechanisms through which food literacy influences nutrition. Pleasure, certainty and choice are often end-points in themselves for service providers and individuals. They are also more likely than nutritional status to be the motivation for developing one's food literacy. The Young People Study reinforced that for food literacy to improve nutrition, it must travel through one of these mechanisms. Attendance, participation and engagement with an intervention relied on it addressing one or all of these mechanisms.

The health sector's role is to work in partnership with those service providers who specialize in these mechanisms to extend their work to include a nutrition outcome. In many cases, these service providers are better placed to address these mechanisms than those working in health. For example, the use of the gastronomy sector to engage people in food literacy programmes which promote healthy eating with a pleasure focus may be more successful than programmes being conducted within health-care settings with a nutrition focus. This may explain the popularity of celebrity chefs in health promotion programmes.

In the first model, values were included as a moderator of the relationship between food literacy and nutrition. These might, however, better describe the mechanisms of choice, certainty and pleasure. Schwartz has identified nine domains to universally define values (Schwartz 1994). The value domains are useful in describing individuals, groups and populations. Botonaki applied these domains to explain convenience orientation in food consumption (Botonaki & Mattas 2010). In mapping values and convenience food seeking, the study found that those who favoured convenience valued power, achievement and hedonism. Those that favoured food preparation, shopping in specialized stores and the sensory appeal of food valued security and conformity. These mechanisms, therefore, may represent different motivations through which to engage individuals in food literacy and may help to explain the different emphasis that nations place on population level food literacy development.

Moreover, these three mechanisms are representative of key elements of the new modernity described by contemporary social theorists. In his work *Modernity and Self-Identity*, Giddens (1991) describes the inter-connection between certainty and choice in modern society. He describes a 'post-traditional order' in which key institutions that have guided society, such as religion, have broken down. In their place, individuals are left to determine their own identity from a greater choice of options but less certainty than these key institutions provided. Here he describes the complexity of this task:

> Modernity institutionalises the principle of radical doubt and insists that all knowledge takes the form of hypotheses: claims which may very well be true, but which are in principle always open to revision and may have at some point to be abandoned.
>
> (Giddens 1991: 3)

Giddens goes on to describe this as then occurring amid a 'puzzling diversity of options and possibilities' (Giddens 1991: 3). The certainty of tradition and habit has been replaced by the need to make decisions based on rational knowledge. He refers to trust as being crucial to personality development. He asserts that a small number of simple decisions are based on past experience but others requiring a more critical knowledge rely on trust. In describing how trust is used in modern society, he refers again to the fluidity and lack of certainty around knowledge and how experts have replaced traditional institutions in providing this. For those excluded from key social systems and institutions, this trust is likely to be diminished.

The emergence of food literacy as a relatively new construct may be explained by Giddens's modernity. He describes the pace, scope and profoundness of social change as greater than in any prior system. Food systems and our interaction with them are part of this. The individual's knowledge and trust of these systems cannot keep up with this pace of change.

The emergence of food literacy may be an attempt to make sense of it all, try to order the choice and restore trust and certainty. It may be that, like personality development, this trust is a crucial element of developing a healthy relationship with food. Giddens describes this as being difficult in a global modern society which re-orders time and space in everyday life. Food is available in more different forms, places and times than ever before. Eating, consequently, also includes more options than ever before.

Gabriel and Lang highlight the commodification of food and eating (Gabriel & Lang 2006). They describe the consumer as a 'god-like figure' for whom pleasure is the ultimate pursuit. Choice is central to consumerism. More choice is associated with more pleasure and greater consumer power. They too describe a breakdown of traditional institutions, now replaced with the market.

It is perhaps not surprising, therefore, that the results of these studies identified the mechanisms of certainty, choice and pleasure. They are, perhaps, more a modern representation with an everyday event, eating, rather than being unique to the application of food literacy. Regardless, these mechanisms help to explain the emergence of the construct of food literacy in policy, practice and society. More importantly, they help to describe how the practical elements of day to day eating relate to nutrition in contemporary society.

Nutrition outcomes

Results of the Young People Study and a review of food literacy interventions reinforced that nutrition outcomes are broadly defined. The nature of the nutrition outcome sought should be articulated in programme planning and will influence the depth of knowledge and skill in each food literacy component. The term 'diet quality' can be used to broadly describe a range of nutrition outcomes. Measures of diet quality typically capture the extent to which food intake meets both dietary guidelines and food group intake recommendations (McNaughton et al. 2008). Dietary patterns may also be a useful end measure as they can be used to describe more contemporary styles of eating (Cunha et al. 2010). At the individual level, food literacy could be targeted with a specific food component as the outcome. For example, a dietitian may work with a client to improve planning and management, selection and preparation domains for the purposes of avoiding gluten.

It is useful to consider different levels of nutrition end-points and their application in practice across the health-care continuum from primary prevention, to chronic disease risk management, to medical nutrition therapy. This could be used as a framework to inform a multi-strategic 'model of care' for food literacy. For example, food literacy programmes targeting the well population might aim for outcomes at the level of dietary guidelines and be the responsibility of population health services, whereas those targeting the management of a chronic condition may focus on specific nutrients and be the responsibility of those working in acute, rehabilitation and extended care. Using the model in this way would help practitioners determine which components of food literacy they could support the development of, in which settings, for which populations and to what purpose. It also inherently describes food literacy supported at national, community, household and individual levels.

The research findings acknowledge that food literacy will lead to additional outcomes beyond nutrition; examples include, but are not limited to, social connectedness, ethical and sustainable food choices, and food security. For this reason, they have been included in the final model. This research, however, was designed to explore its relationship to nutrition. Insufficient data was collected on these other outcomes to generate a model of their relationship to food literacy. This is represented in the model by a greater emphasis on nutrition outcomes. The model acknowledges that they may be primary outcomes for other sectors delivering food literacy interventions and would therefore be included in evaluation frameworks as appropriate.

Context

Both studies revealed the relative importance of the components of food literacy and that its capacity to influence nutrition is highly contextual. In the Expert Study model, this was represented by the mediators of food supply and values and their influence on the nature and emphasis of food literacy components. The influence of context was then further explored through a case study of young people and disadvantage. The life-course style of interviewing and analysis in the Young People Study allowed the exploration of these contextual factors over time. Disadvantage was described in terms of poverty, social exclusion, social support, geography and transport. These are consistent with the social determinants of health identified by the World Health Organization (Wilkinson & Marmot 2003). These in turn influenced the nature of the local food supply and early childhood development of food literacy. This is represented in the model by two concentric circles.

Disadvantage influenced the capacity of food literacy to contribute to choice, certainty and pleasure, and ultimately, nutrition and other outcomes. These determinants influenced the relative importance and depth of knowledge or skills for individual components. This is described in quotes presented in the preceding chapter from participants across a spectrum of disadvantage. Two concentric circles were chosen as best representing that the influence of disadvantage is not direct or linear but rather affects the relationship between food literacy and nutrition in a range of ways.

The findings of the Young People Study indicate that people from all backgrounds were capable of demonstrating the components of food literacy and working towards meeting nutrition recommendations. However, the depth of knowledge, skill and behaviour required in each component and the extent to which food literacy was capable of influencing nutrition were determined by social exclusion, poverty, social support, geography and transport. For example, for a person without transport, determining how to access food is more complex; for a single mother on welfare payments and without social support, feeding her family may require more planning and management.

Disadvantage can be defined by the restriction of choice. The emergence of the theme of choice and its related themes of certainty and pleasure in the findings of this study is particularly noteworthy in the context of disadvantage. In a society in which its members are described as consumers rather than citizens, advantage is defined by one's capacity to consume, choose what to consume and derive pleasure from it (Gabriel & Lang 2006). Conversely, those with limited capacity to do so are marginalized and excluded. This very society which boasts empowerment and self-actualization for some creates suppression for others (Giddens 1991). In exploring the meaning of the term food literacy, empowerment was a key theme, but so too was that of fundamental life skills. This perhaps reflects the multiple purposes for which practitioners invest in food literacy interventions. At a whole population level, food literacy may empower citizens to enhance their diet quality, navigate a food supply with greater autonomy and engage in a dialogue over their food system. When working with disadvantaged groups, rather, it may empower through the expansion of choice and inclusion in food and social systems that were otherwise inaccessible.

Components which specifically described critical consumerism and informed food citizenship were not identified as core components of food literacy in the Expert Study (see Chapter 3). This was supported by the results of the Young People Study in which knowing where food comes from and other more critical aspects of selection were not described by participants. It may be difficult to consider a food literacy which empowers without this. These results may be due to the nature of case study. The profound level of disadvantage experienced by some young people may have overemphasized the immediate needs which food was required to meet. However, its lack of identification by both Expert Study participants and more advantaged participants in the Young People Study could also indicate a more general lack of awareness of the impact of social, cultural, economic and environmental systems on individual food intake, their capacity to influence it or demand that it changes.

In the model developed following the Expert Study, food supply and values were thought to be mediators. However, following the Young People Study, it became clear that these were a manifestation of the social determinants of health rather than existing separately on their own. Food literacy, for example, has an influence on nutrition, irrespective of food supply, because being able to work within the local food supply is part of it. However, for those who live in a remote area, have no transport and little income, the planning and management required to routinely access healthy food may be a more important component of food literacy than it is for a wealthy urban dweller living in an apartment above a supermarket. This further highlights the increased complexity of choosing healthy foods for those experiencing disadvantage and the need for efforts to improve nutritional status to extend beyond the individual. Embedding the food literacy and nutrition relationship within the social determinants of health helps to consider where it might sit within broader health, education and social services plans.

Implications for practice and a framework for evaluation

The purpose of the model is to describe the relationship between food literacy and nutrition; to identify elements to include in the planning, implementation and evaluation of interventions including the identification of target populations, settings and partners. This model can guide process, impact and outcome evaluation frameworks and measures.

- The components represent process evaluation constructs.
- The mechanisms box containing choice, pleasure and certainty represents impact level evaluation constructs.
- The hierarchy of nutrition end-points can be used to define outcome evaluation measures.

When the model was tested in the review of interventions, it revealed that most looked at these elements. For example, process evaluation examined behaviour change in preparing food, impact evaluation measured increased enjoyment in eating healthy food, and outcome evaluation measured food intake.

The two outer circles in the model help practitioners to consider the context of their intervention. This, together with mechanisms, will help practitioners to determine who their practice partners may be. These need to be considered and articulated in service policy and planning, monitoring and evaluation.

Food literacy and health

Throughout both studies and in the literature, themes of food insecurity, body weight and chronic disease risk, and their relationship with food literacy emerged. For this purpose, a second model was developed. It is presented in Figure 4.3. The model proposes the contribution of food literacy to each of these health risk factors.

The research identified that food literacy includes multiple components, the exact nature of which is contextually driven. Additionally, these studies suggested that food literacy is likely to influence health in a range of ways. The literature regarding the relationship between various components of food literacy and dietary intake is inconclusive. This relationship is particularly weak when extended to examine body weight (Crawford et al. 2007; Kenny et al. 2008; Larson et al. 2006; Smith et al. 2010). It is likely, therefore, that food literacy is an enabler to healthy eating and health overall, rather than a risk factor per se. That is, focusing on food literacy alone is unlikely to influence health outcomes, rather it is an important adjunct to other strategies which address health and wellbeing.

Due to its multi-component, contextual nature, strategies that address food literacy are likely to influence health in a range of ways, making them a good investment. This model proposes the points of influence of food literacy along the causal pathway to chronic disease. Confounder arrows show where food literacy could link into broader frameworks which address disadvantage, food insecurity, nutritional status, body weight and chronic disease risk. While a focus on food literacy may buffer against an obesogenic or food insecure environment,

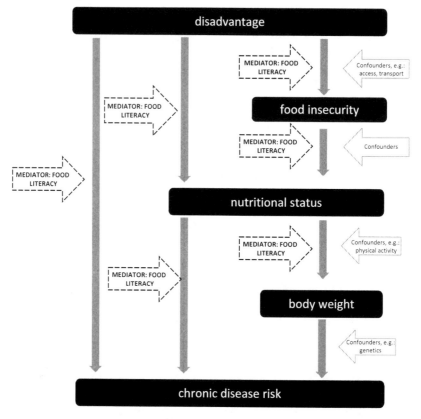

Figure 4.3 A conceptual model of the role of food literacy in food security, nutritional status, body weight and chronic disease

multi-strategic plans still need to continue to work towards influencing them. If food literacy is the scaffolding that empowers individuals, households, communities or nations to protect diet quality through change and support dietary resilience over time, then it follows that it acts to protect health and wellbeing at various points along the causal pathway to chronic disease.

This second model helps to position food literacy within broader health plans, particularly those addressing chronic disease. It guides evaluation in articulating the likely contribution of food literacy along a risk factor pathway. At times, food literacy related interventions have been expected to more directly affect food insecurity, body weight and chronic disease risk than can reasonably be expected from such interventions. This is evidenced by some of the outcome measures used by existing interventions. When the intervention fails to do so, investment ceases and work in the area is abandoned. This model, together with food literacy and the nutrition model in Figure 4.2, should be used to articulate expectations of food literacy work, including evaluation frameworks, to judge their effectiveness.

Conclusions

This research used an assets-based philosophy to formulate protective rather than risk factor pathways for health. This approach shifts nutrition promotion out of its current punitive paradigm and reinstates it as being focused on well-being, nourishment and sustainability in the full sense of those terms. The Expert Study asked best-selling cookbook authors, food historians, food producers, school text book writers, food relief agencies and other food experts what was needed to meet food needs. This represented the diversity of needs food fulfils for all of us and the biological, social, cultural and economic systems it exists within. In the Young People Study, participants described what being good with food and meeting food needs meant. Neither of these studies applied a health end-point, rather they used constructivist grounded theory to let the protective factors of healthy eating emerge.

In describing the relationship between food literacy and nutrition and other health outcomes, the models presented in this chapter can inform practice and investment decisions. They describe what to do and why, what to measure and the nature of performance indicators at each point. The involvement of practitioners in the presentation of these models has contributed to their translation into practice.

References

Botonaki, A. & Mattas, K. 2010, 'Revealing the values behind convenience food consumption', *Appetite*, vol. 55, no. 3, pp. 629–638.

Crawford, D., Ball, K., Mishra, G.D., Salmon, J. & Timperio, A. 2007, 'Which food-related behaviours are associated with healthier intakes of fruits and vegetables among women?', *Public Health Nutrition*, vol. 10, no. 3, pp. 256–265.

Cullerton, K., Vidgen, H. & Gallegos, D. 2012, *A Review of Food Literacy Interventions Targeting Disadvantaged Young People*, Queensland University of Technology, Brisbane, Queensland, viewed 10 December 2015, <http://eprints.qut.edu.au/53753/>.

Cunha, D.B., de Almeida, R.M.V.R., Sichieri, R. & Pereira, R.A. 2010, 'Association of dietary patterns with BMI and waist circumference in a low-income neighbourhood in Brazil', *British Journal of Nutrition*, vol. 104, no. 06, pp. 908–913.

Gabriel, Y. & Lang, T. 2006, *The Unmanageable Consumer*, 2 edn, Sage, London.

Giddens, A. 1991, *Modernity and Self-Identity*, Stanford University Press, Stanford, California.

Kenny, D., Denney-Wilson, E., Nelson, P. & Hardy, L. 2008, 'Eating habits of young offenders on community orders and associations with overweight and obesity', *Nutrition and Dietetics*, vol. 65, pp. 198–204.

Larson, N.I., Story, M., Eisenberg, M.E. & Neumark-Sztainer, D. 2006, 'Food preparation and purchasing roles among adolescents: associations with sociodemographic characteristics and diet quality', *Journal of the American Dietetic Association*, vol. 106, no. 2, pp. 211–218.

McNaughton, S., Ball, K., Crawford, D. & Mishra, G.D. 2008, 'An index of diet and eating patterns is a valid measure of diet quality in an Australian population', *Journal of Nutrition*, vol. 138, no. 1, pp. 86–93.

Prime Minister's Science Engineering and Innovation Council 2010, *Australia and Food Security in a Changing World*, Department of Prime Minister and Cabinet, Canberra, viewed 26 June 2011, <http://www.chiefscientist.gov.au/wp-content/uploads/Food Security_web.pdf>.

Queensland Public Health Forum 2009, *Eat Well Queensland: Are we Half Way there Yet?: Midpoint Implementation Review*, Queensland Public Health Forum, Brisbane, viewed 22 September 2010, <http://www.health.qld.gov.au/qphf/>.

Schwartz, S.H. 1994, 'Are there universal aspects in the structure and contents of human values?', *Journal of Social Issues*, vol. 50, no. 4, pp. 19–45.

Smith, K., McNaughton, S., Gall, S., Blizzard, L., Dwyer, T. & Venn, A. 2010, 'Involvement of young Australian adults in meal preparation: cross-sectional associations with abdominal obesity and body mass index', *Journal of the American Dietetic Association*, vol. 110, no. 9, pp. 1363–1367.

Wilkinson, R. & Marmot, M. (eds) 2003, *The Social Determinants of Health: The Solid Facts*, 2 edn, World Health Organization, Centre for Urban Health, Copenhagen, viewed 10 December 2015, <http://www.euro.who.int/__data/assets/pdf_file/0005/98438/e81384.pdf>.

5 Using a health literacy frame to conceptualize food literacy

Doris E. Gillis

Introduction

Food literacy is one of multiple literacies needed to function in today's world. Its emergence underscores the importance of context in understanding how people engage with information about food in various situations and settings, and the challenges they face in meeting their goals for health, wellness and quality of life. The lack of a universal understanding of the term 'food literacy', with several definitions emerging in the growing literature, parallels to a large extent the lively debate over recent decades on the meaning of health literacy. Like health literacy, understandings of food literacy stem from different disciplines, epistemologies and experiences relevant to evolving practice and policy concerns.

In this chapter, the less well developed concept of food literacy is examined as it reflects aspects of health literacy drawing upon well recognized definitions and frameworks. Food literacy's interplay with health literacy and related social determinants of health, including links to health disparities and concerns about equitable access to food and nutrition information, is explored. Implications for its application in practice and policy contexts, which illustrate alignments with health literacy, are also offered.

Connections between education and health outcomes have been well established with calls for public health interventions that promote health equity through upstream efforts (Hahn & Truman 2015). Literacy, the cornerstone of education, is recognized as an important determinant of health and is closely associated with health literacy (Ronson & Rootman 2004). Understanding the concept of health literacy, and by extension food literacy, begins with an introduction to the core concept, literacy.

Literacy as social practice

Most definitions of literacy centre on the basic need for people in a literate society to have command over the written word, emphasizing the value of literacy in supporting people's ability to use information in carrying out their daily lives. Rather than depicting a distinct set of skills, such as reading and writing, recent understandings of literacy reflect its more dynamic nature 'based on manifold communicative and social practices' (UNESCO 2004: 29).

Conceptualizing literacy as social practice, and less as an ability which one has or not, shifts the focus away from acquisition of technical skills. Situated within the context of economic, political and social trends in today's complex, pluralistic and information-dense society recognizes 'many practices of literacy embedded in different cultural processes, personal circumstances and collective structures' (UNESCO 2004: 6). Thus, being literate in today's society requires not one but multiple literacies appropriate to various situations and contexts across the life course. Common examples include computer literacy, financial literacy, media literacy, health literacy and, most recently, food literacy.

The idea of multiple literacies as social practice has the potential to challenge practitioners to shift their thinking away from what literacy *does to* people towards what people *can do with* literacy in their daily lives. It places importance on building capacity for individuals to engage in their communities and the society in which they live – a premise central to the field of adult education. This rethinking of literacy from a deficit-based to a strength-based approach is reminiscent of similar shifts in the field of health promotion, with the reframing of health from merely the absence of disease to a resource for everyday living. Health is explicitly described as social practice in the Ottawa Charter for Health Promotion (WHO 1986) statement, 'Health is created in the context of everyday life – where people live, love, work and play'. Viewing both health and literacy as resources for everyday living underpins the notion of health literacy as an asset (Nutbeam 2008), thereby opening up many opportunities for its application and for reflecting upon the emerging concept of food literacy from the perspective of social practice. As noted by Coveney, 'food is never just "food", but it is always symbolic of other capabilities and capacities, depending on the lens used' (2013: 6). Beyond being essential for human health, food is embedded within the interrelated socio-cultural, economic, political, and environmental concerns of the everyday lives of people (Began et al. 2012).

Given the fundamental problem in establishing a set of values common to all people in a pluralistic society, it is not surprising that defining literacy, and its associated concepts, is contentious. Some authors argue that literacy and health literacy are separate concepts, while others contend that health literacy is simply literacy within the health context (Rootman 2004). Recently, food literacy has been described as a sub-set of health literacy (Howard & Brichta 2013). Recognizing the ambiguous nature of literacy appears central to appreciating the diverse approaches to defining health literacy – and other literacies – and, more specifically, to identifying how practitioners engage with these various notions.

The evolving concept of health literacy

Situated at the nexus of individual and broader social system-wide factors, health literacy is a multidimensional way of thinking about timely health concerns. Increasingly, health literacy is referred to as a 'vital resource for everyday living, a key determinant of health, and a critical aspect of health disparities' (Gillis, Begoray & Rowlands 2012: 2). It is recognized as a key determinant of population health as concerns grow about health inequalities and social inequities, with efforts to enhance health literacy shown to improve health outcomes relevant to addressing health inequities (Kickbusch et al. 2013). People with limited levels of literacy are more likely to have difficulty accessing health services, engaging in self-care as well as seeking and understanding information to make informed health-related decisions, including tasks related to accessing food and nutrition services, managing diet-related conditions and making healthy food choices. Those who struggle most in daily life because of limited health literacy tend to be older adults, recent immigrants, members of ethnic minorities, and those with lower levels of education and/or low language proficiency. Proficiency in applying basic literacy skills is closely associated with health literacy (Neilson-Bohlman, Panzer & Kindig 2004).

Defining health literacy

The core processes of accessing, understanding and using health pertinent information are reflected in most definitions of health literacy. However, such definitions reflect various notions of literacy emanating from the fields of literacy and education, as well as differing perspectives on health debated within the health field. Two disciplinary approaches to defining and addressing health literacy have emerged (Pleasant & Kuruvilla 2008). On the one hand, the biomedical or clinical approach focuses on patients' basic literacy skills and ability to understand information in order to comply with recommendations and expert advice from health professionals. Derived from a medical model of practice, this approach tends to privilege scientific knowledge and expert advice over the experiential knowledge of those served. Moreover, a need to determine 'clinical risk' suggests screening of individuals for low literacy, thereby identifying their limitations. Practices which emphasize literacy deficits further stigmatize and marginalize individuals who are already facing many hardships. In contrast, the public health approach highlights personal autonomy and empowerment, suggesting that professionals can build capacity for individuals to act on information within the circumstances of their daily lives.

Health literacy is framed as a personal asset, drawing from theoretical concepts in the fields of literacy, adult education and health promotion which value multiple ways of knowing, including learning through experience and critical reflection. This approach emphasizes the capacities of people in a manner that can empower them to exert greater control over their health within their life conditions, including addressing the social determinants of their health (Nutbeam 2008).

Despite an abundance of research and commentary on the meaning of health literacy in the literature, there is no universally shared definition. Its international emergence presents particular challenges as the term 'health literacy' is not easily translated across different languages. However, in their comparison of translations of health literacy from five selected European reports, Sørensen and Brand (2013) found evidence of a coherent notion of health literacy, despite numerous translations of the term. They concluded that 'it is clear that the translations clarify the notion and illustrate how it forms part of language as an organic phenomenon, ever growing and changing' (Sørensen & Brand 2013: 9). In thinking of the recent widespread appearance of 'food literacy', exploration of nuances across various languages and international contexts is warranted to determine the extent to which a coherent concept is indeed unfolding.

Australia was a front runner in framing health literacy as a priority health issue in its 1993 national goals for population health (Nutbeam et al. 1993). In 2000, the United States *Healthy People 2010* report (Department of Health and Human Services 2000) called for improving the health literacy of persons with inadequate or marginal literacy skills as a national objective. Early American definitions of health literacy reflected a need for reading and numeracy skills for patients to engage with health information in clinical settings. Growing concern that low health literacy contributed to less adherence with medical advice, poorer health status and less engagement with preventative services prompted the 2004 Institute of Medicine (IOM) report, *Health Literacy: A Prescription to End Confusion* (Neilson-Bohlman, Panzer & Kindig 2004). This landmark document framed health literacy as a mediator between individuals and the health context, defining it as 'the degree to which individuals have the capacity to obtain, process, and understand basic health information and services needed to make appropriate health decisions' (Neilson-Bohlman, Panzer & Kindig 2004: 2). Although widely used, this definition has been questioned because of its emphasis on the skills of individuals in clinical situations with less attention paid to the broader contextual barriers and facilitators that impact people's access and engagement with information for their health (Rudd, McCray & Nutbeam 2012).

A definition of health literacy more aligned with health promotion and public health was included in the World Health Organization's (WHO) health promotion glossary: 'Health literacy represents the cognitive and social skills which determine the motivation and ability of individuals to gain access to, understand and use information in ways which promote and maintain good health' (WHO 1998: 10). Whereas most definitions tended to focus on skills and abilities of individuals, this one extended to what people can do with these capacities to change their lifestyles and the conditions in which they live. It positioned health literacy as critical to empowerment and crucial to participating fully in society – a central assumption underpinning health promotion. The WHO definition further stated that by 'improving people's access to health information and their capacity to use it effectively, health literacy is seen as critical to personal empowerment' (WHO 1998: 10). Health promotion was also reflected in the way health literacy was framed by the Canadian Expert Panel on Health Literacy as 'the ability to access, understand, evaluate and communicate information as a way to promote, maintain and improve health in a variety of settings across the lifecourse' (Rootman & Gordon-El-Bihbety 2008: 11). Not only is importance placed on the many contexts where people engage with information, including and beyond the health-care system, but also on abilities to evaluate and communicate information relevant to one's health across the lifecourse.

Taking action to make environments easier to navigate for access to information, resources and services in support of health and wellbeing requires people from many settings and sectors to work together for system-wide change. This ideal is reflected in Kickbusch, Maag and Saan's (2005) definition highlighting the diversity in settings and contexts within which people, in their various roles as family members, citizens, employees, health-care providers, consumers and decision makers, engage with information related to addressing health concerns and daily wellbeing.

> Health literacy is the ability to make sound health decisions in the context of everyday life – at home, in the community, at the workplace, the health care system, the market place and the political arena. It is a critical empowerment strategy to increase people's control over their health, their ability to seek out information and their ability to take responsibility.
>
> (Kickbusch, Maag & Saan 2005: 10)

Notably, many such settings and roles are highly relevant to food concerns and dietary practices.

According to Nutbeam (2000), education practices need to move beyond *transmitting* information to ones which enable individuals to develop the knowledge and skills required to actually *use* information for improving health at the individual, community and societal levels. He contended that the potential of education for social change can be easily overlooked as interventions tend to be 'done "on" or "to" people, rather than "by" or "with" people' (Nutbeam 2000: 265). Understanding health literacy as a way to make health education more effective in reaching positive health outcomes positions health literacy as an asset (Nutbeam 2008). To this end, Nutbeam (2000) introduced a typology for health literacy which has relevance to health promotion practice, including implications for framing food literacy.

Types of health literacy

Nutbeam's well-known typology distinguishes between three types of health literacy – functional, communicative/interactive and critical health literacy. He claimed that together they 'progressively allow for greater autonomy and personal empowerment' (Nutbeam 1999: 50). Stemming from Freebody and Luke's (1990) classification of literacy, each domain reflects a different way of knowing. Habermas (1968), a critical theorist, has argued that people relate to the world and to one another through three distinct forms of knowledge: empirical or technical knowing, hermeneutic or communicative knowing, and critical or self-reflective knowing.

Functional health literacy is characterized as 'sufficient basic skills in reading and writing to be able to function effectively in everyday situations' (Nutbeam 2000: 263). It is needed to access services and information required to support one's health, such as reading nutrition information on a food label.

Communicative/interactive health literacy refers to 'more advanced cognitive and literacy skills which, together with social skills, can be used to actively participate in everyday activities, to extract information and derive meaning from different forms of communication, and to apply new information to changing circumstances' (Nutbeam 2000: 263–264). Here experiential learning is valued, in contrast to forms of learning which depend mainly on basic literacy skills. In practice, an interactive health literacy approach enhances individuals' capacity to act independently on knowledge, in particular through improvement in their motivation and self-confidence. Closely tied to the idea of supporting self-efficacy, emphasis is on the development of personal skills in a supportive environment; for example, by gathering inner-city families together to grow, prepare and share food through a community-driven food project. Whereas outcomes of efforts to enhance interactive health literacy primarily accrue to individuals through their improved capacity to act independently on knowledge, there may also be social benefits through improved capacity to influence norms and interact with social groups.

Critical health literacy encompasses 'advanced cognitive skills which, together with social skills can be applied to critically analyse information, and to use this information to exert greater control over life events and situations' (Nutbeam 2000: 264). Critical appraisal of information is vital to being health literate in today's society; however, critical health literacy moves beyond communication to the development of skills needed to effect social change to support health. Nutbeam's idea of critical health literacy is emancipatory in nature, rooted in the Freirean notion of 'critical consciousness' which invites interaction, participation and critical analysis directed to improving individual and community capacity to address social and economic determinants of health. A relevant example would be engaging local residents in critical analysis of deep rooted concerns related to household and community food insecurity, and advocating for upstream policy interventions aimed at enhancing health equity.

Examining health promotion practices through Nutbeam's health literacy typology can help practitioners identify inherent tensions in their practice (Gillis & Gray 2012). Complex issues, such as the growing prevalence of childhood obesity and early onset related disease, call for efforts which can address underlying causes rather than providing information directed to individual-level lifestyle change. Government health policies tend to be 'stuck' on promoting healthy lifestyles through behaviour change with emphasis on individual responsibility for health, often failing to recognize living conditions which create barriers to practices such as healthy eating (Alvaro et al. 2011). Reframing problematic issues is needed to shift to upstream interventions focusing on policy change (Dorfman & Wallack 2007). Applying a critical health literacy lens may help elucidate the relative emphasis on individual responsibility for healthy lifestyle behaviours based on informed choice versus social responsibility calling for social action on the broader social determinants of health (Gillis & Gray 2012).

Addressing challenging issues related to food and the public's health requires engaging diverse stakeholders. Bryant (2002) applied these three ways of knowing in understanding how to engage both experts and community citizens in building a case for policy change. She described instrumental knowledge as 'usually created by experts and systematically developed through "scientific" methods' (Bryant 2002: 92) whereas interactive knowledge derived from 'lived experience acquired through dialogue and information sharing among members of a community' (Bryant 2002: 92). In addressing the powerful socio-economic and political forces on society, critical knowledge 'considers questions of right and wrong, analyses existing social conditions, and outlines what can be done to alter social conditions to improve quality of life' (Bryant 2002: 92). Bryant has suggested that together they can build capacity for policy change.

Notably, critical health literacy is not a well developed concept (Chinn 2011). Although a distinct concept important to public health and health promotion efforts, it is not consistently understood nor used by practitioners or researchers. Based on their conceptual analysis, Sykes et al. (2013) identified the need for its further exploration in various contexts. Given the complex food environment and unique situations in which people make food choices, now may be an appropriate time for fruitful debate on the place of critical health literacy in food literacy – or perhaps more precisely development of the notion of critical food literacy. For instance, being food literate in today's supermarket setting requires one to decipher conflicting claims promoting supplemented and highly processed food products which in many cases have been transported from across the globe. In pointing to the relevance of critical health literacy in engaging citizens in policy change, Kickbusch et al. (2013: 40) contend that 'A political debate about health literacy is a debate about power and transparency: it is about a citizen's right to know about the origin and composition of food'. Making food choices within the context of today's complex corporate driven food system may indeed call for critical ways of knowing to challenge current 'taken for granted' food provision practices and develop policies to address power inequalities between providers and consumers of food.

Zarcadoolas, Pleasant and Greer (2006) introduced a framework incorporating four domains of literacy that is well aligned with food literacy. *Fundamental literacy* compares to functional literacy and refers to basic skills such as those needed to read a recipe or food label. *Scientific literacy* entails competence with science and technology and could be seen as central to understanding the body's use of food or how the concept of risk is applied in food safety. *Civic literacy* encompasses abilities that enable citizens to become engaged in public issues through civic action and leadership, such as advocating for affordable access to local food with less dependence on food banks. Lastly, *cultural literacy* speaks to the ability to recognize customs, world-views and social identities in interpreting and acting on information. For example, how can practitioners support new immigrants in developing their capacity to assess local culturally appropriate food and information channels to satisfy their food needs and preferences? Using this framework, Gillis, Gray and Murphy (2012) identified each of these four domains of health literacy reflected in practices of lay leaders and health professionals across the perinatal continuum of care who were engaged in promoting and supporting breastfeeding in a rural health district. This framework shed light on ways that practices could extend beyond transmitting information promoting breastfeeding to consider how to effect social change to better enable women to act upon advice, recognizing cultural barriers and civic opportunities.

Towards an integrated model for health literacy

Through a systematic review of the literature, Sørenson and colleagues (2012) identified key dimensions of the concept of health literacy embedded in prevalent definitions and frameworks. From their analysis, they incorporated both medical and public health perspectives in the following definition.

> Health literacy is linked to literacy and entails people's knowledge, motivation and competences to access, understand, appraise, and apply health information in order to make judgments and take decisions in everyday life concerning healthcare, disease prevention and health promotion to maintain or improve quality of life during the life course.
>
> (Sørenson et al. 2012: 3)

Consistent with understanding literacy as social practice, the above definition reflects health literacy as both a means and an outcome of actions. It informed an integrated model of health literacy intended to guide the development of individual and population level interventions within health care, disease prevention and health promotion settings as well as in developing measurement tools (see Figure 5.1). This framework invites application of the notion of

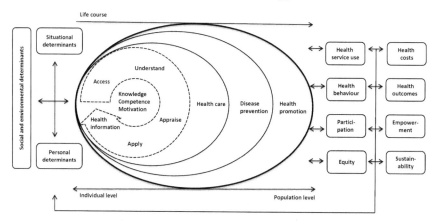

Figure 5.1 Integrated model of health literacy
Source: Sørensen et al. 2012

health literacy within varied contexts addressing many health relevant issues. Applying this integrated model within the context of food related interventions could be useful, for example, in identifying if and how certain population groups access information about food, its preparation, nutritional value etc., as well as determining to what extent they understand, appraise, and ultimately apply it within the context of their daily lives. Importantly, this framework urges consideration of both individual and situational determinants of health literacy as well as the numerous social and environmental determinants influencing capacity to apply food related information to support health relevant actions.

Rootman, Frankish and Kaszap (2007: 61) asserted that health literacy reflects a revitalized way of thinking about health promotion, which can impact 'the way in which people organize their work within the field'. Perhaps the same can be said about food literacy. It is not surprising that food literacy is making its appearance amidst mounting concerns about apparent gaps in food knowledge and skills that people need to make healthy food choices in an increasingly complex food environment. The term 'food literacy' is becoming embedded in the discourse of health practitioners and policy makers as they attempt to address challenging issues in a society where people are overloaded with information about all aspects of food with many paradoxes related to benefits and risks of daily food practices.

The nexus of health literacy and food literacy

The context in which people interact with food information today is multifarious and dynamic. Food and nutrition messages are directed to the public in numerous settings through various channels by a multitude of food 'experts'. Food issues are not simple; they require people to make decisions drawing on all levels of literacy and complementary ways of knowing. Some examples include teasing out the benefits and risks of novel 'super' foods, assessing the credibility and applicability of food and nutrition information messages from celebrity food gurus, assessing contradictory findings reported in the media on the latest diet, determining how to provide an affordable diet for a family on a fixed income, and seeking advice on preventing and managing serious health concerns such as obesity and chronic diseases which impact people across their life course. Food issues infiltrate household conversations, workplace practices and popular media. In everyday life, people confront contradictory messages about what 'healthy' foods to eat and dietary patterns to follow. Engaging with information about food demands knowledge and skills, along with an understanding of the broader contexts in which this information is provided.

Some may argue that food literacy is not a unique concept, but rather a subconcept of health literacy applied within the food and nutrition context. However, its prevalent application in practice and its appearance in the literature suggest that food literacy is emerging as a relevant concept in its own right, and one of the multiple literacies needed to function in today's society. How food literacy is conceptualized is important both in understanding its relationship to health literacy and in determining its potential for application to practice and policy in ways that impact the health and wellbeing of individuals and population groups. Understanding the meaning of food literacy is essential if, like health literacy, its application can foster new ways of thinking about how professionals and policy makers go about their work in more effective ways and the extent to which they can be accountable for their health promotion efforts.

Food literacy as a sub-set of health literacy

'As a subset of health literacy, food literacy affects health outcomes in several ways' (Howard & Brichta 2013: ii.). This statement, in a recent report by the Conference Board of Canada, suggests a conceptualization of food literacy that may reflect constructs embedded in health literacy. Howard and Brichta broadly defined food literacy 'as an individual's food-related knowledge, attitudes, and skills' (2013: 2), incorporating 'household perception, assessment, and management of the risk associated with their food choices' (2013: 2). Food literacy is viewed as the ability of people to select and purchase nutritious foods and meals, safely store and prepare food, interpret food labels and claims, and plan and budget for meals. The authors contend that food literacy skills are important in enabling people to make food related decisions that ultimately impact their diet and their health, as well as their environment.

Increasingly, enhancing food literacy is positioned as a necessary response to offset the perceived deficits in Canadians' food and nutrition knowledge and skills, with the assumption that individuals' food literacy level will influence their food related decisions, thereby impacting their diet and health as well as the broader environment. Interest in promoting efforts to build food literacy is largely driven by the apparent need to address gaps in the public's knowledge about food, nutrition and health which is considered necessary for making healthy food choices, adopting healthy dietary behaviours, and engaging in culinary practices with less dependence on processed foods and away from home eating (Chenhall 2010; Engler-Stringer 2010). The importance placed on the impact of individuals' knowledge, skills and personal behaviours on health reflects a deficit approach in justifying the food literacy agenda.

Framing food literacy as predominantly a set of distinct competencies that determines the ability of the individual to engage with food in a way that meets nutrition needs may minimize the importance of understanding the context and circumstances of 'food getting' in daily living. An overemphasis on the role of personal knowledge and skill as a key determinant of food choice behaviour reinforces the ideological stance which places priority on individual responsibility for health practices and health outcomes. Travers (1997: 58) has argued that a behavioural model that emphasizes 'individualistic, behaviour change strategies negates the role of the social context in shaping behaviour, and thus implies a separation of people and their environment'. Individualization of the concept of food literacy may discount the challenges of the contemporary food getting environment and the constraints of social, cultural, economic and political forces in society on individuals' capacity to act on knowledge and advice, such as that related to healthy eating.

This narrower view is also implicit in the concept of nutrition literacy which is emerging in a somewhat parallel timeline with food literacy. Like food literacy, some authors have referred to nutrition literacy as an extension or sub-set of healthy literacy. Garnweidner and colleagues (2013) suggest that 'Nutrition literacy may be a subordinated concept within health literacy, specified towards nutrition-related information in order to make appropriate dietary decisions' (Garnweidner et al. 2013: 136). According to Blitstein and Evans (2006), nutritional literacy is a form of health literacy, requiring skills in both basic literacy and numeracy. Nutrition literacy tends to align with a clinical approach to health literacy, emphasizing one's capacity for making decisions for health within medical rather than health promotion contexts. Silk and colleagues (2008) crafted a definition of nutrition literacy from the IOM definition for health literacy: 'Nutrition literacy can be defined similarly to health literacy as the degree to which individuals can obtain, process, and understand the basic health (nutrition) information and services they need to make appropriate health (nutrition) decisions, with the qualification that the definition is nutrition specific' (Silk et al. 2008: 4). Zoellner and colleagues (2009) defined nutrition literacy simply as 'the degree to which people have the capacity to obtain, process, and understand basic nutrition information' (Zoellner et al. 2009: 1). It is not surprising to see the emergence of nutrition literacy as an offshoot of health literacy, given the importance placed on individual responsibility for healthy eating as part of healthy lifestyle behaviour change strategies central to the prevention and management of obesity and long term illnesses.

While these definitions of nutrition literacy tend to emphasize a concrete set of technical skills and competencies, years ago Kent (1988) took a broader view more consistent with an understanding of literacy as social practice. 'Nutritional literacy means more than knowing the technical aspects of nutrition…teaching of nutrition should include examination of the world which generates nutrition problems' (Kent 1988: 195). His idea of nutrition literacy reflects aspects of critical health literacy, in particular the importance of critically analysing the root causes of health problems and paying heed to the social determinants of health. In applying Nutbeam's health literacy typology to nutrition, Guttersrud, Dalane and Pettersen (2014: 877) described critical nutrition literacy as 'being proficient in critically analysing nutrition information and advice, as well as having the will to participate in actions to address nutritional barriers in personal, social and global perspectives', with the suggestion that this broader understanding is increasingly relevant to public health nutrition practice.

Dietitians in the USA have been called to integrate health literacy into their practice. Carbone and Zoellner (2012: 263) claim that 'As the field of health literacy matures, dietetics practitioners should seek opportunities to improve their health literacy knowledge and skills, enhance research, and provide more effective interactions with the public'. Gibbs and Chapman-Novakofski (2012) report that health literacy has received limited attention in the nutrition literature, and contend that nutrition professionals should focus more on the nutrition and food related skills that people need in addressing the nutrition implications of disease. A number of barriers to integrating health literacy into practice were identified by dietitians participating in a qualitative study in Canada (Wood & Gillis 2015). Although they shared no common definition of health literacy, all said that health literacy extended beyond basic literacy skills. All three dimensions of health literacy in Nutbeam's model were reflected in their description of practices, with most focusing on functional health literacy and the least on critical health literacy. Notably there was little mention of food literacy.

Food literacy as social practice

Given the complexity of contemporary food getting and eating practices, it seems worth considering the framing of food literacy as social practice, in contrast to a distinct set of knowledge, skills and behaviours. According to Sumner (2013), a new form of food literacy is needed which extends beyond technical knowledge and skills – one which captures the need for individual and social change. Using Nutbeam's three levels of health literacy in reflecting on food literacy, she reiterated that all three forms of knowledge are needed by humans. In supporting the value of including the interactive and critical levels of health literacy, Sumner (2013: 85) states, 'Without including historical-hermeneutic and critical-emancipatory forms of knowledge, food literacy is doomed to remaining a shallow, apolitical, individualistic conceptualization that will contribute little, if anything, to social change'. The significance of critical health literacy to food literacy is underscored in this comment.

Sumner sees food literacy playing an important role 'by encouraging people to read the world in terms of food' (2013: 87). The idea of food literacy as social practice builds on the well established understanding that people's interaction with food is essentially a form of social practice and part of being human (Coveney 2014). Delormier, Frohlich and Potvin (2009) explored food choice as social practice, by applying concepts of 'agency' and 'social structure'. Exploring the influence of rules and resources on routine food practices of families, they identified enabling and constraining conditions affecting food choices, thereby illustrating how integral social structure is to food choice behaviour. Whereas agency is thought of as one's capacity to act, this capacity may be limited by structural constraints limiting food access and choice, as well as ability to act on information and advice promoting healthy eating.

Thinking of food literacy as social practice has implications for planning and implementing interventions aimed at improving eating patterns in population groups in ways that support capacity to act. Whereas individuals may want to act on food information in ways that are health enhancing through their sense of agency, they may live in conditions where they have insufficient income to afford healthy food, lack transportation to get it, and have limited utensils and resources for its preparation. Issues relevant to social and health equity, such as food insecurity, become unveiled when food literacy is framed as social practice, not only a set of technical skills and knowledge. Applying a wider lens of food literacy in designing public health nutrition strategies for addressing such issues may help move practices beyond information provision and food skills training to advocating for improvements in policy and social change to reduce the barriers people face that prevent them from engaging with food in ways that support their health, and that of their communities.

It is this potential for defining food literacy as social practice that has captured the interest of Sumner (2013) who draws her understandings of food literacy from the field of adult education. She states that '[t]o effect positive change in a globalizing world, food literacy must move beyond individualized prescription and notion of blame to become a concept that can analyse current foodscapes and model sustainable alternatives' (Sumner 2013: 84). Given the many challenges to health and equity emanating from the evolving global food system, food literacy is recognized as a timely concept. Sumner's definition of food literacy strives for both individual and social change by encouraging people to 'read the world' in terms of food.

> Food literacy is the ability to 'read the world' in terms of food, thereby recreating it and remaking ourselves. It involves a full-cycle understanding of food – where it is grown, how it is produced, who benefits and who loses when it is purchased, who can access it (and who can't), and where it goes when we are finished with it. It includes an appreciation of the cultural significance of food, the capacity to prepare healthy meals and make healthy decisions, and the recognition of the environmental, social, economic, cultural, and political implications of those decisions.
>
> (Sumner 2013: 86)

Through this description of food literacy, Sumner reminds us of the need to look beyond the knowledge and technical skills of individuals to the social context in which people engage with food in everyday life. This entails an understanding of food literacy as social practice, recognizing that the contemporary world of food getting involves navigating through complex systems in order to access food relevant information and supportive services.

Conclusions

Whether one considers food literacy as a sub-set of health literacy or a unique concept, much can be learned about the nature of food literacy from insights into health literacy gained over the last decades. The emergence of food literacy, like health literacy, underscores the importance of context in understanding how people engage with information about food in various situations and the constraints they face in meeting their personal goals related to food and health. Like literacy and health literacy, food literacy can be viewed as social practice, implying that it reflects more than a concrete set of technical skills. An understanding of food literacy as social practice places importance on the context of everyday living in which people engage with food and with information relevant to food and health, while respecting different types of knowledge and ways of knowing.

Looking at food literacy through an interactive and critical health literacy lens warrants more attention. Critical health literacy is a domain of health literacy that appears to have considerable relevance to food literacy, particularly in addressing current issues related to structural barriers to accessing food for health, and to growing concerns about social inequities and health inequalities. In this regard, further examination and reflection are needed to determine how a notion of critical food literacy might be constructed, applied in practice and guide policy development.

Adoption of the concept of health literacy has been motivated largely by a call for greater accountability among providers of health information with the goal of improving health outcomes. If accountability for food literacy is to be considered a driver for change in practice, it is imperative that outcomes of food literacy interventions can be assessed in terms of their impact on health outcomes. Provision of valuable assessment data should enable practitioners and organizations to better tailor their programmes so that food literacy interventions meet the needs of the intended individuals and population groups. Such data is also useful to inform policy change. Measures of food literacy are needed. Much can be learned from the development and validation of measures of health literacy which is a rapidly advancing field with new scales being designed for application with individuals, groups or populations.

Finally, as one of multiple literacies needed to function in today's world, food literacy appears to call for more exploration both in concept and in practice, with the multifaceted concept of health literacy appearing to be a useful lens for moving forward.

References

Alvaro, C., Jackson, L.A., Kirk, S., McHugh, T.L., Hughes, J., Chircops, A. & Lyons, R.F. 2011. 'Moving Canadian governmental policies beyond a focus on individual lifestyle: some insights from complexity and critical theories', *Health Promotion International*, 26(1), 91–99.

Began, L., Chapman, G.E., Johnston, J., McPhail, D., Power, E.M. & Vallianatos, H. 2012. *Acquired Tastes: Why Families Eat the Way they Do.* Vancouver, BC: UBC Press.

Blitstein, J.L. & Evans, W.D. 2006. 'Use of nutrition facts panels among adults who make household food purchasing decisions', *Journal of Nutrition Education and Behaviour*, 38(6), 360–364.

Bryant, T. 2002. 'Role of knowledge in public health and health promotion policy change', *Health Promotion International*, 17(1), 89–98.

Carbone, E.T. & Zoellner, J.M. 2012. 'Nutrition and health literacy: a systematic review to inform nutrition research and practice', *Journal of the Academy of Nutrition and Dietetics*, 112(2), 254–265.

Chenhall, C. 2010. 'Improving cooking and food preparation skills: a synthesis of the evidence to inform program and policy development' (P.-CPH Network, Trans.), Public Health Agency of Canada, Vancouver, BC, viewed 1 April 2015, http://www.hc-sc.gc.ca/fn-an/nutrition/child-enfant/cfps-acc-synthes-eng.php.

Chinn, D. 2011. 'Critical health literacy: a review and critical analysis', *Social Science & Medicine*, 73(1), 60–67.

Coveney, J. 2014. *Food*. New York: Routledge.

Delormier, T., Frohlich, K.L. & Potvin, L. 2009. 'Food and eating as social practice: understanding eating patterns as social phenomena and implications for public health', *Sociology of Heath & Illness*, 31(2), 215–228.

Department of Health and Human Services. 2000. *Healthy People 2010*, DHHS, Washington, DC.

Dorfman, L. & Wallack, L. 2007. 'Moving nutrition upstream: the case for reframing obesity', *Journal of Nutrition Education and Behavior*, 39(2), S45–50.

Engler-Stringer, R. 2010. 'Food, cooking skills, and health: a literature review', *Canadian Journal of Dietetic Practice and Research*, 71(3), 141–145.

Freebody, P. & Luke, A. 1990. 'Literacies' programs: debates and demands in cultural context', *Prospect*, 5(3), 7–16.

Garnweidner, M., Sverre, L., Pettersen, K. & Mosdol, L. 2013. 'Experiences with nutrition-related information during antenatal care of pregnant women of different ethnic backgrounds residing in the area of Oslo, Norway', *Midwifery*, 29(12), e130–137.

Gibbs, H. & Chapman-Novakofski, K. 2012. 'A review of health literacy and its relationship to nutrition education', *Topics in Clinical Nutrition*, 27(4), 325–333.

Gillis, D.E., Begoray, D. & Rowlands, G. 2012. 'Introducing health literacy in context', in Begoray, D., Gillis, D.E. & Rowlands, G. (eds) *Health Literacy in Context: International Perspectives* (pp. 1–12), Hauppauge: Nova Science Publishers.

Gillis, D.E. & Gray, N.J. 2012. 'Health literacy and healthy lifestyle choices', in Begoray, D., Gillis, D.E. & Rowlands, G. (eds) *Health Literacy in Context: International Perspectives* (pp. 33–56), Hauppauge, NY: Nova Science Publishers.

Gillis, D.E., Gray, N.J. & Murphy, E. 2012. 'Multiple domains of health literacy as reflected in breastfeeding promotion practice: a Canadian case study', *Journal of Health Psychology*, 18(8), 1023–1035.

Guttersrud, Ø., Dalane, J.Ø. & Pettersen, S. 2014. 'Improving measurement in nutrition literacy research using rasch modelling: examining construct validity of stage-specific "critical nutrition literacy" scales', *Public Health Nutrition*, 17(04), 877–883.

Habermas, J. 1968. *Knowledge and Human Interests*, Boston, MA: Beacon Press.

Hahn, R.A. & Truman, B.I. 2015. 'Education improves public health and promotes health equity', *International Journal of Health Services,* 45(4), 657–678.

Howard, A. & Brichta, J. 2013. 'What's to eat? Improving food literacy in Canada', Ottawa: Conference Board of Canada, viewed 30 June 2015, http://www.conferenceboard.ca/e-library/abstract.aspx?did=572.

Kent, G. 1988. 'Nutrition education as an instrument of empowerment', *Journal of Nutrition Education*, 20(4), 193–195.

Kickbusch, I., Maag, D. & Saan, H. 2005. 'Enabling healthy choices in modern health societies', paper presented at Eighth European Health Forum, Bad Gastein, Austria, 5–8 October 2005, viewed 22 July 2015, http://old.ilonakickbusch.com/health-literacy/Gastein_2005.pdf.

Kickbusch, I., Pelikan, J.M., Apfel, F. & Tsouros, A.D. (eds). 2013. *Health Literacy: The Solid Facts*, Copenhagen, DM: World Health Organization, viewed 22 July 2015, http://www.euro.who.int/__data/assets/pdf_file/0008/190655/e96854.pdf.

Neilson-Bohlman, L., Panzer, A.M., Kindig, D.A. & Institute of Medicine. 2004. *Health Literacy: A Prescription to End Confusion*. Committee on Health Literacy. Washington, DC: The National Academies Press.

Nutbeam, D. 1999. 'Literacies across the lifespan: health literacy', *Literacy and Numeracy Studies*, 9(2), 47–56.

Nutbeam, D. 2000. 'Health literacy as a public health goal: a challenge for contemporary health education and communication strategies into the 21st century', *Health Promotion International*, 15, 259–267.

Nutbeam, D. 2008. 'The evolving concept of health literacy', *Social Sciences & Medicine*, 67(12), 2072–2078.

Nutbeam, D., Wise, M., Bauman, A., Harris, E. & Leeder, S. 1993. *Goals and Targets for Australia's Health in the Year 2000 and Beyond*, AGPS, Canberra.

Pleasant, A. & Kuruvilla, S. 2008. 'A tale of two health literacies: public health and clinical approaches to health literacy', *Health Promotion International*, 23(2), 152–159.

Ronson, B. & Rootman, I. 2004. 'Literacy: one of the most important determinants of health', in Raphael, D. (ed.), *Social Determinants of Health: Canadian Perspectives* (pp.139–169), Toronto, ON: Canadian Scholars' Press.

Rootman, I. 2004. 'Health promotion and literacy: implications for nursing', *Canadian Journal of Nursing Research*, 36(1), 13–21.

Rootman, I. & Gordon-El-Bihbety, D. 2008. *A Vision for a Health Literate Canada: Report of the Expert Panel on Health Literacy*, Ottawa, ON: Canadian Public Health Association.

Rootman, I., Frankish, J. & Kaszap, M. 2007. 'Health literacy: a new frontier', in O'Neill, M., Peterson, A., Dupere, S. & Rootman, I. (eds) *Health Promotion in Canada: Critical Perspectives* (pp. 61–73) (2nd edn), Toronto, ON: Canadian Scholars' Press.

Rudd, R.E., McCray, A.T. & Nutbeam, D. 2012. 'Health literacy and definitions of terms', in Begoray, D., Gillis, D.E. & Rowlands, G. (eds) *Health Literacy in Context: International Perspectives* (pp. 13–32), Nova Science Publishers, Hauppauge, NY.

Silk, K.J., Sherry, J., Winn, B., et al. 2008. 'Increasing nutrition literacy: testing the effectiveness of print, web site, and game modalities', *Journal of Nutrition Education and Behavior*, 40, 3–10.

Sørensen, K. & Brand, H. 2013. 'Health literacy lost in translations? Introducing the European Health Literacy Glossary', *Health Promotion International*, 29(4), 634–644. doi:10.1093/heapro/dat013.

Sørenson, K., van den Broucke, S., Fullam, J., Doyle, G., Pelikan, J., Slonska, Z. & Brand, H. 2012. 'Health literacy and public health: a systematic review and integration of definitions and models', *BMC Public Health*, 12, 80. doi:10.1186/1471-2458-12-80.

Sumner, J. 2013. 'Food literacy and adult education: learning to read the work by eating', *Canadian Journal for the Study of Adult Education*, 25(2), 79–92.

Sykes, S., Wills, J., Rowlands, G. & Popple, K. 2013. 'Understanding critical health literacy: a concept analysis', *BMC Public Health*, 13, 150. doi:10.1186/1471-2458-13-150.

Travers, K.D. 1997. 'Nutrition education for social change: critical perspectives', *Journal of Nutrition Education*, 29, 57–62.

UNESCO (United Nations Educational, Scientific, and Cultural Organization). 2004. *The Plurality of Literacy and its Implications for Policies and Programmes*, UNESCO Education Sector Position Paper ED-2004/WS/31. Paris: UNESCO

Wood, J. & Gillis, D.E. 2015. 'Exploring dietitians' engagement with health literacy: concept and practice', *Canadian Journal of Dietetic Practice and Research*, 76, 1–5. doi:10.3148/cjdpr-2015–2003.

World Health Organization (WHO). 1986. *Ottawa Charter for Health Promotion*. Geneva: WHO.

World Health Organization (WHO). 1998. *Health Promotion Glossary*. Geneva: WHO.

Zarcadoolas, C., Pleasant, A. & Greer, D.S. 2006. *Advancing Health Literacy: A Framework for Understanding and Action*, San Francisco, CA: Jossey-Bass.

Zoellner, J., Connel C., Bounds, W., Crook, L. & Yadrick, K. 2009. 'Nutrition literacy status and preferred nutrition communication channels among adults in the lower Mississippi Delta', *Preventing Chronic Disease*, 6(4), A128, viewed 20 June 2015, http://www.cdc.gov/pcd/issues/2009/oct/08_0016.htm.

6 Food literacy and food choice

A constructionist perspective[1]

Carole Bisogni, Stephanie Bostic, Jeffery Sobal and Margaret Jastran

Introduction

Food literacy is a recent term, and parallels other concepts like financial literacy, technological literacy, and health literacy. Food literacy is 'composed of a collection of interrelated knowledge, skills and behaviours required to plan, manage, select, prepare, and eat foods to meet needs and determine intake' (Vidgen & Gallegos 2014: 54). Food literacy is multifaceted and multidimensional, and has four major domains (plan and manage, select, prepare, eat) that each include several components (Vidgen & Gallegos 2014). The food literacy of individuals is diverse and dynamic, and varies in extensiveness and scope. A review of evidence about food literacy and dietary intake finds positive associations between food literacy and healthier food choices (Vaitkevicute, Ball & Harris 2015).

This chapter examines food literacy from the perspective of the Food Choice Process Model (Furst et al. 1996; Sobal & Bisogni 2009), a framework that represents food choice as multilevel, contextual, multifaceted, dynamic, integrated, and diverse (Sobal, Bisogni & Jastran 2014). This model defines food choice as people's thoughts, feelings and actions related to food and eating. The model takes a constructionist perspective by viewing people as perceiving, creating, interpreting, negotiating, managing, enacting, and reflecting about many aspects of food and eating (Sobal et al. 2006). While people execute many food activities in mindless ways, they also carry out many food and eating activities thoughtfully within the contexts in which they live.

Food choice is considered to be multi-level because it can be examined at different levels of analysis from individuals to populations, from an aggregate view of overall food and eating to particular situation-specific eating events (Sobal, Bisogni & Jastran 2014). Food choice is contextual because people's thoughts, feelings and actions are dependent upon the macro-environments and micro-environments in which they live. Food choice is multi-faceted because it reflects the many different phenomena involved in how and why people think, feel and act as they do when it comes to food and eating. Food choice is dynamic as illustrated by the many ways that food choice changes over time and situations. While many aspects of food choice are stable, people encounter changes in their environments and across their life course that cause them to adjust and adapt their ways of thinking, feeling, and acting related to food and eating. Food choice is integrated because the different aspects of food and eating are connected to each other and to other parts of people's lives. Diversity in food choice is illustrated by the many different ways that populations, communities, households, and individuals think, feel and act related to food and eating.

This Food Choice Process Model was developed inductively using interviews with adults to generate the model as grounded theory. Originally published in 1996 (Furst et al. 1996), the model has been revised and elaborated upon as a result of many follow-up studies (Food Choice Research Group 2015). Although the model was developed using data from a specific region in one time period of the United States, the key constructs are relevant to other areas and other eras. The model takes an emic (insider) perspective in that it was developed to reflect people's own experiences with food and eating. While the model shares many concepts and themes with other frameworks developed by experts using an etic (outsider) approach, the model is generally more comprehensive and includes several original components. In this way, the model offers some unique perspectives about the topic of food literacy. The model emphasizes people's own views about how well they are achieving their goals in food and eating and whether or not they have the resources to achieve their goals. The model emphasizes people's own standards and values for food choice rather than what experts think people should value and choose.

The Food Choice Process Model has four main components (Figure 6.1): 'Life Course', 'Influences', 'Personal System', and 'Activities' (Furst et al. 1996; Sobal et al. 2006). Life course encompasses how people develop, construct, and experience food choice over time, including how food choice is shaped by the macro and micro contexts in which people deal with food and eating. Influences

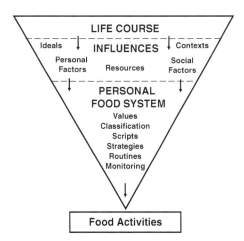

Figure 6.1 Food Choice Process Model

include a broad set of factors that shape food choice including ideals, personal factors, resources, social factors, and contexts. The personal system encompasses many processes that people construct to interpret influences and execute food activities. The personal system includes food choice values (key considerations a person has about food choice) and value negotiations, and also how people classify foods and situations, establish scripts, develop strategies, create routines, and monitor how things are going. Activities include the many actions, decisions, and behaviours people carry out as they handle food, including acquiring, preparing, eating, and cleaning up food. Food activities also include the actions related to providing resources, gathering information, interacting with other people, and managing one's health and wellness. The following sections discuss how each of these components (life course, influences, personal system, and activities) provides insight about the topic of food literacy.

Life course

The life course component focuses upon how people experience food choice across time, through life stages and life events, and within the historical and socio-cultural contexts of their lives (Devine 2005; Devine et al. 1998). People also consider food choice in terms of expected future time (Jabs & Devine 2006). This forethought and anticipation of the future suggests that people develop knowledge and skills for food literacy from infancy to the present time and also consider the knowledge and skills that they may use in some time yet to come, like an adolescent who may state 'I'm learning to cook now so that I will be able to take care of myself when I leave home'.

Considering the many aspects of food and eating that people must learn, the sphere of food literacy is vast. Experiences early in the life course establish some of the basic components of food literacy. Children must learn to distinguish food from non-food, and they also learn to feed themselves, chew and swallow, handle basic utensils, identify when they are hungry, recognize foods that are nourishing, and act in socially acceptable ways during meals. Although parents explicitly teach children to eat and instruct them about how to handle food over the life course, food literacy is mostly acquired in informal, interpersonal ways as people are educated by family members or others and also learn by observing other people in their social world. For example, someone might explain 'We eat salad after the main dish because that is how my family ate it'.

The knowledge and skills that people need for food literacy to manage food activities shift over time as their circumstances change. Adulthood and independent living require expanded sets of shopping, cooking, and cleaning up skills. Grown children often contact friends and family for advice about cooking and shopping. Becoming a parent or caregiver requires that a person learn how to feed dependents, which can be learned from family, friends, print or electronic media, and professionals. People may have different needs for food literacy for their own personal eating that differ from the food literacy that they need in providing food for others. Individual standards and ideals vary between roles, affecting food literacy. A parent who eats mostly snack food at work may describe family meals at home as 'I really want my children to grow up liking vegetables and eating balanced meals so I cook a green vegetable most nights and try to eat dinner with them'.

Over time people may become interested in different aspects of food and eating, expanding their food literacy to learn how to cook new cuisines, how to garden, how to preserve food, or how to become vegetarian (Jabs et al. 1998a). People may move to new environments that change access to food. External factors like rising food prices, food shortages, access to local foods, new food products, or new food contaminants may require people to find and use new information about food and eating. People may develop health problems or experience increases or decreases in income or household size, which may change what they need to know to manage food and eating. Older adults who have less involvement in cooking may need label reading skills but less food preparation skill. A person might assert 'I don't need my roasting pan any more because I don't really cook that much'.

A life course perspective positions the food literacy a person has as changing over time and as acquired in both implicit and explicit ways. The person may assimilate knowledge and skills with little consciousness or be an active agent in modelling what others have done, in identifying what they need to know for their circumstances, and in constructing ways to get it from available sources.

Influences

Food literacy is shaped by several influences, including ideals, personal factors, resources, social factors, and contexts (Furst et al. 1996). Influences are factors that shape the personal system and food activities. Influences provide structure within which food choices are made, and these influences are often assets and constraints that shape food literacy. The next sections discuss these major categories of influences.

Ideals

Ideals are ideas that are collectively constructed, shaped, and used by cultures and sub-cultures. Ideals provide values and norms that offer expectations and reference points for food activities, offering cultural literacy about 'the right way' or 'inappropriate ways' for engaging with food, and are some of the major influences on food choice (Falk, Bisogni & Sobal 1996). Ideals are learned through socialization into a culture, and enable people to have food literacy for that particular culture. For example, someone learns what constitutes culturally appropriate foods and when, where, with whom, and how to eat them as they grow up by being socialized to select, prepare, and consume foods that their family and community find 'proper'. One community might consider a 'proper' breakfast to be coffee, eggs, and bacon while another may see an appropriate breakfast as mint tea and chickpea stew.

Ideals provide 'cultural capital' that constitutes resources for engaging in eating and demonstrating to others that a person has food literacy for a particular group. The extent of an individual's cultural capital may vary, with some people being highly food literate about manners and eating but not having invested the time and effort to be very literate about shopping and cooking. Such a person might proclaim 'We had lobster on vacation, so I know how to eat it, but I never learned to cook it'.

In contemporary Western societies, many cultures and subcultures co-exist and offer a variety of cultural food choices within the food environment. This cultural diversity leads to considerable cultural pluralism, where many cultural, ethnic, and regional foods can be acquired, prepared, and consumed (Devine et al. 1999). Individuals are increasingly challenged to become more culturally aware and less 'culture bound' in their food choices, which gives food literacy broader scope. People increasingly combine food cultures, and draw upon a variety of 'cultural tool kits' (Swidler 1986) as they use components of culture to construct food choice activities. A cook may affirm 'I learned to make rice the Korean way, but it works just fine to use leftover rice to make Italian-style arancini stuffed with Korean barbecued pork'. Food environments are dynamic and evolve, and interact and blend in ways that offer interested individuals the challenge of adapting and adopting new practices to keep their food literacy current in a diverse and shifting food environment. Such a changing and multicultural food environment challenges shoppers, cooks, and eaters to increasingly greater levels of food literacy to eat in a healthy manner.

Personal factors

Personal factors are a person's needs, preferences, and capabilities that affect how they manage food and eating. When individuals enact food choices, their physiological condition and health characteristics, medications, taste sensitivity, allergies, personality, gender, and responsibilities are important influences. Individuals possess 'health capital' as an asset which ranges from high levels of fitness to physical capabilities that decline with poor health or age. An elderly individual might lament 'I can no longer stand up at the stove long enough to stir fry my vegetables and meat so I use the slow cooker or microwave'.

Personal factors include the internalized roles that people play and their personal eating identities (Bisogni et al. 2002). These personal factors provide capabilities and boundaries that are considered in food choices, like the management of vegetarian identities in selecting foods (Jabs et al. 2000). Someone may claim 'I'm a picky eater, and I like what I eat. I'm not going to try anything else'.

Feeling especially hungry or ill on a particular day may shape food choice. Health and wellness are personal factors (health capital) affecting food choices and the development of food literacy. For example, a person who has been diagnosed with a nutrition-related disease, like diabetes, requires new skills and knowledge to navigate recommended food and eating routines. Discovering new food intolerances may cause someone to learn how to shift cooking methods like announcing 'We rarely prepare soups with milk or other dairy products now since my wife has become lactose intolerant over the years'. With a need for dietary changes comes a need for changes in skills and eating patterns. Old food preferences may no longer be met and new sources of eating enjoyment may need to be found. Food literacy often develops and shifts in response to these changes.

Personal factors are seen as 'human capital', which constitutes the knowledge, skills, and personal attributes that a person possesses as a resource. The four domains of food literacy (Vidgen & Gallegos 2014) depend heavily on the development of food related human capital through a person exercising judgement based on knowledge, incorporating cognitions with sensory information, and manually manipulating objects. Some of the varied food management related activities depending on human capital include maintaining foods at safe temperatures, selecting ripe produce, smelling when a food is done and removing it from the heat before it burns, and planning a food budget. Like food choice, human capital is dynamic; it may increase through experience or formal learning or decrease through decreased physical capability. Greater human capital in one domain may allow someone to compensate for a lack of other resources. A mother might declare 'Knowing how to prepare the inexpensive bruised fruit and vegetables helps me stretch my budget so I can feed my kids fruits and vegetables through the whole month'.

Resources

Resources are assets that can be used in food choice. Resource availability enables and constrains what people consider in making food choices. Some food options may be viewed as being 'out of bounds' because they require unavailable assets, although greater food literacy may help some people cope with limited resources in food choice. Major forms of assets include tangible financial assets and time availability.

Financial assets include a person's current income as well as saved wealth that constitute 'financial capital' which can limit and/or enhance food literacy. People with more money can pay for more food, higher quality foods and access to foods they desire, while those with less money must more carefully consider finances in making food decisions. Money also facilitates exposure to new foods and the variety of settings where food literacy can be learned. Financial resources can be exchanged for the services of others if someone has low food literacy, such as paying for grocery delivery or prepared foods if someone does not have the time, skills and knowledge to shop or cook. Processed foods also have 'value added' in the form of preparation work performed by the food industry, and people with low food preparation literacy often pay for corporations to do their food preparation for them.

Time availability is an asset that would seem to be equally accessible for everyone, with 24 hours in a day and 168 hours and seven days in a week. However, social and economic obligations may create 'time poverty' for many people, where they believe they must give higher priority to activities other than the foodwork that constitutes all of the tasks involved in dealing with food (Bove & Sobal 2006). Employment is a major influence upon food choice, and it requires food literacy for people to manage work tasks at their jobs and foodwork tasks at home (Devine et al. 2003). People with greater food literacy have the capability to engage in planning and management of foodwork, which permits them to more efficiently use their available time assets. For example, someone may reveal 'I've figured out what foods I can put in the oven, then go do chores, and later come back and serve, so it doesn't seem like cooking takes much time'.

Social factors

Social factors are the relationships of a person that shape their food choice and constitute their 'social capital'. People consider others when they eat, and modify where, when, how, and what they consume depending on who is jointly involved in a particular food choice. For example, people shop, cook and serve foods with their family, friends, co-workers, and others in mind. Someone may disclose 'I'd like to eat smaller meals, but to please everybody at home I need to make lots of food and lots of types of food'.

People consume most of their food in commensal units, where they eat with others. Family members are the most frequent commensal partners, with meals and snacks frequently eaten at home with relatives. Individuals shop, cook, serve, and clean up foods in light of other family members, with family partners negotiating and managing family meals (Bove, Sobal & Rauschenbach 2003). Families bring in ideas, skills, and foods to the household unit, and jointly develop and maintain family food literacy together. Children and other family members are socialized into becoming more (or sometimes less) food literate by means of participating in household food activities together. The family serves as a unit that has developed social capital, with family relationships offering food knowledge and support. Even if one family member cannot perform a food task, often another family member has the knowledge and time to engage in food planning, selection, and preparation.

In addition to families, people draw upon social capital from others in their social networks (Jabs et al. 1998b). Other people offer social support in food choice, where they share information, materials, empathy, and feedback about food. People use their network connections as a resource to learn and practise their food literacy, like when someone reports 'I didn't know how to cook salmon, but my friend did, showed me how, and now I make salmon every week'.

Contexts

Contexts are the settings in which people live. Contexts involve the ever-changing environments that individuals experience. Several important dimensions of contexts include the physical environment, the food system, and the media. All of these contexts represent 'material capital' as tangible things that shape and are used as resources in food choice.

The physical environment is composed of spaces and objects that influence food choice (Sobal & Wansink 2008). Large scale aspects of the environment like climate and infrastructure such as transportation shape food choices, and food literacy can assist people in dealing with these structures. Someone may be highly food literate in selecting foods, declaring 'I know where to shop for any kind of cuisine that you would like in this city'. People navigate their environment and engage in eating patterns that can be represented by eating maps (Sobal et al. 2012). Smaller scale built objects can greatly enhance food choice, with household spaces like cupboards, furniture and appliances like stoves, cooking implements like good knives, and eating containers like appropriately sized plates facilitating the way people plan, select, prepare, and eat foods (Sobal & Wansink 2007). Food literacy helps acquire useful objects and know how to use them, like professing 'I took a cooking class to learn which knife to use, and now I eat types of food that I never did before'.

The food system is the set of processes involved in growing and transforming raw materials into foods and nutrients used by the body (Sobal, Khan & Bisogni 1998). People engage with food systems to produce, process, distribute, acquire, prepare, and consume foods (Griffin & Sobal 2014), and vary in the levels of food system literacy (Widener & Karides 2014) they have about different stages in the food system. For example, one person may be knowledgeable about accessing food by gardening and shopping but not know much about cooking, while someone else may be a skilled cook who can easily cook meals from whatever foods are available but knows little about where her food comes from.

Another important context for food is the media. Media ideas and information about food are used to establish food literacy and engage in food choice (Wadsworth & Thompson 2005). Print, broadcast, and electronic media provide information, values, and resources about food that are incorporated into food literacy. The media are one of the most important sources of food and nutrition information that people use in food choice, and media literacy (knowledge and understanding of the media) is related to food literacy: individuals who consume more news media are more likely to consume healthier foods (Kean et al. 2012). High access to electronic media offers an important source for deciding what and how to eat. For example, people may easily view videos about food shopping, cooking, and serving on their handheld electronic devices as they make food plans and food decisions. When explaining how she decides what to make for dinner, someone may express 'I'll look in the refrigerator to see what I have, and then I'll search the internet for a main ingredient, or maybe look at some blogs for a recipe idea'.

Personal systems

In personal systems, people actively construct the meanings, understandings, and skills they use to manage food activities related to food literacy in their circumstances according to how they perceive them (Furst et al. 1996). People develop and negotiate food choice values (e.g. health, taste, price, convenience, relationships), classify foods and situations, and construct scripts and routines to achieve their values related to food literacy (Connors et al. 2001). Several important personal food systems processes are highly relevant for food literacy and will be discussed in this section, including values, classification, scripts, strategies, routines, and monitoring.

Constructing and managing food choice values

Values are meanings that people consider and weigh in food choice (Furst et al. 1996), and the most common values that are taken into account in food choice are taste, price, convenience, health, and relationships (Furst et al. 1996; Sobal & Bisogni 2009). For a particular food decision, these values may be congruent or conflict with each other, such as a food being tasty and convenient but expensive and unhealthy. People manage values in food choice (Connors et al. 2001), and the extent of their food literacy is important in constructing values and negotiating them in particular eating episodes (Bisogni et al. 2007). The importance of food choice values may vary over time in response to situations, with some people valuing taste more highly in some seasons of the year and health more in other seasons (Smart & Bisogni 2001).

   Taste is a crucial value in food choice, and more extensive food literacy helps people identify and prepare good tasting foods. Price is often a limiting factor in food choice, and food literacy can provide knowledge that is useful for making less expensive food choices (Vidgen & Gallegos 2014). Convenience is a crucial value, and food literacy is required to make efficient food choices (Jabs et al. 2007). People value healthy food choice and establish and employ many meanings for healthy foods (Bisogni et al. 2012) that are enhanced with greater food literacy. Relationships with others are established and valued in food choice, and people weigh these relationships in food choice and become more skilled at managing relationships over time (Bove et al. 2003). In addition to these core food choice values, additional values are also considered including ethics, ecology, religion, and others (Jabs et al. 1998a).

   Food literacy shapes value negotiations in complex ways. Food literacy is multifaceted, and people are more or less food literate in combining taste, cost, convenience, health, relationships, and other values in food choice.

Classifying foods and situations

Classification is a fundamental task in all realms of life, including food choice. People are socialized into one or more cultures and social worlds that have rules for classifying foods and food related items (Furst et al. 2000). Learning, remembering, and applying food classification in a complex world is a fundamental aspect of food literacy. People need to know what items are classified as foods and what is not food, what is appropriate food for a particular place/time/person, what food will be easiest or hardest to prepare, and what is a healthy and unhealthy food or a reasonably priced food (Bisogni et al. 2012; Falk et al. 2001). For example, a young person may be scolded for not being literate in classifying insects as non-food in one culture, while in another culture children may be encouraged to eat crickets as tasty foods whenever they are encountered.

Classification of food activities is important in food literacy (Blake et al. 2007). People develop complex cognitive 'schema' that mentally represent the many factors involved in types of foods available, sources of food, preparation techniques and cooking equipment, and eating practices (Blake & Bisogni 2003). Having broader and more developed classifications offers options and alternatives that make people more literate in food choice options and the conditions under which particular options apply in specific situations.

Most food choice is situational, with different foods and eating activities represented as appropriate and inappropriate for particular situations that involve when, where, and who is involved (Sobal et al. 2010). Being sufficiently literate to competently make food choices requires knowing classifications for which foods are appropriate for which meals, which preparation and storage procedures are acceptable and unacceptable, and which eating practices are customary or deviant. For example, in contemporary USA eating baked potatoes for a formal breakfast may be nutritionally adequate, but would not be culturally, socially, or personally classified as appropriate for someone with extensive food literacy.

Constructing and enacting scripts

Food choice scripts (Bisogni et al. 2011; Blake et al. 2008) offer procedural knowledge for enacting values in making food choices. While food choice schema offer ideas about food choice, it requires considerable mental effort to weigh values and make choices in every eating episode. To save mental effort, people make their food choices more efficient by constructing scripts for repeated food choices (Blake et al. 2008) so they can more easily engage in eating activities. Having a set of scripts available for a variety of food choice settings and episodes provides a person with flexibility and improved food literacy. For example, someone with high script scope (consideration of many factors) and script flexibility (including many options) may have worked out scripts for a fast and efficient meal, a safe and healthy meal, and a meaningful and social meal that they can perform when the need arises.

Developing strategies and tactics

Strategies are heuristics that people use in food choice decisions (Sobal et al. 2006). Food choice strategies draw upon food choice values and goals to implement values in particular situations (Lynch & Bisogni 2014). These strategies expedite food choice by providing underlying principles for making decisions, thus requiring less mental effort. General strategies include the use of elimination, limitation, substitution, addition, modification, and routinization as rules for making food decisions (Sobal et al. 2006). In addition to these broader strategies, more specific and concrete food choice tactics are employed to make specific food selections (Lynch & Bisogni 2014), such as always eating the healthiest foods on a plate first and then eating less healthy foods later. Individuals with more extensive food literacy have broader repertoires of strategies and tactics they can employ in food choice.

People tend to use multiple strategies in food choice decisions, and most develop a set of personal food choice procedures that constitute a repertoire (Falk, Bisogni & Sobal 1996). These food choice repertoires may focus on a primary strategy, use different strategies sequentially, or conditionally employ selected strategies in specific situations. People with more comprehensive food literacy have more fully developed strategies, tactics, and repertoires cognitively available to enact food values, achieve food goals, and make food choices.

Establishing and performing routines

Food choice routines are elaborated scripts that are developed over time for regular and established food choice activities (Bisogni et al. 2011; Jastran et al. 2009). Routines become ritualized to achieve solutions for the best fit of factors that satisfy food choice values and meet food choice goals in particular repeating sequences of situations. Food routines provide structure, schedules, and predictability for individuals as well as for the people with whom they shop, cook, and eat. Routines become embedded in everyday food culture and facilitate food choice with minimal mental and physical effort.

Food choice routines can positively contribute to food literacy by meeting basic requirements of food safety, efficiency, health, and sociability as people may meet for lunch in the same place with the same people most workdays. Food choice routines can negatively limit food literacy by restricting food patterns, routinizing unhealthy food events, or repeatedly choosing unhealthy foods. Some routines have a rigid scope. For example, going to a pub after work most Fridays can result in an unhealthy dietary intake. Rigid routines can limit flexibility and adaptability to new life circumstances such as someone who may assert 'I have always eaten a meat and potatoes type of dinner but now that I am retired, I can no longer afford it. I don't know how to cook many meatless meals and I don't think they are very satisfying'.

Monitoring and revision

People engage in self-monitoring of their food choice activities (Lynch & Bisogni 2012, 2014) as they try out and reflect about their food choices. This contributes to food literacy by regularly reconstructing their personal food systems to adjust to a variety of settings and situations. For example, people evaluate how well their food selection, preparation, and eating fit with their values and goals and may adjust where they shop, how they cook, and whom they eat with over time. Monitoring and revision change over the life course. Changes related to life course transitions and turning points are perceived, interpreted, and reacted to by individuals as they complete their education, change jobs, engage and disengage with family, and experience health problems from adolescence (Vaitkevicute et al. 2015) to late adulthood (Falk, Bisogni & Sobal 1996).

Food activities

Food activities are what people do, think, and feel related to food, and are guided by the personal food system, shaped by influences, and embedded within life course conditions and experiences. The scope of individual and household food activities includes acquiring, preparing, serving, eating, storing, sharing, and cleaning up food (Sobal & Bisogni 2009). Each of these activities requires particular kinds of knowledge that correspond with the domains of food literacy identified by Vidgen and Gallegos (2014) as planning and managing, selecting, preparing, and eating.

Food activities occur within particular eating episodes, which are events when people deal with food (Bisogni et al. 2007). Eating episodes are multi-dimensional and include the overlapping and interacting features of food and drink, location, time, activities, social setting, mental processes, physical condition, and recurrence. People consider these features as they decide about food choice, and engage in food activities based on those considerations. Individuals with more extensive food literacy can consider more dimensions and manage them better than those with more limited food literacy. Changing circumstances are part of life for most people and learning to adapt expectations and strategies is critical to being satisfied. Thus, for example, a person with greater food literacy can invoke their skills, experience, and strategies to more quickly and confidently navigate food and eating in a disaster situation that leaves them with limited water or food access.

Conclusions

Food literacy is an important concept that has wide-ranging implications and applications. Food choice and food literacy intersect and interact in a variety of complementary ways, with food choice concepts and processes linking with the different dimensions of food literacy. As people construct food choice, they draw upon the knowledge and skills they established in developing their food literacy.

The processes of food choice yield the food and meals people eat; however, people also reflect about their results. The concept of food choice capacity is the person's evaluation of how well they are managing food and eating (Bisogni et al. 2005). Three components underlie food choice capacity: the person's circumstances, their food management skills, and their standards (expectations for food quality, types, and preparation). All three components shift over the life course, with experiences informing development of standards and food management skills. Someone may express 'Until I went to that workshop, I didn't know how much fruit to eat but now I plan to eat two cups of fruit every day'. When they are able to meet their standards, the person has high food choice capacity. If they are unable to meet their standards, they have low food choice capacity. Food choice capacity reflects the person's overall satisfaction with their food activities. A key contrast between food literacy and food choice capacity is that food choice capacity is based on the person's own emic standards, while food literacy incorporates broader etic perspectives about health, such as wellbeing and safe food handling practices.

People with low food choice capacity may be limited by their circumstances, food management skills, or both. Many people with low food choice capacity have limited food literacy. Improving the ability to adapt to circumstances or food management skills can improve both food literacy and food choice capacity. People with low food choice capacity are one group who may be motivated to seek improved knowledge or skills and benefit from efforts to improve food literacy. In contrast, people with high food choice capacity may have widely varying levels of food literacy as one person's standards may not incorporate health and wellbeing while another person's standards do. Those with minimal interest in food, or those with low standards, may have both high food choice capacity and low food literacy. Due to their satisfaction with how they are managing food and eating, people with high food choice capacity may have less motivation to seek or develop greater food literacy.

Food literacy is a durable set of knowledge and skills that can empower a person to adapt to their circumstances and make food choices that promote health and wellbeing. The Food Choice Process Model emphasizes the dynamic and evolving experience of the eater as they interpret changes within their personal situation as well as within the macro-context, from changes in food and agricultural systems to new types of popular media. As social and individual standards shift, the knowledge and skills needed to be food literate will also need to transform to effectively and responsively promote public health.

Note

1   The authors would like to thank the Division of Nutritional Sciences at Cornell University for support in preparing this chapter.

References

Bisogni, C.A., Connors, M., Devine, C.M. & Sobal, J. (2002). Who we are and how we eat: A qualitative study of identities in food choice. *Journal of Nutrition Education and Behavior*, 34(3), 128–139.

Bisogni, C.A., Falk, L.W., Madore, E., Blake, C.E., Jastran, M., Sobal, J. & Devine, C.M. (2007). Dimensions of everyday eating and drinking episodes. *Appetite*, 48(2), 218–231.

Bisogni, C.A., Jastran, M. & Blake, C.E. (2011). The construction of eating episodes, food scripts and food routines. In V. Preedy, R.R. Watson & C.R. Martin (eds) *Handbook of Behavior, Food and Nutrition* (pp. 987–1009). New York: Springer.

Bisogni, C.A., Jastran, M., Seligson, M. & Thompson, A. (2012). How people interpret healthy eating: Contributions of qualitative research. *Journal of Nutrition Education and Behavior*, 44(4), 282–301.

Bisogni, C.A., Jastran, M., Shen, L. & Devine, C.M. (2005). A biographical study of food choice capacity: Standards, circumstances, and food management skills. *Journal of Nutrition Education and Behavior*, 37(6), 284–291.

Blake, C.E. & Bisogni, C.A. (2003). Personal and family food choice schemas of rural women in Upstate New York. *Journal of Nutrition Education and Behavior*, 35(6), 282–293.

Blake, C.E., Bisogni, C.A., Sobal, J., Devine, C.M. & Jastran, M. (2007). Classifying foods in contexts: How adults categorize foods for different eating situations. *Appetite*, 49(2), 500–510.

Blake, C.E., Bisogni, C.A., Sobal, J., Jastran, M. & Devine, C.M. (2008). How adults construct evening meals: Scripts for food choice. *Appetite*, 51(3), 127–136.

Bove, C.F. & Sobal, J. (2006). Foodwork in newly married couples: Managing family meals. *Food, Culture, and Society*, 9(1), 69–89

Bove, C.F., Sobal, J. & Rauschenbach, B.S. (2003). Food choices among newly married couples: Convergence, conflict, individualism, and projects. *Appetite*, 40(1), 25–41.

Connors, M., Bisogni, C.A., Sobal, J. & Devine, C.M. (2001). Managing values in personal food systems. *Appetite*, 36(3), 189–200.

Devine, C.M. (2005). The life course perspective: Understanding food choices in time, social location, and history. *Journal of Nutrition Education and Behavior*, 37(3), 121–128.

Devine, C.M., Connors, M., Bisogni, C.A. & Sobal, J. (1998). Life-course influences on fruit and vegetable trajectories: A qualitative analysis of food choices. *Journal of Nutrition Education*, 31(6), 361–370.

Devine, C.M., Connors, M., Sobal, J. & Bisogni, C.A. (2003). Sandwiching it in: Managing food and work in low and moderate income urban households. *Social Science & Medicine*, 56(3), 617–630.

Devine, C.M., Sobal, J., Bisogni, C.A. & Connors, M. (1999). Food choices in three ethnic groups: Interactions of ideals, identities and roles. *Journal of Nutrition Education*, 31(2), 86–93.

Falk, L.W., Bisogni, C.A. & Sobal, J. (1996). Food choice processes of older adults. *Journal of Nutrition Education*, 28(5), 257–265.

Falk, L.W., Sobal, J., Bisogni, C.A., Connors, M. & Devine, C.M. (2001). Managing healthy eating: Definitions, classifications, and strategies. *Health Education and Behavior*, 28(4), 425–439.

Food Choice Research Group. (2015). Cornell Food Choice Research Group Homepage. Division of Nutritional Sciences, Cornell University, Ithaca, NY 14853, viewed 20 December 2015, http://www.human.cornell.edu/dns/foodchoice/index.cfm.

Furst, T.M., Connors, M., Bisogni, C.A., Sobal, J. & Falk, L.W. (1996). Food choice: A conceptual model of the process. *Appetite*, 26(3), 247–265.

Furst, T.M., Connors, M., Sobal, J., Bisogni, C.A. & Falk, L.W. (2000). Food classifications: Levels and categories. *Ecology of Food and Nutrition*, 39(5), 331–355.

Griffin, M.K. & Sobal, J. (2014). Consumer food system participation: A community analysis. *Ecology of Food and Nutrition*, 53(6), 579–595.

Jabs, J.A. & Devine, C.M. (2006). Time scarcity and food choices: An overview. *Appetite*, 47(2), 196–204.

Jabs, J.A., Devine, C.M., Bisogni, C.A., Farrell, T.J., Jastran, M. & Wethington, E. (2007). Trying to find the quickest way: Employed mothers' constructions of time for food. *Journal of Nutrition Education and Behavior*, 39(1), 18–25.

Jabs, J.A., Devine, C.M. & Sobal, J. (1998a). A model of the process of adopting vegetarian diets: Health vegetarians and ethical vegetarians. *Journal of Nutrition Education*, 30(4), 196–202.

Jabs, J.A., Devine, C.M. & Sobal, J. (1998b). Maintaining vegetarian diets: personal factors, social networks, and environmental resources. *Canadian Journal of Dietetic Practice and Research*, 59(4), 183–189.

Jabs, J.A., Sobal, J. & Devine, C.M. (2000). Managing vegetarianism: Identities, norms and interactions. *Ecology of Food and Nutrition*, 39(5), 375–394.

Jastran, M., Bisogni, C.A., Blake, C.E., Sobal, J. & Devine, C.M. (2009). Eating routines: Embedded, value based, modifiable, and reflective. *Appetite*, 52(1), 127–136.

Kean, L.G., Prividera, L.C., Boyce, A. & Curry, T. (2012). Media use, media literacy, and African American females' food consumption patterns. *Howard Journal of Communications*, 23(3), 197–214.

Lynch, A. & Bisogni, C.A. (2012). Understanding self-monitoring and weight loss after gastric bypass surgery: An exploratory study. *Obesity Surgery*, 22(12), 1818–1826.

Lynch, A. & Bisogni, C.A. (2014). Gastric bypass patient's goal-strategy-monitoring networks for long-term dietary management. *Appetite*, 81(Oct), 138–151.

Smart, L.R. & Bisogni, C.A. (2001). Personal food systems of male college hockey players. *Appetite*, 37(1), 57–70.

Sobal, J., Beckman, L., Pham, A., Croy, M. & Marquart, L. (2010). Situational food choices: Social representations of where, when, and who consumes whole grain foods. *Topics in Clinical Nutrition*, 25(1), 75–83.

Sobal, J. & Bisogni, C.A. (2009). Constructing food choice decisions. *Annals of Behavioral Medicine*, 38(Supplement 1), S37–46.

Sobal, J., Bisogni, C.A., Devine, C.M. & Jastran, M. (2006). A conceptual model of the food choice process over the life course. In R. Shepherd & M.M. Raats (eds) *Psychology of Food Choice* (pp. 1–18). Oxfordshire, UK: CABI Publishing.

Sobal, J., Bisogni, C.A. & Jastran, M. (2014). Food choice is multifaceted, contextual, dynamic, multilevel, integrated, and diverse. *Mind, Brain, and Education*, 8(1), 6–12.

Sobal, J., Blake, C.E., Jastran, M., Lynch, A., Bisogni, C.A. & Devine, C.M. (2012). Eating maps: Places, times, and people in eating episodes. *Ecology of Food and Nutrition*, 51(3), 247–264.

Sobal, J., Khan, L.K. & Bisogni, C.A. (1998). A conceptual model of the food and nutrition system. *Social Science and Medicine* 47(7), 853–863.

Sobal, J. & Wansink, B. (2007). Kitchenscapes, tablescapes, platescapes, and foodscapes: Influences of micro-level built environments on food intake. *Environment & Behavior*, 39(1), 124–142.

Sobal, J. & Wansink, B. (2008). Built environments and obesity. In E. Blass (ed.) *Obesity: Causes, Mechanisms, Prevention, and Treatment* (pp. 281–299). Sunderland, Massachusetts: Sinauer Associates.

Swidler, A. (1986). Culture in action: Symbols and strategies. *American Sociological Review*, 51(2), 273–286.

Vaitkevicute, R., Ball, L.E. & Harris, N. (2015). The relationship between food literacy and dietary intake in adolescents: A systematic review. *Public Health Nutrition*, 18(4), 649–658.

Vidgen, H.A. & Gallegos, D. (2014). Defining food literacy and its components. *Appetite*, 76(1), 50–59.

Wadsworth, L.A. & Thompson, A.M. (2005). Media literacy: A critical role for dietetic practice. *Canadian Journal of Dietetic Practice and Research*, 66(1), 30–36.

Widener, P. & Karides, M. (2014). Food system literacy: Empowering citizens and consumers beyond farm-to-fork pathways. *Food, Culture & Society*, 17(4), 665–687.

7 Food literacy beyond the individual

The nexus between personal skills and victim blaming

Martin Caraher

Introduction

> It's the cheapest form of luxury you'll ever get. The thing that stops people eating well is lack of knowledge, not money ... Nowadays, food is so cheap. Even if you're on the dole, you can eat like a king – but you need the knowledge.
>
> (Alex James in Lewis 2011)

> I'm not judgmental, but I've spent a lot of time in poor communities, and I find it quite hard to talk about modern-day poverty. You might remember that scene in [a previous series] *Ministry of Food*, with the mum and the kid eating chips and cheese out of Styrofoam containers, and behind them is a massive fucking TV. It just didn't weigh up.
>
> The fascinating thing for me is that seven times out of 10, the poorest families in this country choose the most expensive way to hydrate and feed their families. The ready meals, the convenience foods.
>
> (Jamie Oliver in Deans 2013)

The concern with low levels of cooking skills among populations is not new and in fact can be seen in the cycle of news with newspapers carrying headlines every three to four years on how young people cannot cook, do not recognize vegetables or families do not eat together (Murcott 2010). The two views expressed above from celebrities are illustrative of the concern I am raising: that those who do not or cannot cook are seen as problematic, in some ways perverse, in some ways just lacking knowledge, and should know better. This of course goes against at least three decades of evidence which shows that information on its own is not sufficient to bring about changes in behaviour.

Concerns with a lack of cooking skills in the population can be traced back to the 1780s coinciding with the start of urbanization of rural classes with the *Times of London* calling for young women to be educated in the skill of domestic economy. Likewise public health has long had a relationship, albeit uneasy, with cooking, seeing it as a way to influence healthy eating. Edwin Chadwick, the great public health reformer, called for cooking education among the labouring classes as he claimed in 1842 that: 'ignorance of domestic economy leads to ill health by the purchase of unsuitable and at the same time expensive food' (Chadwick 1842: 140), a view not dissimilar to the two which started this chapter and a plea reiterated in the *Journal of the American Medical Association* in 2010 (Lichtenstein & Ludwig 2010).

Modern concerns with the lack of cooking skills, since the 1980s, have focused on the links to healthy food choice and preparation. The Obama administration has heavily endorsed cooking, mainly through the First Lady and Cooking Matters, as a means of addressing the US obesity problem (http://cookingmatters.org/). Despite this long history of concern, the situation has not stimulated serious policy debate or discussion over the role of cooking in the population. This chapter will not deal with the myriad influences on cooking such as the food industry, new technologies, and so on; these arguments can be found in other works (see for example: Lang & Caraher 2001; Short 2006; Vileisis 2008; Wrangham 2009). Here the focus is on a critique of cooking and food literary which locates the individual as the centre and solution to the problem. This fits closely with the critiques offered by Crawford in the 1970s and 1980s in his descriptions of healthism and victim blaming. He defined healthism as 'a pre-occupation with personal health as a primary – often *the* primary – focus for the definition and achievement of personal well-being, a goal which is to be attained primarily through the modification of life styles' (Crawford 1980: 368). This focus on healthism at the individual level can lead to blaming those who do not conform and are thus the victims of their own inaction. There has been a shift in emphasis from teaching individuals and communities to eat healthily through the mechanism of culinary skills and food literacy to a situation where the emphasis is on cooking skills (Herbert et al. 2014; Hollows & Jones 2010; Pike & Kelly 2014). The assumption seems to be that culinary skills or the narrower focus on cooking skills results in healthier, leaner populaces. According to Collins (2009) many television reality shows dealing with obesity also focus on cooking skills as the 'real driver of the series' (Hollows & Jones 2010: 310). The same can be said of community initiatives where the focus on food literacy or culinary nutrition is often forfeited in favour of a narrow emphasis on cooking skills. Bear this distinction in mind as you read the rest of this chapter. The emphasis for practical issues such as space will focus on community cooking initiatives, although a similar critique can be applied to school-based cooking initiatives.

The changing cooking scene

Since the 1980s there has been much promotion of cooking projects and initiatives in the UK, the USA and Australia (Caraher & Cowburn 2004; Caraher & Dowler 2007; Condrasky & Helger 2010; Huntley 2008, 2014; National Food Alliance 1993; Royal Society for the Encouragement of Arts, Manufacturers and Commerce 1997). This has occurred alongside changes in the way cooking is taught in schools and as a generation turned to ready-made and processed meals (Belasco 2008; Caraher & Lang, 1999). The main emphasis has been the *supposed* contribution of cooking to healthy eating. Concerns with cooking can also be located within what is being called the 'new austerity' movement in the developed world or global north. This 'new austerity' is characterized by behaviours that are voluntarily undertaken or adopted and which have an underpinning ecological basis. These choices, in other circumstances, might be seen as limiting. So choosing not to eat imported food, spurn supermarkets, eat locally, grow your own or buy foods which are local or organic, cook from scratch, are all activities which fit into this category (see Roep & Wiskerke 2006). These can be seen as part of the attempt to 'save the world'. All are worthy and notable, and actions many reading this chapter would aspire to. These are not up for debate here, but what is being questioned is the use of these motivations and behaviours for application to a wider population.

Choice or necessity?

The choices that people are making in the name of what might be called the new concerns with ecological health mirror the facts of life of those who live with 'want' – that is, restricted choice and diets. The distinction is, of course, that of choice – if I choose to eat less meat and consume less or cook food from local sources then that is different than if this consumption is a matter of necessity and lack of choice (for examples of austerity as a lifestyle choice see Kingsolver 2007; Pollan 2009). These initiatives also tend to operate at the individual level of choice (Herbert et al. 2014). They focus on providing people with skills and knowledge but do little to address the circumstances in which they live. Culinary capital is only one aspect of the decision making process around choosing and preparing healthy food (Naccarato & Lebesco 2012).

A structural effect: the nutrition transition?

Changes in dietary and food culture have been influenced by the nutrition transition (Caballero & Popkin 2002). We have argued elsewhere that such structural changes are accompanied by changes in culinary practices (Lang & Caraher 2001). These changes are driven by changes in work and urbanization, not by individual choice per se. The changes in any society are complex and always influenced by local food culture and customs. However, they tend to follow a pattern whereby in the first stages of development, the rich adopt the food habits of the rich first-world countries. This can take the form of consumption of take-away and processed foods, all of which can contribute to chronic diseases such as heart disease and cancers (Egger & Swinburn 2010). The reasons for this are twofold – these lifestyle choices are culturally aspirational but also expensive and only the well off can afford them (Rodrigues et al. 2007). The nutrition transition affects the foods people eat and aligned with this are changes in food sourcing, preparation and eating habits. The second stage of the changes is rooted in the food system becoming more industrial and concentrated so that processed foods and fast food become more affordable to all. Fast food is 'fast' thanks to modern technology and suits modern lifestyles (Schlosser 2001) and in many instances is a viable option for those on low incomes. The dietary impacts of such moves are an increase in the fat, salt and sugar content of these foods with possible long-term consequences for health burdens. Cooking can be viewed as a cultural artefact within these early changes and 'unfashionable' and archaic, especially cooking from scratch and with local produce, although eating local does not mean eating native, as Australians do not eat kangaroos nor do people in the UK eat squirrels or foxes. Such changes can be tracked in the way the Mediterranean diet has changed over time with women liberated from foraging green vegetables in the fields and a move to processed and ready-to-eat meals. In fact, the use of take-away and fast food (or street food) often becomes an important money and labour saving mechanism for many who are engaged in piece-meal work. At the latter stage of the transition, the rich classes return to do eating more basic foods due to the health implications and because they can afford to (Rodrigues et al. 2007). For the poor in emerging economies, eating street food is one way of gaining time and saving money, gaining time by not cooking and saving money by not having to buy fuel and using the time thus saved to do work that generates income. Tinker (1997) in her study of street foods in seven countries in Asia and Africa shows that the poor spend more (relatively) on street foods and have a higher calorific intake from these sources than those on high incomes. Research from Accra in Ghana shows that the lowest quintile groups consumed up to 31% of their total calories outside the home. Far from being a luxury they cannot afford, street and fast food are important in freeing up time for income generating work among the poor (Maxwell et al. 2000). This can be seen as part of the nutrition transition driven by the need to earn income.

Hayden's (1981) historical review of the domestic scene, which reviewed the work of early American feminists such as Charlotte Perkins Gilman, prophesied that true liberation would come with community kitchens and homes without kitchens. Attar (1990) pointed to the enslaving process that domestic cookery imposed and continues to impose on women's lives and said that the removal of compulsory cooking for girls was one of the best moves for liberating them from the kitchen. Dixon and colleagues show that changes in food preparation in the home owe more to employment status and cultural changes in the home (Banwell et al. 2012; Dixon et al. 2014). These are of course paralleled by the production of food and technologies which make it easier. Similar to the studies from Asia and Africa mentioned in the above paragraph, issues beyond food literacy and the possession of culinary capital have an influence on food preparation and consumption. Yet public health nutrition when addressing cooking seems reluctant to take on such influences, demonstrating a distinct lack of public health imagination and capacity (Caraher & Cowburn 2015).

Public health: food security and cooking

What definitions of food security do not capture is the social and cultural aspects of food poverty or food insecurity. The quality and variety of social life around food suffer. Goode (2012) shows how families living on low incomes change their food habits (foodways) to reflect their circumstances. So culinary and cultural capital become subservient to financial capital. This can vary from what is called '*holiday hunger*' (children going without food during school holiday periods) through not having enough to give to visitors, to not entertaining due to embarrassment over the lack of food to offer. The point is that such changes in consumption are not merely the consequence of individual lifestyle choices but of structural changes in both the national and global food systems such as the ready availability and cheapness of foods that are high in fat, salt and sugar. This has shifted the balance of symptoms of food poverty to issues such as over-consumption of processed and take-away foods as well as obesity. So there is a shift from under- to over- or malconsumption, but also the nature and quality of the foods change. These global class divisions can be seen within nation states. In high to middle income countries, the middle and poor groups in a country may have access to the same facilities as the consuming class but be disadvantaged by issues such as price, ease of access and cultural distance. So behaviours are not just the result of individual agency but of large-scale structural change and this equally applies to cooking. By tackling cooking, we are tackling the symptoms not the cause. The skills related to cooking may be important, and if you are living in poverty they may help you manage better, but they do not change your material circumstances.

Healthism under the banner of the new austerity movement

Many low-income groups, as well as facing problems with the price of food, also face problems with the price of fuel to cook it and the competing priorities of whether to spend on food or other necessities that are non-negotiable (All Party Parliamentary Inquiry into Hunger and Food Poverty 2014). Seeking solutions in cooking could be said to ignore the structural influences of the global food system and 'Big Food' (Moodie et al. 2013); it also medicalizes and creates what Crawford (1977, 1980, 1984) calls a form of healthism in that it locates the solution at the individual level. Similarly to Crawford's arguments about self-help and alternative health care movements, it also runs the danger of depoliticizing food and the food system. Food is conceptualized as indivi-dual, not political; the danger of such moves and initiatives is that the message becomes one that you can be responsible for your health and help save the world!

The term 'new austerity' is used here to describe those choices people make in the light of ecological sustainability (Caraher 2009; Caraher & Reynolds 2005). This is different from the austerity experienced in, for example, Europe after the Second World War (Fearnley-Whittingstall 2010; Kynaston 2007), when many of the choices and behaviours were imposed and controlled through legislation and rationing. The 'new austerity' is different in that it is closely related to concerns about ecological sustainability, peak oil and a genuine desire to make things 'better' and make a difference (Hopkins 2008; Pinkerton

& Hopkins 2009). A new generation of food campaigners has arisen who see denial and lifestyle choice as a solution to the global problems of over-industrialization of the food system and concentrations of power within that system. Many of these new austerity projects are individually focused and assume the power of the individual to make changes in the system (Belasco 2007), whether as a participant in an alternative project or as a consumer. Pollan (2008, 2009, 2013) can be seen as one of the key advocates of this new austerity. He has listed a number of rules for a food manifesto that typifies this approach to the problems, the vast majority being based on the individual making choices. However, the poor often do not have the option to adopt alternative food behaviours. Initiatives based on growing often ignore the fact that one of the major limitations on the poor is space – space to live and space to grow. So, for some, the new austerity is a lifestyle choice while for other groups it is a fact of life constrained by the lack of capital assets of which culinary capital is only a minor part.

This emerging group of 'new austerity' initiatives and behaviours centres around ecological sustainability, alternative supply chains and local food, with many of this new generation of 'alternative food' networks being rooted in choice and lifestyle. This is not to demean or diminish these new approaches based on lifestyle choice, but to point out that the opportunity to exercise choice is not an equal opportunity for all (Troy, Miller & Oslor 2011). My point here is that such approaches do not compensate for the influences at a structural or corporate level on communities, not that cooking initiatives are wrong, have no impact or are not needed.

There are many reasons to support cooking in the home but we need to be careful of our choice and rationales. For example, the promotion of cooking at an individual level is ecologically not sustainable; there might be many reasons to support and promote home cooking but it is not efficient. During the Second World War the UK government nationalized the food service sector in order to ensure adequate nutrition but also based on the fact that individual household cooking was wasteful and inefficient, bulk cooking was much more efficient. In the developing world (first stages of the nutrition transition) as populations move to urban areas, they cease or cut down on cooking related to three factors: the loss and lack of access to biomass to cook on; the nature of work; and a loss of cooking modelling over time. Of the three, it is the last we turn to as the solution. This is not just true of the developing world as Dixon and colleagues in various publications have shown; it is also that the commodified environment and labour market policies, such as zero hour contracts, are as good at indicting the cooking that occurs in the home as the absence or presence of cooking skills (Banwell et al. 2012; Dixon et al. 2014). Short (2003, 2006) notes that the skills it takes to run a home and put food on the table have changed, and what is clear from the work of Dixon and colleagues as well as that of Dowler (1995) is that a new form of domestic economy is being practised.

For health campaigners and even celebrities such as Jamie Oliver who may express mystification over why people value food so little (see opening quotes), the issues are complex. Work we are carrying out in a deprived area in the north west of England shows families are adept at stretching their food dollar and other resources (Caraher et al. 2011). One family involved in the study had attended a cooking class and described stocking their store cupboard following a shopping trip to the supermarket. The bottom shelf is loaded with 'pot noodle', to which boiling water is added to reconstitute it. The story behind this shopping shows an admirable sense of domestic economy, which related to a concern with feeding the family and not letting them go hungry, managing on a limited budget and buying food that can store and keep without enormous associated costs for reheating or cooking. The family was on an income below the UK median income of £240/week. The family cook had attended a cooking class and could cook, did identify how this had helped them make changes to the family diet, but also reported that buying fresh fruit and vegetables posed domestic problems: buying fruit meant that it was likely to be eaten quickly and vegetables were difficult to store and were less likely to be acceptable to hungry children and adults. This is an austerity that comes from enforced circumstances, not choice.

This new austerity movement and its promotion of cooking also run the risk of stigmatizing and alienating those who live in deprived circumstances as it is premised on the principles of choice and availability, options not equally available to all. Food and heating costs rose during the global financial crisis that occurred between 2007 and 2013, thus making cooking less of an option for some (Huntley 2008). So families had to choose between 'eating and heating' (All Party Parliamentary Inquiry into Hunger and Food Poverty 2014). This was a new concern with 'bio-mass' in the first world. Food prices increased as well as fuel at the same time that wages remained static or in real terms decreased. Eating fast food became a real option and in fact remained steady among low-income groups as it declined among middle-income ones between 2008 and 2014 (Caraher, O'Keefe, Lloyd & Madelin 2013).

Blaming the victim

The irony, or what campaigners and advocates such as Oliver and James (see quotes at the beginning of this chapter) fail to understand, is that choice based on limiting your choice requires other resources, such as time, land or skills such as food literacy. Cooking requires time, knowledge and skills but also access to economic capital. Of course, those in reduced circumstances can grow their own food but with greater resource demands and fewer returns for their inputs. Additionally, if the solutions are seen to lie in self-choice then such approaches run the danger of distracting attention from the structural determinants of culinary capital and food literacy and reinforcing the victim blaming. As a result, food poverty can be reduced to an issue of choice or management. 'Hunger' equally may be reduced to a matter of individual choice and a consequence of the wrong choice of lifestyle – that is, if only you produced your own food or cooked from scratch you would not be hungry or wanting (see

Lewis 2011 for an example of this argument). In a similar vein, Pollan (2009) calls eating an agricultural act and calls for us all to be involved in growing at least some of our own food. Yet such a laudable aim is subject to the availability of resources and social capitals and indeed power in a market economy (Caraher 2009; Caraher & Carey 2010, 2011). Pollan (2013) in his book *Cooked* is almost pornographic in his focus on food and the means of transforming it; it certainly does not meet with his 2009 call for action and a food manifesto based on parsimony. This is in contrast to Huntley's (2014) skilful exposé of cooking in Australia.

Our research in 1999 showed a population with low levels of skills with the rich having higher levels of a skills deficit (Caraher et al. 1999; Lang & Caraher 2001). Most of the more recent research does not contradict this position. Adams & White (2015) found that amongst women, older age, not being in employment, lower social class, greater education, and living with other adults or children were positively associated with time spent cooking while for men few differences in time spent cooking were seen. So those living on low incomes may be no worse in terms of skills than the rich, but the rich can buy their way out of ill health and into healthy food preparation and consumption, yet the solutions often seem to lie in targeting the '*poor*'. A 2007 study among low-income households showed cooking confidence was universally high and that over 80% of the low-income population lived in a household where the 'main food provider' had well-developed cooking skills (Nelson et al. 2007). Since then there has been an increase in activities to teach cooking in schools and to adults in community settings.

The most important source for learning about cooking and the handing on of skills was and is the family, specifically mothers; but schools are also identified as important sources of learning about cooking – especially for men. In 2010 commercial research from the *BBC Food Magazine* and the French magazine *Madame Figaro* showed 72 per cent of the British cooks were at home daily, compared to 59 per cent of the French, and that 50 per cent of British cooks spent more than 30 minutes preparing a meal while only a quarter of the French respondents reported spending that long. Perhaps it takes more time to open the packages! The French were more likely to cook from basics and to sit down to consume the meal in a group. Also more detailed examination of the findings suggests that the UK 'cook' prepares two or three meals for different members of the family, whereas the French prepare one family or household meal. The social capital, in the UK, around households and kitchens has shifted from the 1990s, when the indicator of success was having a kitchen which was rarely used, to having two kitchens preferably with a double oven and six cooking plates (see Figure 7.1). This has been driven by the influence of TV programmes where one kitchen is now either an outdoor one or a baking kitchen (Collins 2009).

The evidence suggests that those on low incomes manage their households with dignity and parsimony; they may not cook from scratch or even purchase the amounts of fresh fruit and vegetables that those on higher incomes do but

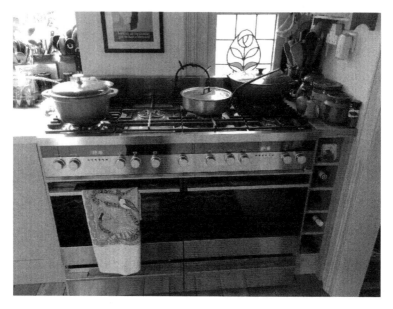

Figure 7.1 The new affluence

they manage against almost impossible odds. Jamie Oliver, Alex James and Michael Pollan (2013) in his book *Cooked* show little understanding of the ways that people actually live, work and prepare food. Those on low incomes manage well and within their resources; what Oliver, James and Pollan fail to recognize is how people on low incomes source and prepare food, which is with difficulty, but in most cases skilfully and imaginatively. Dowler (1995) in her study of single parent families shows how they managed well within their limited resources. Our own work in Liverpool shows similar results with those on restricted incomes opting for energy dense/processed foods which store well. Alex James, in the opening quotes, contends that eating is a 'form of luxury', but unlike for him who sends his children to fee-paying schools this is a luxury not all can afford!

Discussion

All the above comes from someone who has supported cooking as a necessary life-skill and campaigned for the retention of cooking in school curricula. However, the ways in which cooking is now being used and abused to lay blame on low-income communities and those who are poorly skilled or those who choose not to cook worries me, hence the critical examination of how cooking can be used and perhaps inadvertently come to blame the victim. I have been in too many meetings where campaigners make unjustifiable claims as to the efficacy of cooking. In one meeting it was claimed compulsory cooking in schools along with gardens would 'cure' obesity. While I am willing to admit to cooking contributing to a sense of healthy and sustainable living, I am unwilling to allow its elevation to a cure all or magic bullet. The evidence on cooking is emerging based on the assumption that providing cooking skills can tackle the burden of unhealthy eating; this assumption remains unproven and debatable in the wider scheme of people's lives. From this two issues arise. The first is the relationship of cooking skills to health outcomes; research on Taiwanese elderly showed that women benefited more from cooking more frequently than did men, and that those 'who cooked most frequently (>5 times/week, compared with never) had only 59% of the mortality risk' (Chia-Yu Chen et al. 2012). The second issue is how to ensure that households engage in the activity of cooking and eating, remembering that cooking and eating are not solitary activities and can involve households in activities beyond eating and nutrition (Goode 2015). Assuming from the above and other work that cooking skills do contribute to health, two questions are raised for those wishing to promote cooking in the home: how to ensure skills are passed on from one generation to another at a time of increasing food chain complexity and how to help people cook at a time where there is such a reliance on processed foods (Erlich, Yngve & Wahlqvist 2012). Other research explores how to transmit cooking skills where a generation of families and individuals have not been exposed to this skill in the home setting, or cooking skills are not taught in the classroom setting (Caraher, Wu, Seeley & Lloyd 2013; Cowan & Devine 2012).

Various charities and local community civil society groups have run and supported cooking in community settings (Caraher & Cowburn 2004). These remain popular if unproven ways of delivering skills or maybe of changing home practices (Rees et al. 2012). The Rees et al. (2012) systematic review of teaching adults '*home cooking*' found only one initiative had been properly evaluated.

> The courses that have been looked at in evaluation studies appear broadly similar to one another. They all introduce participants to practical cooking skills, with some courses emphasizing food safety and hygiene, and others shopping on a budget. They tend to be offered to existing community groups, rather than to individuals, and are usually run in community settings, which range from all-purpose centres to purpose-built community kitchens.
>
> (Rees et al. 2012: 2)

The consequences of the approaches described above, aided and abetted by the emergence of the celebrity chef campaigner, all contribute to a climate of healthism and victim blaming (Rousseau 2012). The taking on board of responsibility for teaching cooking by civil society groups allows governments to abdicate responsibility for the demise of cooking and the contribution of a 'Big Food' agenda which encourages dependency. Albritton (2009) argues that capitalism creates hunger and obesity and disengagement, and that these dialectics of the new poverty, including changes in cooking skills, are the result of control of the food system by a small number of global companies right through the food chain. For many food is something that is sourced in supermarkets, comes in packets and from take-aways.

Such beliefs often chime with political agendas and explain why people such as Jamie Oliver are invited to give evidence on inequality to a select Parliamentary committee despite his declaration that he does not understand modern-day poverty (http://www.gponline.com/jamie-oliver-gives-evidence-mps-health-inequalities/article/934569). Yet his 'quite hard to talk about modern-day poverty' (see quote at beginning of chapter) attitude does not stop him putting forward solutions based on individual approaches such as growing food or cooking it. We are in danger of returning to a 'Thoreauvian' view of simple living (Thoreau 1854) where the underlying assumption is that there are spiritual dangers in not owning a farm which lead one to suppose that 'breakfast comes from the grocery store' (Leopold 1966: 6). Many people in the public health and sustainability movements seem to view the supposed absence or demise of cooking in a similar vein of nostalgia.

Veblen's (1994) 'theory of the leisured class' and the ways of demonstrating conspicuous consumption through one's sophistication around fine food has shifted to criteria unheard of a few decades ago. Yes the cooking climate has changed: the 'poor' used to source food locally and cook their own, while the rich sourced food from many lands and ate out; now the rich source locally and the 'poor' eat food, albeit processed, from many lands. The capital assets required to live a local and sustainable life have shifted. My colleagues and I in 1999 questioned the basis of what constitutes cooking skills and the importance of possessing skills to deal with new foods and the necessity of learning new skills for new technology and processed foods (Caraher et al. 1999). Short (2003, 2006) has argued that what is occurring is a restructuring of skills and not a demise in skills per se. Whatever the arguments over what constitutes cooking, the general view as espoused by Stitt and others was that some core cooking skills are necessary as the base of this pyramid of skills (Stitt et al. 1997; see also Caraher et al. 1999).

The real heroes are those who continue to feed their families in the face of shrinking family income and the condemnation of the professional classes for being feckless and uncaring. Poverty and its consequence food poverty are not isolated from other forms of poverty; poverty is not about managing occasionally in straitened circumstances but debilitating in its week in/week out regularity. Poverty is relentless and grinds you down; it is for many not a one-off event but a continual drudge (Seabrook 2013; Tonybee 2013).

Some seek ways to redress that disenfranchisement through food initiatives based around growing and cooking and this results in, for some, a reconnection to food. This is among the reasons why many embrace alternative food networks and supply systems as an attempt to escape such control by outside factors; a lack of trust in the conventional food system drives people towards a sense of localism and control of food through cooking in their personal lives. We have argued elsewhere that the pedagogy of imparting cooking skills can be empowering, by giving people skills and knowledge not just about healthy cooking and food preparation but also by making them aware of the 'politics' in food (Caraher & Reynolds 2005).

So what can be learned from the above? As one interested in policy, I suggest a number of things. Firstly, the activity of reintroducing cooking back into schools and communities never resolved the dilemma over tensions concerning the role of the state. Secondly, the energy of the 'cooking movement' was dissipated and became focused on delivering a series of projects as opposed to ensuring that they were built into educational and health policies. This also resulted in the various groups ending up being competitors for the delivery of services as government at national and local levels contracted out many of the services. The tensions over why we should teach people to cook have still not been resolved. The main drives have come from the health sector which believes this is a way forward to deliver healthy eating (Lang & Caraher 2001). Many celebrity chefs have connected to this, the most obvious being Jamie Oliver (others are Stephanie Alexander in Australia and Alice Waters in the USA). Yet the agendas, while overlapping, are not always in perfect alignment. Cooking can be fun and deliver on taste and social agendas as well as health, but it can also encourage unhealthy eating. What happens, for example, when a chef or instructor promotes butter over lower fat spreads, adds sugar to a recipe or uses processed meat products rather than fresh meat? Of course, there are ways of resolving these dilemmas. One of the problems has been that many of those promoting cooking see it as a panacea for nutrition, family life, obesity and longevity.

There has been insufficient focus on food culture and the role of cooking within it or vice versa. This has partially happened because the health sector has funded much of the work and even celebrity chefs have promised to deliver better health outcomes. A narrow focus on health runs the danger of being too utilitarian and joyless. There is a parallel danger in the various programmes making commitments to deliver on health outcomes in order to obtain short-term funding. As noted earlier, cooking can be a powerful tool to help improve health status, but it cannot deliver in isolation.

Conclusions

Food austerity is the 'new rock and roll' – eating local food and cooking it are the new badges of lifestyle choice. What people sought to hide during the Great Depression is now a public badge of alternativeness – growing your own food, being frugal and denying yourself certain foods – albeit through choice as opposed to necessity (Kingsolver 2007); a modern-day version of Thoreau's *Walden* (1854). With the popularity of the new austerity movement, there come some potential downsides. The thrust of this argument is alluring but worrying as it runs the risk of victim blaming and of allowing the behaviours to be closely associated with values that assume self-help is the answer.

Many of these new austerity projects are individually focused and assume the individual has the power to make changes in the system (Belasco 2007), whether as a participant in an alternative project or as a consumer. Pollan (2008, 2009) can be seen as one of the key advocates of this new austerity. He has listed a number of rules for a food manifesto that typifies this approach to the problems, the vast majority being based on the individual making choices not structural changes. However, those living in reduced circumstances often do not have the option to adopt alternative food behaviours. Initiatives based on growing and cooking often ignore that the major limitations on those living in poverty are space and resources – space to live and space to grow, poor cooking equipment and access to means of cooking (Stead et al. 2004). So, for some, the new austerity is a lifestyle choice while for other groups it is a fact of life.

References

Adams, J. & White, M. (2015) Prevalence and socio-demographic correlates of time spent cooking by adults in the 2005, UK Time Use Survey. Cross-sectional analysis. *Appetite*, 92: 185–191, viewed 20 December 2015, http://dx.doi.org/10.1016/j.appet.2015.05.022.

Albritton, R. (2009) *Let them Eat Junk: How Capitalism Creates Hunger and Obesity*. Pluto Press: London.

All Party Parliamentary Inquiry into Hunger and Food Poverty (2014) *Feeding Britain: A Strategy for Zero Hunger in England, Wales, Scotland and Northern Ireland. The Report of the All-Party Parliamentary Inquiry into Hunger in the United Kingdom*. The Children's Society: London.

Attar, D. (1990) *Wasting Girls' Time: The History and Politics of Home Economics*. Virago: London.

Banwell, C., Broom, D., Davies, A. & Dixon, J. (2012) *Weight of Modernity: An Intergenerational Study of the Rise of Obesity*. Springer: New York.

Belasco, W. (2007) *Appetite for Change: How the Counterculture took on the Food Industry and Won*. 2nd edn. Cornell University Press: New York.

Belasco, W. (2008) *Food: The Key Concepts*. Bloomsbury: London.

Caballero, B. and Popkin, B. (2002) *The Nutrition Transition: Diet and Disease in the Developing World*. Academic Press: London.

Caraher, M., (2009) Food and fairness through ecological public health? A critical analysis. *Journal of the Home Economics Institute of Australia*, 16(2), 2–6.

Caraher, M. & Carey, D. (2010) Issues on food sustainability in Australia. *Nutridate*, 21(4), 2–6.

Caraher, M. & Carey, D. (2011) Issues on food sustainability in Australia: Part II. *Nutridate*, 22(2), 2–5.

Caraher, M. & Cowburn, G. (2004) A survey of food projects in the English NHS regions. *Health Education Journal*, 63(3), 197–219.

Caraher, M. & Cowburn, G. (2015) Guest commentary: Fat and other taxes, lessons for the implementation of preventive policies. *Preventive Medicine*, 77, 204–206, viewed 20 December 2015, http://dx.doi.org/10.1016/j.ypmed.2015.05.006.

Caraher, M. & Dowler, E. (2007) Food projects in London: lessons for policy and practice – A hidden sector and the need for 'more unhealthy puddings…sometimes', *Health Education Journal*, 66(2), 188–205.

Caraher, M. & Lang, T. (1999) Can't cook, Won't cook: a review of cooking skills and their relevance to health promotion. *International Journal of Health Promotion and Education*, 37(3), 89–100.

Caraher, M. & Reynolds, J. (2005) Sustainable food futures: Lessons for home economics pedagogy and practice. *Journal of the Home Economics Institute of Australia*, 12(2), 2–15.

Caraher, M., Lang, T., Dixon, P. & Carr-Hill, R. (1999) The state of cooking in England: The relationship of cooking skills to food choice. *British Food Journal*, 101(8), 590–609.

Caraher, M., Lloyd, S., Seeley, A., Davison, R. et al. (2011) *Report of a Cooking Initiative in Liverpool: A study of the Activities of Can Cook, CIC*. Centre for Food Policy, City University: London.

Caraher, M., O'Keefe, E., Lloyd, S. & Madelin, T. (2013) The planning system and fast food outlets in London: Lessons for health promotion practice. *Revista Portuguesa de Saude Publica*, 31(1), 49–57.

Caraher, M., Wu, M., Seeley, A. & Lloyd, S. (2013) When chefs adopt a school? An evaluation of a cooking intervention in English primary schools. *Appetite*, 62:50–59. DOI:10.1016/j.appet.2012.11.007.

Chadwick, E. (1842) *Report on the Sanitary Condition of the Labour Population and on the Means of its Improvement*. May: London.

Chia-Yu Chen, R., Meei-Shyuan, L., Yu-Hung, C. & Wahlqvist, M.L. (2012) Cooking frequency may enhance survival in Taiwanese elderly. *Public Health Nutrition*, 15(7), 1142–1149. DOI:10.1017/S136898001200136X.

Collins, K. (2009) *Watching What We Eat: the Evolution of Television Cooking Shows*. Continuum: New York.

Condrasky, M. & Helger, M. (2010) How culinary nutrition can save the health of nation. *Journal of Extension*, 48(2). Article Number 2COM1.

Cowan, J.A. & Devine, C.M. (2012) Process evaluation of an environmental and educational nutrition intervention in residential drug-treatment facilities. *Public Health Nutrition*, 15(7), 1159–1167. DOI:10.1017/S1368980012000572.

Crawford, R. (1977) You are dangerous to your health: The ideology and politics of victim blaming. *International Journal of Health Services*, 7(4), 61–680.

Crawford, R. (1980) Healthism and the medicalisation of everyday life. *International Journal of Health Services*, 10(3), 365–387.

Crawford, R. (1984) A cultural account of 'health': control, release and the social body. In McKinlay, J.B. (ed.) *Issues in the Political Economy of Healthcare*. Tavistock: New York, 60–103.

Deans, J. (2013) Jamie Oliver bemoans chips, cheese and giant TVs of modern-day poverty. The Guardian, Tuesday 27 August, viewed 20 December 2015, http://www.theguardian.com/lifeandstyle/2013/aug/27/jamie-oliver-chips-cheese-modern-day-poverty.

Dixon, J., Woodman, D., Strazdins, L., Banwell, C., Broom, D. & Burgess, J. (2014) Flexible employment, flexible eating and health risks. *Critical Public Health*, 24(4), 461–475. DOI: 10.1080/09581596.2013.852162.

Dowler, E. (1995) *Factors Affecting Nutrient Intake and Dietary Adequacy in Lone-parent Households*. Ministry of Agriculture, Food and Fisheries: London.

Egger, G. & Swinburn, B. (2010) *Planet Obesity: How We're Eating Ourselves and the Planet to Death*. Allen and Unwin: NSW.

Erlich, R., Yngve, A. & Wahlqvist, M.L. (2012) Cooking as a healthy behavior (Editorial). *Public Health Nutrition*, 15(7), 1139–1140. DOI:10.1017/S1368980012002662.

Fearnley-Whittingstall, J. (2010) *The Ministry of Food: Thrifty Wartime Ways to Feed your Family Today*. Hodder & Stoughton/Imperial War Museum: London.

Goode, J. (2012) Feeding the family when the wolf's at the door: The impact of over-indebtedness on contemporary foodways in low-income families in the UK. *Food and Foodways: Explorations in the History and Culture of Human Nourishment*, 20(10), 8–30. DOI: 10.1080/07409710.2012.652016.

Hayden, D. (1981) *The Grand Domestic Revolution*. MIT Press: Cambridge, MA.

Herbert, J., Flego, A., Gibbs, L., Waters, E., Swinburn, B., Reynolds, J. & Moodie, M. (2014) Wider impacts of a 10-week community cooking skills program – Jamie's Ministry of Food, Australia. *BMC Public Health*, 14: 1161, viewed 20 December 2015, http://www.biomedcentral.com/1471-2458/14/1161.

Hollows, J. & Jones, S. (2010) 'At least he's doing something': Moral entrepreneurship and individual responsibility in Jamie's Ministry of Food. *European Journal of Cultural Studies*, 13(3), 307–322.

Hopkins, R. (2008) *The Transition Handbook: From Oil Dependency to Local Resilience*. Green Books: Devon.

Huntley, R. (2008) *Eating between the Lines: Food and Equality in Australia*. Black Inc.: Melbourne.

Huntley, R. (2014) *Does Cooking Matter?* Penguin Special (Australia): Melbourne.

Kingsolver, B. (2007) *Animal, Vegetable, Miracle: Our Year of Seasonal Living*. Harper Collins: London.

Kynaston, D. (2007) *Austerity Britain 1945–51*. Bloomsbury: London.

Lang, T. & Caraher, M. (2001) Is there a culinary skills transition?: Data and debate from the UK about changes in cooking culture. *Journal of the Home Economics Institute of Australia*, 8(2), 2–14.

Leopold, A. (1966) *A Sand Country Almanac*. Ballantine: New York.

Lewis, H. (2011) The NS Interview: Alex James. *The New Statesman*, 27 June 2011, p 30–31, viewed 28 May 2015, http://www.newstatesman.com/music/2011/06/interview-food-cheese-nice.

Lichtenstein, A.H. & Ludwig, D.S. (2010) Bring back Home Economics education. *Journal of the American Medical Association*, 303(18), 1857–1858. DOI:10.1001/jama.2010.592.

Maxwell, D., Levin, C., Armar-Klemesu, M., Ruke, M., Morris, S. & Ahiadeke, C. (2000) *Urban Livelihoods and Food and Nutrition Security in Greater Accra, Ghana. Research Report no 112*. International Food Policy Research Institute: Washington, DC.

Moodie, R., Stuckler, D., Monteiro, C. et al. (2013) Profits and pandemics: Prevention of harmful effects of tobacco, alcohol, and ultra-processed food and drink industries. *Lancet*, 381, 670–679.

Murcott, A. (2010) *Family Meal; Myth, Reality and the Reality of Myth*. Presentation at the British Library as part of the Myths and Realities: a New Series of Public Debates, 9 March 2010. The British Library: London.

Naccarato, P. & Lebesco, K. (2012) *Culinary Capital*. Berg: London.

National Food Alliance (1993) *Get Cooking!* National Food Alliance, Department of Health and BBC Good Food: London.

Nelson, M., Erens, B., Bates, B., Church, S. & Boshier, T. (2007). *Low Income Diet and Nutrition Survey* (Vol. 3). *Nutritional Status; Physical Activity; Economic, Social and other Factors*. Food Standards Agency: London.

Pike, J. & Kelly, P. (2014) *The Moral Geographies of Children, Young People and Food*. Palgrave Macmillan: Basingstoke.

Pinkerton, T. & Hopkins, R. (2009). *Local Food: How to Make it Happen in your Community*. Green Books: Devon.

Pollan, M. (2008). *In Defence of Food*. Penguin: London.

Pollan, M. (2009). *Food Rules: An Eater's Manual*. Penguin: London.

Pollan, M. (2013). *Cooked: A Natural History of Transformation*. Penguin: London.

Rees, R., Hinds, K., Dickson, K., O'Mara-Eves, A. & Thomas, J. (2012) *Communities that Cook: A Systematic Review of the Effectiveness and Appropriateness of Interventions to Introduce Adults to Home Cooking*. EPPI Centre, Social Science, Research Unit, Institute of Education, University of London: London.

Rodrigues, S.S.P., Caraher, M., Trichopoulou, A. & de Almeida, M.D.V. (2007) Portuguese households' diet-quality – adherence to Mediterranean food pattern and compliance with Who population dietary goals. *European Journal of Clinical Nutrition*, 62, 1263–1272.

Roep, D. & Wiskerke, H. (eds) (2006) *Nourishing Networks: Fourteen Lessons about Creating Sustainable Food Supply Chains*. Rural Sociology Group of Wageningen University and Reed Business Information: Doetinchem.

Rousseau, S. (2012) *Food Media: Celebrity Chefs and the Politics of Everyday Interference*. Bloomsbury: London.

Royal Society for the Encouragement of Arts, Manufacturers and Commerce (RSA) (1997) *Focus on Food: The Appreciation, Design, Production, Cultural and Social Importance of Food*. RSA: Dean Clough, Halifax, UK.

Schlosser, E. (2001) *Fast Food Nation: The Dark Side of the All-American Meal*. Houghton Mifflin: Boston, MA.

Seabrook, J. (2013) *Povertyland: Poverty and the Poor in Britain*. Hurst and Company: London.

Short, F. (2003) Domestic cooking skills. *Journal of the Home Economics Institute of Australia*, 10(3), 13–22.

Short, F. (2006) *Kitchen Secrets: The Meaning of Cooking in Everyday Life*. Berg: London.

Stead, M., Caraher, M., Wrieden, W., Longbottom, P., Valentine, K. & Anderson, A. (2004) Confident, fearful and hopeless cooks: Findings from the development of a food-skills initiative. *British Food Journal*, 106(40), 274–287, viewed 20 December 2015, http://dx.doi.org/10.1108/00070700410529546.

Stitt, S., Jepson, M., Paulson-Box, E. & Prisk, E. (1997) Schooling for capitalism: Cooking and the national Curriculum. In Köhler, B.M., Feichtinger, E., Barlösius, E. & Dowler, E. (eds) *Poverty and Food in Welfare Societies*. WZB: Berlin.

Thoreau, H.D. ([1854] 2004) *Walden*. Collector's Library: London.

Tinker, I. (1997) *Street Foods: Urban Food and Employment in Developing Countries*. Oxford University Press: New York.

Tonybee, P. (2013) *Hard Work: Life in Low-pay Britain*. Bloomsbury: London.

Troy, L.M., Miller, E.A. & Oslor, S. (2011) *Hunger and Obesity: Understanding a Food Insecurity Paradigm; Workshop Summary*. National Academies Press: Washington.

Veblen, T. (1994) *Theory of the Leisure Class: An Economic Study in the Evolution of Institutions*. Penguin Classics Edition: London.

Vileisis, A. (2008) *Kitchen Literacy: How We Lost Knowledge of Where Food Comes from and Why we Need to Get It Back*. Shearwater: Washington DC.

Wrangham, R. (2009) *Catching Fire: How Cooking Made Us Human*. Profile Books: London.

8   The nexus between food literacy, food security and disadvantage

Danielle Gallegos

Introduction

Internationally, there is a strong focus on hunger reduction and eradication (United Nations 2015). In low income countries, where agricultural, transport and health infrastructures are weakest, malnutrition, stunting and micronutrient deficiency rates are highest as a direct result of insufficient quantities of quality food. High income countries such as Australia, New Zealand, Canada and the United States pride themselves on their robust agricultural systems and ability to produce food for their own populations and for export. These countries are products of the Green Revolution, where the advancement of science in relation to agriculture, animal husbandry and food production has purportedly created self-sufficient nation states who have permanently removed any spectre of hunger from within their populations (Lang, Barling & Caraher 2009).

It could be argued that in these countries there is a surfeit of foods available for consumption and yet parts of the population still struggle to put food on the table; they continue to be food insecure. In high income countries these households are using strategies that may change the quality (as well as the quantity) of foods consumed to ensure that the promise of hunger is minimized. As a result, their health is usually compromised (Robaina & Martin 2013). Food systems are complex and as such require navigation and negotiation. In high income countries the complex food systems that supply a surfeit of food (in terms of quantity) mean that the ability to navigate these systems has become paramount to health. This chapter will explore the concepts of food security within a high income country context, it will map the constructs of food security with those of food literacy and finally it will describe a reconfiguration of food literacy.

Food security and the right to food

Food security has been framed, defined and contested depending on the prevailing political and social discourses (Jarosz 2011). As a key concept, food security has ostensibly shifted from a focus on agricultural productivity at a national level to a more micro-level approach that encompasses rights-based, equitable access to affordable food at the household and individual level (Jarosz 2011; MacMillan & Dowler 2012). In reality, food security continues to be framed as a problem of inadequate agricultural productivity – with the under-lying urgency being that the world will need to double global food production by 2050 (Tomlinson 2013). Most high income countries heeded the post-Second World War imperative for increasing agricultural production at any cost, but the sustainability of these measures is being called into question (Lang, Barling & Caraher 2009). Attention is now turning to a focus on climate change and the potential changed conditions that will significantly limit food supply. This in turn is driving a call for innovation in food production and processing, and an investment in research to reverse declining production (PMSEIC 2010). Sustained agricultural intensification (that is, producing enough quantity) combined with market liberalization remains an economic goal for high income countries in order to increase global market share with value-added agricultural commodities (Department of Agriculture 2012; Kirwan & Maye 2013). This increase is framed as a national contribution to gross domestic product, employment and viable agricultural and food manu-facturing systems that will offset any underlying 'poverty' (Department of Agriculture 2012; PMSEIC 2010).

Ensuring sustainable, equitable food production internationally has to remain on the global agenda. However, to think that a macro-economic approach will 'trickle down' to ensure incomes and a level of livelihood that will enable ongoing household access to enough food that maximizes health is naïve. The latest international definition of food security encompasses the complexity of the situation by highlighting the tension between production and consumption as well as quantity and quality of the food supply with not just the absence of hunger as the end goal but the maximization of health.

> Food and nutrition security exists when all people at all times have physical, social and economic access to food, which is safe and *consumed* in sufficient *quantity and quality* to meet their dietary needs and food preferences, and is supported by an environment of adequate sanitation, health services and care, allowing for a *healthy and active* life.
>
> (Committee on World Food Security 2012: 8; emphasis added)

What are the elements of food security?

Underpinning this definition of food security is a framework that employs four pillars: availability, access, stability, and utilization (Committee on World Food Security 2012b). These pillars take into consideration a range of elements contributing to food security including food sufficiency (quantity); nutrient adequacy (quality); cultural acceptability; safety; certainty and stability (Coates 2013). In summary, availability implies that foods are available to be consumed; at the household level this means that foods are available due to agricultural endeavour at a local or national level and/or are available for purchase. As poverty advocates have acknowledged, availability does not ensure predictable access (Sen 2000). Access acknowledges the resources or entitlements required to bring that food to the table; this could be economic or physical (transport), it could also include legal and social entitlements (Carletto, Zezza & Banerjee 2013).

Stability recognizes that a food supply needs to be able to transcend adverse weather and civil or economic conditions at a broader national as well as household level. The utilization umbrella is broad and includes the resources (physical, human and social) to transform food items into meals. From a human capital perspective this element includes knowledge, skills and socio-cultural dimensions that influence decisions about food choices. It also refers to the conditions under which the food is prepared; there is a growing recognition of the role of sanitation and the potential for unhygienic practices to limit the food available and also to reduce the biological utilization of nutrients (Ngure 2014).

Is food insecurity an issue in high income countries?

The measurement and reporting of food insecurity in high income countries is distinguished by the fact that, in the main, the tools are only taking into consideration one element of food security – economic access. Minimal consideration is given to physical and social access, cultural acceptability, and nutritional quality of food available, safety of food available, the stability of the food supply or the aspects of utilization, all of which impinge on household food security. There is growing recognition that food security cannot be measured by a single construct and that its complexity requires a multiplicitous tool

Food security monitoring and surveillance in countries such as Canada and the United States is undertaken on a regular basis utilizing validated multi-item scales. In the United States the prevalence of food insecurity is collected annually and for the last three years has been between 14.3% and 14.9% of households, with very low food security, where children in the household may be going hungry, steady at around 5.7% (Coleman-Jensen, Gregory & Singh 2014). In Canada, prevalence is at 8.3% of households, of which 2.5% were experiencing hunger (Statistics Canada 2013). Monitoring of food security in Australia is done poorly, there is no regular collection of data and there is a reliance on a single question which underestimates prevalence and fails to identify severity (Ramsey et al. 2012). The most recent data is from the Australian National Aboriginal and Torres Strait Islander Health Survey (2012–2013) and the National Nutrition and Physical Activity Survey (2011–2012) which utilized two questions: 'In the past 12 months was there any time when you or members of your household ran out of food and couldn't afford to buy more?' and for those who responded yes, 'When this happened did you or members of your household go without food? (Australian Bureau of Statistics 2015). For non-Indigenous households prevalence is at 3.7%, with 1.4% going without food (Australian Bureau of Statistics 2015). This is considered an underestimation, with prevalence of food insecurity in lower income areas or groups identified as being approximately 25% when a more sensitive tool is used (Nolan et al. 2006; Ramsey et al. 2012).

There is growing recognition of the consequences of food insecurity in high income countries and its contribution to the burden of disease. Food insecure households self-report poorer health and increased health service utilization (Ramsey et al. 2012). These households are typically consuming diets lower in quality (Leung et al. 2014) leading to greater risk of obesity in children and adults (particularly women) and cardiovascular disease due to changed food choices and variation in food consumption patterns (Ford 2013; Kaur, Lamb & Ogden 2015). The literature, however, as well as the models for alleviation of food insecurity still have a tendency to polarize those experiencing food insecurity into either passive victims of the system with little agency, or irresponsible consumers who have failed to make informed choices and continue to practise poor dietary habits (Crotty, Rutishauser & Cahill 1992). In Australia, the consistently low numbers of households in the general population that are identified as being food insecure have meant that consecutive governments have argued for the success of maintaining a strong economy that supports employment growth alongside a social welfare safety net (Department of Agriculture 2012). Food insecurity remains largely invisible, the consequences attributed to the failure of the individual, making a focus on strategies focused on the consumer much more palatable than systemic change (Dowler & O'Connor 2012; Lambie-Mumford & Dowler 2014).

Food insecurity and disadvantage

Food insecurity in high income countries disproportionately affects those experiencing a higher level of relative disadvantage. Invariably disadvantage within a food insecurity framework is conflated to mean low income and these households are more likely to be food insecure. Increasingly, however, in high income countries, poverty is not measured by an absolute income standard, that is the poverty line; relative poverty is identified by comparing living standards against a socially defined set of necessities. This list of necessities is determined by experts but ratified through social consensus (Gannon & Bailey 2014) and forms the basis of an income that provides a living wage. A living wage will allow a family to secure food, shelter, education, clothing, healthcare, transport and other necessities of modern living (Werner & Lim 2015). In the United Kingdom both quantity and quality of food are identified as a necessity: two meals a day for adults and three meals for children; fresh fruit and vegetables every day; meat, fish or equivalent every other day for adults and every day for children; and roast joint or equivalent once a week (Gordon et al. 2013). In Australia this is limited to a single subjective quantity construct: 'a substantial meal at least once a day' (Saunders & Wong 2012: 38).

As is typical of most neoliberal governments, there continues to be an emphasis on individual responsibility and mutual obligation; that is, in order to receive income support individuals need to demonstrate 'citizenship' by actively seeking employment and participating in the process (Brackertz 2014). In addition, this is reinforced through the ideology that low income families could do better if they simply managed their household finances more efficiently – hence a focus on budgeting and financial literacy (Brackertz 2014). This fails to acknowledge that for many low income families their situation is not a result of irresponsible spending or poor budgeting but is rooted in 'complex and intertwined personal, environmental and structural factors' (Brackertz 2014: 390).

While low income is an important cause of poor living, it is not necessarily the only contributor (Saunders & Wong 2012). Hence, describing poverty or disadvantage has moved to identifying other elements of deprivation, social exclusion and capabilities that can lead to impoverished lives (Hick 2012; Sen 2000). Capabilities do not refer to internal abilities; rather they indicate a failure of society to provide opportunities or freedom and are not related to individual deficits (Burchardt 2000). Likewise Hick (2012) indicates that deprivations are enforced; they are not caused by voluntary non-participation. From within a food context, the lack of availability and access to healthy food choices represents a failure to provide the opportunities to enable health. There is a conundrum, however, in that as consumption of poorer food choices becomes adaptive, the argument could be made that the line between deprivation and voluntary non-participation becomes blurred. That is, that those on lower incomes choose foods they can afford based on status, which over time becomes a cultural taste aesthetic and preference (Maillot, Darmon & Drewnowski 2010).

What is the response to food insecurity in high income countries?

In the absence of providing a living wage that ensures economic access to a quantity and quality of food that is required for an active and healthy life, the primary response by governments to the alleviation of food security in high income countries is based on a charitable approach. In this model, households need to actively source foods from a variety of emergency food relief agencies in the form of food banks, food rescue and other sources. The state therefore effectively has shifted the onus of responsibility in food provisioning from government to charitable organizations and as such is able to ignore food insecurity as an issue of social justice and a fundamental human right (MacMillan & Dowler 2012; Tarasuk & Eakin 2003).

In Canada, it is estimated that only 20–30% of those who identify as being food insecure use emergency food relief and that this usage is more an act of desperation rather than a protective strategy. The 'pure' charitable model is a needs-based approach that assumes recipients are passive – that is, assistance is provided without 'expectation of action from the recipient, without obligation and without legal protections'. The charitable model, therefore, does not necessarily fit with a rights-based approach, primarily because it fails to return beneficiaries to a state of food self-reliance and fails to maintain human dignity. In attempting to adopt a more rights-based approach organizations have moved to creating more enabling environments which they have interpreted as building personal skills. As such, organizations assume knowledge and skills deficits and link access to food with nutrition education, budgeting and cooking skills that could be seen as either an attempt to empower individuals or as a neoliberal attempt to resolve food insecurity through individualizing responsibility. Such approaches still fail to acknowledge that diet quality is mediated by diet cost and that education alone will not change food prices (Aggarwal et al. 2011).

The move by charitable agencies to provide programmes that attempt to improve personal skills is a forerunner to the next model adopted largely by the public health sector. The household improvement and support model was a response to the charitable model and an attempt to provide less stigmatizing programmes that focused on improving conditions for vulnerable communities (Collins, Power & Little 2014). These programmes, which include community kitchens, good food boxes, community gardens as well as the ubiquitous cooking skill workshops, seek to increase participant knowledge in a more digni-fied way. While well-meaning, they fail to reach the intended target group, and are not a long-term solution to food insecurity (Engler-Stringer & Berenbaum 2007). The common thread to these approaches to alleviating food insecurity is a focus on food literacy.

Where does food literacy fit in?

If we use the definition of disadvantage described here, then food security is providing appropriately distributed, sustainable opportunities to access the funda-mental commodity – food; while food literacy is being able to, at an individual and community level, take advantage of these opportunities. From a capabilities perspective, food literate individuals living in food insecure situations are potentially more likely to be able to reach certainty, choice and pleasure out-comes for longer periods of time, until resources are so depleted that it is no longer possible. Food literacy therefore has the potential to ameliorate some aspects of food insecurity, by increasing resilience and maximizing the use of available resources. Food literacy could be the key to maximizing food security for a limited amount of time. The cautionary caveat is that food literacy is not independent of context. In situations of deprivation and disadvantage, food literacy will be unable to improve the quality or quantity of food, where this food or the means to grow or acquire it are simply not present. A focus on food literacy could therefore mask underlying food security systems failures.

Food literacy has been empirically defined as the framework that empowers individuals, households, communities and nations to protect diet quality through change (Vidgen & Gallegos 2014). In other words it is about knowl-edge, skills and behaviours that promote the adaptability of diets in order to maintain quantity and quality despite circumstances and challenges. If we interrogate food insecurity, resilience is a key feature. Food secure individuals, households, communities and nations have an ongoing supply, access to and utilization of food in sufficient quantities and of a quality that maximizes health.

This supply, if stable and predictable, is independent of the context, be that physical, social or economic.

The next section will look at individual elements of food literacy and how they integrate with food security. It will go on to describe how food literacy and food security tenets can be combined to create a food literate nation where all its citizens have access to a safe food supply that provides a diet of sufficient quantity and quality for a healthy and active life.

Planning, management and selection

Food security has been described as a 'managed process' whereby predominantly women utilize a range of coping strategies to avoid or delay hunger for their families and in particular for their children (Martin & Lippert 2012). Undertaking this level of management, in particular where chronic food insecurity is present, takes a high level of food literacy.

For those experiencing disadvantage, prioritizing money for food is not a simple feat. Individuals and households need to balance a range of competing priorities including ensuring access to one of the other fundamental human rights – shelter. In Australia it is estimated that over 50 per cent of Australians spend more than 30 per cent of their disposable income on housing options and therefore experience household affordability stress (Wood, Ong & Cigdern 2014). Those on low incomes not only spend a higher proportion of their incomes on housing, they also spend more of their income proportionately on food (Kettings, Sinclair & Voevodin 2009; Palermo 2011). Insecure housing is identified as one of the primary triggers for the uptake of food aid (Lambie-Mumford & Dowler 2014). Accepting food aid, via foodbanks and other emergency relief food agencies, is often the strategy of last resort and is not an alternative acceptable coping strategy (Lambie-Mumford & Dowler 2014; Loopstra & Tarasuk 2015). In other words, before relying on food aid, food insecure households utilize a range of strategies that either enable them to stretch money further in order to source food, or minimize costs within the food budget to enable more food to be purchased. With household expenses fixed and a priority, the food budget is often the only flexible item, requiring household managers to make often daily decisions about payments and food choices (Lambie-Mumford & Dowler 2014).

With a smaller proportion of income available for food purchasing, a range of other strategies are employed that involve adaptation to local food environments within personal financial constraints (Cannuscio et al. 2014). Households experiencing food insecurity will prioritize the cost of food over any other factors; that is, they will seek out foods that will enable them to stretch their money further, sacrificing convenience (Cannuscio et al. 2014). In this case price is prioritized over time. However, this perhaps simplifies a complex web of negotiation, where households weigh up and offset distance travelled, time involved and cost as well as quality of foods available (Zachary et al. 2013).

Typically, when income is constrained then dietary decisions are driven by the need to maximize energy value for money spent, resulting in energy dense, nutrient poor diets (Brimblecombe & O'Dea 2009; Drewnowski & Darmon 2005; Ramsey et al. 2012). Compromising food quality (in terms of overall health as well as safety) is a recognized coping strategy and, in order to ameliorate the effects of hunger (in the short term), energy dense foods that are cheaper per kilojoule are consumed in higher quantities (Drewnowski 2004) in anticipation of food scarcity (Walker & Kawachi 2012). Consumption of fruits and vegetables that are less energy dense and more costly per kilojoule subsequently decreases (Robaina & Martin 2013).

This is borne out in estimates from the USA and Australia where low income households, in order to meet the dietary guidelines, must spend anywhere between 30% and 70% of their budget on fruit and vegetables and healthy food items (Cassady, Jetter & Culp 2007; Palermo et al. 2008). Given the pressure on the household budget, these figures belie the primary argument that emerges from government and charitable agencies, that is, not being able to 'eat properly' is a fundamental failure of the individual to budget appropriately and cook (Garthwaite, Collins & Bambra 2015; Stewart et al. 2011). This implies that food insecure households do not exhibit food literacy. However, given the coping strategies employed, the reverse could be argued; that is, food insecure households exhibit high levels of food literacy that is contextualized to the prevailing conditions.

Planning takes a variety of forms depending on the level of disadvantage and where households are in the food insecurity trajectory. Changing types of foods consumed to more energy dense, nutrient poor choices is often the first step. For many families who have lived with poverty, this may no longer be a conscious decision but a way of life, and these households may not even consider themselves food insecure – they are after all able to put food on the table. Other coping strategies that can become adaptive, in other words so ingrained that they are no longer overt ways to ameliorate food security, include identifying where to shop and shopping at different stores based on price; buying in bulk; catching foods on sale as a collective; choosing what items to purchase in a fortnightly pay cycle based on need; prioritizing food items based on children's needs and/or preferences and, in the USA, utilizing food coupons with maximum effect (Crotty, Rutishauser & Cahill 1992; Rose 2011; Wiig & Smith 2008). There is growing evidence that families experiencing food insecurity have a detailed understanding of healthy eating; however, external conditions mean that they need to prioritize quantity and satiety over quality.

At a deeper level of disadvantage, food literate management could be seen as being able to manipulate charitable food supplies to ensure a regular supply of food whether on a daily or a weekly basis. Manipulation of charitable food supplies could be described as an adaptive strategy. The dependence on charitable food suppliers by those experiencing significant disadvantage is indicative of the failure or dismantling of the social welfare safety net (Tarasuk & Eakin 2003). The adaptive strategy to utilize these resources is a testament to individual resilience and resourcefulness in ensuring 'that food can be regularly accessed through the same source, irrespective of changes in circumstances or environment' (Vidgen & Gallegos 2014: 55).

Preparation and eating

The preparation and eating domains of food literacy involve being able to make a good tasting meal from whatever food is available, applying basic principles of food safety, as well as understanding the impact of food on wellbeing, including the nutritional elements related to quality, quantity and frequency of food items. Finally, they also encompass the act of eating as a commensal, social act. Within the food security domain, preparation of food, food safety, and food and nutrition knowledge and diet diversity fall under the umbrella of 'utilization' (Committee on World Food Security 2012b).

Assumptions are generally made that levels of skill around cooking and food preparation and the concomitant knowledge around nutrition, health and wellbeing are generally low among those on low incomes or experiencing disadvantage. Agencies embrace these assumptions and rely on the implementation of cooking programmes and advice on meal planning because their clients are 'largely unaware of how to cook properly, more typically relying on unhealthy convenience foods' (Garthwaite, Collins & Bambra 2015: 42). There is evidence, however, that low income households are more likely to cook foods at home (McLachlan, Gilfillan & Gordon 2013; Smith, Ng & Popkin 2014) and that these households deploy a high level of food literacy in order to put food on the table. Such strategies at the preparation end include cooking dishes that are cheap and filling; eating nutritionally sound but socially devalued foods; making use of foods that can be frozen and stored; storing and using leftovers; stretching the food to make it last longer; removing spoiled areas or insects from food to extend its usability; using foods that were beyond the expiry date; cutting down on the variety of fruits and vegetables to only those that are most affordable, most filling, are the easiest to store and last the longest (Crotty, Rutishauser & Cahill 1992; Kempson et al. 2003; Nielsen, Lund & Holm 2015; Warin et al. 2015). Not all of these strategies would fit with the definition of food security as they fail to meet the social acceptability of food and its procurement.

The relationship between time, food choice, food security and food literacy is complex and underexplored (Lawrence et al. 2009). For low income families time management is in response to the minimal control they may have over their environments which may include insecure, low wage, inflexible jobs and unexpected events (Jabs et al. 2007). There are indications that women will always work hard to prioritize the feeding of their children in order that they do not go hungry (Martin & Lippert 2012; Stevens 2010) but need to do so in the shortest time possible to enable them to move on to other tasks (Jabs et al. 2007). Efforts through organized programmes that therefore privilege 'cooking-from-scratch' on a budget – such as the USA's Thrifty Food Plan and

Australia's FOODCents® – fail to take into consideration the time element (Davis & You 2011). As Rose (2011) has previously indicated such programmes are incongruous with welfare policy that mandates women to look for work within the labour market but then assumes they will be at home to cook from scratch.

While there is evidence that nutrition knowledge among low income families is low, especially around nutrition categories rather than necessarily food categories (Cluss et al. 2013), Coveney (2005) provides a timely reminder regarding interpretation of these results. Low income families tend to relate more to foods and the impact foods have on external appearance, while families on higher incomes relate the nutritional value of foods in terms more likely to be understood by a health professional. The way low income families understand and appreciate the nutritional value of food may be different, but it does not necessarily make it wrong, and care needs to be taken in ensuring that the way low income families make sense of food and health is not devalued (Coveney 2005).

There is no doubt that knowing the nutritional value of foods and how to prepare them are skills that can maximize health, and having such skills may provide practical solutions to extend food security. In other words, food literacy may be a resource that enables individuals to take advantage of the available food opportunities. However, improving these skills will not necessarily alleviate food insecurity, especially if we take into consideration the other important element – time.

Time scarcity is increasingly considered a salient factor for high and low income households that has compressed the time available for meal preparation and given rise to a variety of meal management strategies (Morin et al. 2013). It has also been identified as a potential factor influencing the ability to prepare healthier food (Monsivais, Aggarwal & Drewnowski 2014). Time and money are *both* needed to manage a household where money is lacking. Hence, food insecure families are also potentially time insecure families (Jabs & Devine 2006).

For low income and/or disadvantaged households there are a number of factors to take into consideration including the stressors of role overload, household chaos, and the complex manipulation of time to balance obligations. Decreases in economic security may lead to more frequent moving from one household to another, changes in the size of the household to improve economic viability, demands for childcare at irregular hours, jobs that require longer commutes and heads of households engaged in non-standard employment – all leading to household chaos (Coleman-Jensen 2011; Vernon-Feagans et al. 2012). These households may experience difficulty in managing household and food needs, with work taking precedence; there are indications that households with heads who are in multiple or part-time jobs, or who have varied hours of employment, are more likely to be food insecure (Coleman-Jensen 2011).

In their analysis of the daily rhythm and time organization of working women living in poverty Roy, Tubbs and Burton (2004) identified that women needed to work through a puzzle each day which balanced work with childcare arrangements and transportation. Daily sustenance tasks were allocated to time blocks. In looking at the quotidian allocation of time, the allocation of time to food preparation is one of the few flexible elements over which women may exert some control. Work outside the home is prescribed, commute times are set, and managing childcare is a priority. Using convenience foods or off-setting time by buying pre-prepared food items is a legitimate means by which time can be managed (Roy, Tubbs & Burton 2004). Minimizing meal pre-paration potentially creates time which can lead to moments where the stressors of everyday life can be alleviated and families can relax (Devine et al. 2006; Warin et al. 2015). For families where income is not guaranteed these moments can be hard to come by.

The combination of time and financial poverty intersects with coping strategies surrounding eating together. Mealtimes and family food involvement have been linked with improved diet quality, socialization and child and adolescent outcomes (Anving & Sellerberg 2010; Fulkerson et al. 2014; Leech et al. 2014). However, for many families who are food insecure, occasions where food is eaten together are another example of complex planning and literacy. Creating these social occasions can rely on an array of coping strategies including maximizing food intake from external sources (for example, vis-iting relatives for a meal); pooling of limited food resources in order to feed larger numbers (inviting guests to bring food); or staggering mealtimes in order to facilitate food consumption for part of a household (Tubbs, Roy & Burton 2004).

Conclusions

The goal of food literacy is to protect diet quality through change, and in so doing create more choice, certainty and pleasure (Vidgen & Gallegos 2014). MacMillan and Dowler (2012: 199) remind us of the goal of food security: 'that people should not have to make trade-offs between immediate poor nutritional status and long term livelihood sustainability'. The examples given above provide a clear indication that the discourse needs to shift from a deficit-based individualized response, where the main premise is that the poor have failed in their duty as citizens. The nexus between food literacy and food security is a reminder that the reconfiguration of health, and particularly nutritional health, as a biomedical 'problem' cannot be divorced from the social context (Aronson 1982; Schubert et al. 2011). Nor should what are essentially failures of the political system be turned into 'problems of deviance or moral order' (Aronson 1982: 484).

What this chapter has demonstrated is that food literacy is contextual and that those on low incomes display a range of strategies which would indicate a high degree of food literacy. If we accept that those households on low incomes have agency to make decisions within the food environment, and that it is the interplay of agency and structural factors that needs to be addressed

(Rose 2011), then more upstream approaches that address the root of the issue will be more effective. This means that relying on developing food literacy as the primary strategy for alleviating food insecurity will be inadequate. The focus needs to shift to providing a living wage to all citizens that incorporates in its calculation the means to provide meals of sufficient quality to maximize and promote health, the means to provide affordable housing, and the means to manage food price volatility in order to be able to create food environments where healthy food choices can be made to empower rather than to shame.

References

Aggarwal, A., Monsivais, P., Cook, A.J. & Drewnowski, A. 2011, 'Does diet cost mediate the relation between socioeconomic position and diet quality?', *European Journal of Clinical Nutrition*, vol. 65, pp. 1059–1066.

Anving, T. & Sellerberg, A.-M. 2010, 'Family meals and parents' challenges', *Food, Culture & Society*, vol. 13, no. 2, pp. 201–214.

Aronson, N. 1982, 'Nutrition as a social problem: a case study of the entrepreneurial strategy in science', *Social Problems*, vol. 29, no. 5, pp. 474–487.

Australian Bureau of Statistics 2015, *Australian Aboriginal and Torres Strait Islander Health Survey: Nutrition Results – Food and Nutrients, 2012–13, Cat # 4727.0.55.005* ABS, viewed 30 July 2015, <http://www.abs.gov.au/AUSSTATS/abs@.nsf/DetailsPage/4727.0.55.0052012-13?OpenDocument>.

Brackertz, N. 2014, 'The impact of financial counselling on alleviating financial stress in low income households: A national Australian empirical study', *Social Policy and Society*, vol. 13, no. 3, pp. 389–407.

Brimblecombe, J.K. & O'Dea, K. 2009, 'The role of energy cost in food choices for an Aboriginal population in northern Australia', *Medical Journal of Australia*, vol. 190, no. 10, pp. 549–551.

Burchardt, T. 2000, 'Social exclusion: concepts and evidence', in D. Gordon & P. Townsend (eds), *Breadline Europe. The Measurement of Poverty*, Policy Press, Bristol, pp. 385–406.

Cannuscio, C.C., Hillier, A., Karpyn, A. & Glanz, K. 2014, 'The social dynamics of healthy food shopping and store choice in an urban environment', *Social Science & Medicine*, vol. 122, pp. 13–20.

Carletto, C., Zezza, A. & Banerjee, R. 2013, 'Towards better measurement of household food security: Harmonizing indicators and the role of household surveys', *Global Food Security*, vol. 2, no. 1, pp. 30–40.

Cassady, D., Jetter, K.M. & Culp, J. 2007, 'Is price a barrier to eating more fruits and vegetables for low-income families?', *Journal of the American Dietetic Association*, vol. 107, no. 11, pp. 1909–1915.

Chilton, M. & Rose, D. 2009, 'A rights-based approach to food insecurity in the United States', *American Journal of Public Health*, vol. 99, no. 7, pp. 1203–1211.

Cluss, P.A., Ewing, L., King, W.C., Reis, E.C., Dodd, J.L. & Penner, B. 2013, 'Nutrition knowledge of low income parents of obese children', *Translational Behavioral Medicine*, vol. 3, no. 2, pp. 218–225.

Coates, J. 2013, 'Build it back better: Deconstructing food security for improved measurement and action', *Global Food Security*, vol. 2, no. 3, pp. 188–194.

Coleman-Jensen, A., Gregory, C. & Singh, A. 2014, *Household Food Security in the United States in 2013*, USDA, Washington DC.

Coleman-Jensen, A.J. 2011, 'Working for peanuts: nonstandard work and food insecurity across household structure', *Journal of Family and Economic Issues*, vol. 32, pp. 84–97.

Collins, P.A., Power, E.M. & Little, M.H. 2014, 'Municipal-level responses to household food insecurity in Canada: A call for critical, evaluative research', *Canadian Journal of Public Health*, vol. 105, no. 2, pp. e138–141.

Committee on World Food Security 2012a 'Coming to terms with terminology', Food and Agricultural Organization, Rome, viewed 10 December 2015, <http://www.fao.org/docrep/meeting/026/MD776E.pdf>.

Committee on World Food Security 2012b, *Global Strategic Framework for Food Security and Nutrition*, Food and Agricultural Organization, Rome, viewed 30 July 2015, <http://www.fao.org/fileadmin/user_upload/bodies/CFS_sessions/39th_Session/39emerg/ME498E_CFS_2012_39_5_Add_1_Rev_1.pdf>.

Coveney, J. 2005, 'A qualitative study exploring socio-economic differences in parental lay knowledge of food and health: Implications for public health nutrition', *Public Health Nutrition*, vol. 8, pp. 290–297.

Crotty, P.A., Rutishauser, I. & Cahill, M. 1992, 'Food in low-income families', *Australian Journal of Public Health*, vol. 16, no. 2, pp. 168–174.

Davis, G.C. & You, W. 2011, 'Not enough money or not enough time to satisfy the Thrifty Food Plan? A cost difference approach for estimating a money–time threshold', *Food Policy*, vol. 36, no. 2, pp. 101–107.

Department of Agriculture 2012, *The National Food Plan*, Commonwealth of Australia, Canberra, viewed 30 July 2015, <http://www.agriculture.gov.au/ag-farm-food/food/publications/national_food_plan/white-paper>.

Devine, C.M., Jastran, M., Jabs, J., Wethington, E., Farrell, T.J. & Bisogni, C.A. 2006, '"A lot of sacrifices". Work-family spillover and the food choice coping strategies of low-wage employed parents', *Social Science & Medicine*, vol. 62, pp. 2591–2603.

Dowler, E.A. & O'Connor, D. 2012, 'Rights-based approaches to addressing food poverty and food insecurity in Ireland and UK', *Social Science & Medicine*, vol. 74, no. 1, pp. 44–51.

Drewnowski, A. 2004, 'Obesity and the food environment: Dietary energy density and diet costs', *American Journal of Preventive Medicine*, vol. 27, no. 3, Supplement, pp. 154–162.

Drewnowski, A. & Darmon, N. 2005, 'The economics of obesity: Dietary energy density and energy cost', *American Journal of Clinical Nutrition*, vol. 82, no. 1, pp. 265S–273S.

Engler-Stringer, R. & Berenbaum, S. 2007, 'Exploring food security with collective kitchens participants in three Canadian cities', *Qualitative Health Research*, vol. 17, no. 1, pp. 75–84.

Ford, E.S. 2013, 'Food security and cardiovascular disease risk among adults in the United States: Findings from the National Health and Nutrition Examination Survey, 2003–2008', *Preventing Chronic Disease*, vol. 10, p. E202.

Fordyce-Voorham, S. 2016, 'Preliminary findings of a food literacy program evaluation using a food literacy model', *Journal of the Home Economics Institute of Australia*, vol. 22, no. 3, pp. 2-12.

Fulkerson, J.A., Larson, N., Horning, M. & Neumark-Sztainer, D. 2014, 'A review of associations between family or shared meal frequency and dietary and weight status outcomes across the lifespan', *Journal of Nutrition Education and Behavior*, vol. 46, no. 1, pp. 2–19.

Gannon, M. & Bailey, N. 2014, '"Attitudes to the 'necessities of life": Would an independent Scotland set a different poverty standard to the rest of the UK?', *Social Policy and Society*, vol. 13, no. 3, pp. 321–336.

Garthwaite, K.A., Collins, P.J. & Bambra, C. 2015, 'Food for thought: An ethnographic study of negotiating ill health and food insecurity in a UK foodbank', *Social Science & Medicine*, vol. 132, pp. 38–44.

Gordon, D., Mack, J., Lansley, S., et al. 2013, *The Impoverishment of the UK: PSE UK First Results: Living Standards*, Poverty and Social Exclusion Research United Kingdom, viewed 30 July 2015, <http://poverty.ac.uk/sites/default/files/attachm ents/The_Impoverishment_of_the_UK_PSE_UK_first_results_summary_report_Ma rch_28.pdf>.

Hick, R. 2012, 'The capability approach: Insights for a new poverty focus', *Journal of Social Policy*, vol. 41, no. 2, pp. 291–308.

Jabs, J. & Devine, C. 2006, 'Time-scarcity and food-choices: An overview', *Appetite*, vol. 47, pp. 196–204.

Jabs, J., Devine, C.M., Bisogni, C.A., Farrell, T.J., Jastran, M. & Wethington, E. 2007, 'Trying to find the quickest way: Employed mothers' constructions of time for food', *Journal of Nutrition Education and Behavior*, vol. 39, no. 1, pp. 18–25.

Jarosz, L. 2011, 'Defining world hunger: Scale and neoliberal ideology in international food security policy discourse', *Food, Culture & Society*, vol. 14, no. 1, pp. 117–139.

Kaur, J., Lamb, M.M. & Ogden, C.L. 2015, 'The association between food insecurity and obesity in children – The National Health and Nutrition Examination Survey', *Journal of the Academy of Nutrition and Dietetics*, vol. 115, no. 5, pp. 751–758.

Kempson, K., Keenan, D.P., Sadani, P.S. & Adler, A. 2003, 'Maintaining food sufficiency: Coping strategies identified by limited-resource individuals versus nutrition educators', *Journal of Nutrition Education and Behavior*, vol. 35, no. 4, pp. 179–188.

Kettings, C., Sinclair, A.J. & Voevodin, M. 2009, 'A healthy diet consistent with Australian health recommendations is too expensive for welfare dependent families', *Australia New Zealand Journal of Public Health*, vol. 33, pp. 566–572.

Kirwan, J. & Maye, D. 2013, 'Food security framings within the UK and the integration of local food systems', *Journal of Rural Studies*, vol. 29, pp. 91–100.

Lambie-Mumford, H. & Dowler, E. 2014, 'Rising use of "food aid" in the United Kingdom', *British Food Journal*, vol. 116, no. 9, pp. 1418–1425.

Lang, T., Barling, D. & Caraher, M. 2009, *Food Policy: Integrating Health, Environment and Society*, Oxford University Press, Oxford.

Lawrence, G., Richards, C. & Lyons, K. 2013, 'Food security in Australia in an era of neoliberalism, productivism and climate change', *Journal of Rural Studies*, vol. 29, pp. 30–39.

Lawrence, W., Skinner, C., Haslam, C., Robinson, S., Inskip, H., Barker, D., Cooper, C., Jackson, A. & Barker, M. 2009, 'Why women of lower educational attainment struggle to make healthier food choices: The importance of psychological and social factors', *Psychology & Health*, vol. 24, no. 9, pp. 1003–1020.

Leech, R.M., McNaughton, S.A., Crawford, D.A., Campbell, K.J., Pearson, N. & Timperio, A. 2014, 'Family food involvement and frequency of family dinner meals among Australian children aged 10–12 years. Cross-sectional and longitudinal associations with dietary patterns', *Appetite*, vol. 75, pp. 64–70.

Leung, C.W., Epel, E.S., Ritchie, L.D., Crawford, P.B. & Laraia, B.A. 2014, 'Food insecurity is inversely associated with diet quality of lower-income adults', *Journal of the Academy of Nutrition and Dietetics*, vol. 114, no. 12, pp. 1943–1953.e2.

Loopstra, R. & Tarasuk, V. 2015, 'Food bank usage is a poor indicator of food insecurity: Insights from Canada', *Social Policy and Society*, vol. 14, no. 3, pp. 443–455.

MacMillan, T. & Dowler, E. 2012, 'Just and sustainable? Examining the rhetoric and potential realities of UK food security', *Journal of Agricultural and Environmental Ethics*, vol. 25, no. 2, pp. 181–204.

Maillot, M., Darmon, N. & Drewnowski, A. 2010, 'Are the lowest-cost healthful food plans culturally and socially acceptable?', *Public Health Nutrition*, vol. 13, pp. 1178–1185.

Martin, M.A. & Lippert, A.M. 2012, 'Feeding her children, but risking her health: The intersection of gender, household food insecurity and obesity', *Social Science & Medicine*, vol. 74, no. 11, pp. 1754–1764.

McLachlan, R., Gilfillan, G. & Gordon, J. 2013, *Deep and Persistent Disadvantage in Australia: Productivity Commission Staff Working Paper*, Australian Government Productivity Commission, Canberra, viewed 26 June 2015, <http://www.pc.gov.au/research/completed/deep-persistent-disadvantage/deep-persistent-disadvantage.pdf>.

Monsivais, P., Aggarwal, A. & Drewnowski, A. 2014, 'Time spent on home food preparation and indicators of healthy eating', *American Journal of Preventive Medicine*, vol. 47, no. 6, pp. 796–802.

Morin, P., Demers, K., Turcotte, S. & Mongeau, L. 2013, 'Association between perceived self-efficacy related to meal management and food coping strategies among working parents with preschool children', *Appetite*, vol. 65, pp. 43–50.

Ngure, F.M., Reid, B. M., Humphrey, J.H., et al., 2014, 'Water, sanitation, and hygiene (WASH), environmental enteropathy, nutrition, and early child development: Making the links', *Annals of the New York Academy of Sciences*, vol. 1308, pp. 118–128.

Nielsen, A., Lund, T.B. & Holm, L. 2015, 'The taste of "the end of the month", and how to avoid it: Coping with restrained food budgets in a Scandinavian welfare state context', *Social Policy and Society*, vol. 14, no. 3, pp. 429–442.

Nolan, M., Rikard-Bell, G., Mohsin, M. & Williams, M. 2006, 'Food insecurity in three socially disadvantaged localities in Sydney, Australia', *Health Promotion Journal of Australia*, vol. 17, pp. 247–254.

Palermo, C. 2011, 'The cost of nutritious food: A determinant of health', *Nutrition & Dietetics*, vol. 68, no. 4, pp. 246–247.

Palermo, C.E., Walker, K.Z., Hill, P. & McDonald, J. 2008, 'The cost of health food in rural Victoria', *Rural and Remote Health*, vol. 8, no. 4.

PMSEIC 2010, *Australia and Food Security in a Changing World*, The Prime Minister's Science, Engineering and Innovation Council, Canberra, Australia, viewed 2 November 2012, <http://www.chiefscientist.gov.au/wp-content/uploads/FoodSecurity_web.pdf>.

Ramsey, R., Giskes, K., Gavin, T. & Gallegos, D. 2012, 'Food insecurity among adults residing in disadvantaged urban areas: Potential health and dietary consequences', *Public Health Nutrition*, vol. 15, pp. 227–237.

Robaina, K.A. & Martin, K.S. 2013, 'Food insecurity, poor diet quality, and obesity among food pantry participants in Hartford, CT', *Journal of Nutrition Education and Behavior*, vol. 45, no. 2, pp. 159–164.

Rose, D.J. 2011, 'Captive audience? Strategies for acquiring food in two Detroit neighborhoods', *Qualitative Health Research*, vol. 21, no. 5, pp. 642–651.

Roy, K.M., Tubbs, C.Y. & Burton, L.M. 2004, 'Don't have no time: Daily rhythms and the organization of time for low-income families', *Family Relations*, vol. 53, no. 2, pp. 168–178.

Saunders, P. & Wong, M. 2012, *Promoting Inclusion and Combating Deprivation: Recent Changes in Social Disadvantage in Australia*, Social Policy Research Centre, University of New South Wales, Sydney, viewed 29 June 2015, <https://www.sprc.unsw.edu. au/media/SPRCFile/2012_12_FINAL_REPORT.pdf>.

Schubert, L., Gallegos, D., Foley, W. & Harrison, C. 2011, 'Re-imagining the "social" in the nutrition sciences', *Public Health Nutrition*, vol. 15, no. 2, pp. 352–359.

Sen, A. 2000, *Social Exclusion: Concept, Application and Scrutiny*, Social Development Papers No. 1, Office of Environment and Social Development, Asia Development Bank, Manila, Philippines, viewed 10 December 2015, <http://www.adb.org/sites/ default/files/publication/29778/social-exclusion.pdf>.

Smith, L.P., Ng, S.W. & Popkin, B.M. 2014, 'Resistant to the recession: Low-income adults' maintenance of cooking and away-from-home eating behaviors during times of economic turbulence', *American Journal of Public Health*, vol. 104, no. 5, pp. 840–846.

Statistics Canada 2013, *Household Food Insecurity, 2011–2012*, Statistics Canada, viewed 30 July 2015, <http://www.statcan.gc.ca/pub/82-625-x/2013001/article/11889-eng.htm>.

Stevens, C.A. 2010, 'Exploring food insecurity among young mothers (15–24 years)', *Journal for Specialists in Pediatric Nursing*, vol. 15, no. 2, pp. 163–171.

Stewart, H., Hyman, J., Frazão, E., Buzby, J.C. & Carlson, A. 2011, 'Can low-income Americans afford to satisfy MyPyramid fruit and vegetable guidelines?', *Journal of Nutrition Education and Behavior*, vol. 43, no. 3, pp. 173–179.

Tarasuk, V. & Eakin, J.M. 2003, 'Charitable food assistance as symbolic gesture: An ethnographic study of food banks in Ontario', *Social Science & Medicine*, vol. 56, no. 7, pp. 1505–1515.

Tomlinson, I. 2013, 'Doubling food production to feed the 9 billion: A critical perspective on a key discourse of food security in the UK', *Journal of Rural Studies*, vol. 29, pp. 81–90.

Tubbs, C.Y., Roy, K.M. & Burton, L.M. 2005, 'Family ties: Constructing family time in low-income families', *Family Process*, vol. 44, no. 1, pp. 77–91.

United Nations 2015, *Millennium Development Goals and Beyond 2015*, viewed 30 July 2015, <https://www.un.org/millenniumgoals/>.

Vernon-Feagans, L., Garrett-Peters, P., Willoughby, M. & Mills-Koonce, R. 2012, 'Chaos, poverty, and parenting: Predictors of early language development', *Early Childhood Research Quarterly*, vol. 27, no. 3, pp. 339–351.

Vidgen, H.A. & Gallegos, D. 2014, 'Defining food literacy and its components', *Appetite*, vol. 76, pp. 50–59.

Walker, R.E. & Kawachi, I. 2012, 'Use of concept mapping to explore the influence of food security on food buying practices', *Journal of the Academy of Nutrition and Dietetics*, vol. 112, no. 5, pp. 711–717.

Warin, M., Zivkovic, T., Moore, V., Ward, P.R. & Jones, M. 2015, 'Short horizons and obesity futures: Disjunctures between public health interventions and everyday temporalities', *Social Science & Medicine*, vol. 128, pp. 309–315.

Werner, A. & Lim, M. 2015, 'The ethics of the living wage: A review and research agenda', *Journal of Business Ethics*, pp. 1–15.

Wiig, K. & Smith, C. 2008, 'The art of grocery shopping on a food stamp budget: Factors influencing the food choices of low-income women as they try to make ends meet', *Public Health Nutrition*, vol. 12, pp. 1726–1734.

Wood, G., Ong, R. & Cigdern, M. 2014, 'Housing affordability dynamics in Australia: New insights from the last decade', *Australian Housing and Urban Research Institute Final Report*, Canberra, viewed 10 December 2015, <http://researchbank.rmit.edu.au/view/rmit:29659>.

Zachary, D.A., Palmer, A.M., Beckham, S.W. & Surkan, P.J. 2013, 'A framework for understanding grocery purchasing in a low-income urban environment', *Qualitative Health Research*, vol. 23, no. 5, pp. 665–678.

9 The development of food literacy

Helen Vidgen

Introduction

So far this book has explored food literacy and its various dimensions. It has described a food literacy that has multiple components and is contextually defined. It has described a food literacy that applies at the individual, household, community and national levels to protect diet quality through change and support dietary resilience over time. Chapters have also conceptualized how food literacy influences health, wellbeing, food choice and food security. Within each of these, the interplay between this collection of inter-related knowledge, skills and behaviours to plan, manage, select, prepare and eat foods to meet needs and determine food intake, that is, food literacy, and the broader food supply and determinants of health and wellbeing has been explored. The following four chapters examine the development of food literacy. The first reports the descriptions of young people who reflected on how their food and eating had developed and evolved over time. They describe this at the individual level but in doing so describe the interplay between other key institutions of health, education and food production. These institutions, and the food literacy work that occurs within them, is then explored in more detail in the three chapters that follow. The reader is encouraged to consider these results alongside learning and development theory to propose how food literacy develops, including the role of individuals, households, communities and nations, and in particular, what food literacy at each of these levels might look like.

This chapter reports the findings of the Young People Study, described in Chapters 3 and 4. This was a qualitative study of thirty-seven young people (aged 16–25 years, mean age 19.8 years) who were responsible for feeding themselves. Participants talked about food and eating in their current 'household' and then worked backwards to reflect on different food and eating environments and the contribution of these different stages and situations to their food literacy. They talked about where and from whom they learnt about food, when this happened over their life-course and what factors prompted this learning. All interviews were conducted face to face.

As described in Chapter 3, participants all lived in an Australian capital city and were purposefully sampled across a spectrum of disadvantage ranging from homelessness to university graduates. Young people were recruited through services in order to reach people experiencing different levels of disadvantage. The Red Cross Night Café provides services to young people experiencing homelessness. The Albert Park and Kingston Flexible Learning Centres provide services to young people who have been through a significant period of dis-engagement, e.g. juvenile detention, expulsion from school, homelessness, and are now aiming to re-engage. The services differed in that Albert Park targeted older people (16–25 years) and was located in an area of relative advantage, whereas Kingston serviced younger people (up to 19 years) who tended to still live in a parental type of home but was located in an area of very high dis-advantage. The participants in these three groups either had no income or relied on welfare payments. The Ipswich City Council was used to recruit young people who had completed their schooling and were employed but lived in a geographically defined area of high disadvantage. This is defined by an index derived from Australian census data (Pink 2008). Finally, participants were recruited through a university business school using snowballing. These students had all completed their schooling and were engaged in or had completed a tertiary qualification. All lived in areas of highest advantage (Pink 2008). Additional 'non-disadvantaged' participants were initially recruited through a nutrition service agency, Nutrition Australia Queensland. The young people in these latter three groups predominantly derived their income from wages. The sample included fifteen males and twenty-two females.

When young people developed food literacy

Prior to the commencement of this study, health and education practitioners had anecdotally observed key transition times at which interest in developing food knowledge, skills and behaviours was heightened. Interventions in both of these sectors often assume critical learning opportunities which this research was interested in examining further.

There were few milestones that were common to all participants; more specifically, the significance of these milestones as transition points varied greatly, most often according to level of disadvantage. Exiting school, for example, is considered a standard milestone for all young people; however, for most of the young people experiencing disadvantage, the end of school varied considerably. This included interrupted schooling, lengthy absences, abrupt exiting, not actively participating in their schooling for some time and so then gradually disengaging and then re-engaging years later. For those young people not experiencing disadvantage, finishing school was a fairly standard experience; that is, it happened at the age of 17, at the end of a school year, with a plan of what might happen next, for example further education or employment. Those young people who were most disadvantaged were also least likely to have completed their schooling and had interrupted schooling.

This study originally planned to examine the milestone of leaving the parental home, envisaging that this may have been a key transition point for developing one's relationship and identity with food. Youth service providers, however, suggested that while this might be a significant milestone and potential transition point for the mainstream population, for marginalized young people its significance was less important, and in fact, they may be unable to identify either their parental home or when they left it. The study instead sampled young people who were responsible for feeding themselves, asked questions about when this first began and the different homes and households they had lived in.

Table 9.1 shows the age at which participants first left their parental home and became responsible for feeding themselves. The different participant groups represent increasing levels of disadvantage. Terms were not defined: for example, participants determined what they considered 'leaving home' and 'responsible for feeding themselves' meant. It is clear from the table that as the groups became more marginalized and more disadvantaged, their age for leaving home and being responsible for feeding themselves decreased. In the most disadvantaged groups, girls tended to be made responsible for feeding themselves younger than boys. This responsibility also often included being responsible for feeding other children and adults in the household. The following interview excerpts further describe these experiences.

Silke was interviewed at the Kingston Flexible Learning Centre where she was aiming to complete year 12. She describes her current living situation and her movements over time.

Table 9.1 The age when participants first became responsible for feeding themselves and first left their parental home

Recruitment site	Age when first left parental home		Age when first became responsible for food		Total number of participants
	Mean	*Range*	*Mean*	*Range*	
Australian Red Cross Night Café	15.0★	12–19★	14.6	7–19	7
Albert Park Flexible Learning Centre	15.8	14–18	14.7	7–18	9
Kingston Flexible Learning Centre	16.0★★★	16★★★	12.0	8–16	5
Ipswich City Council	17.0	15–19	17.0	15–19	6
QUT School of Business	19.6★★	17–23★★	19.1	17–24	8
Nutrition Australia Queensland	21.0	20–22	19.5	17–22	2

Source: Young People Study Recruitment Site

Notes: ★one participant had not left their parental home; ★★two participants had not left their parental home; ★★★three participants had not left their parental home

I'm seventeen. I live at McCarthy; it's in Browns Plains. I've been living there for about four months now with my dad and my sister. Before that I lived with my mother in Marsden for eight years in the same place and before that we were everywhere. Forty places, at least. We never – Marsden was the longest we ever stayed put. We were moving constantly, almost every month pretty much. Just within the area – we just changed from Nanango or the coast or Sunshine, everywhere – we couldn't stay still. I was usually with my mum, my sister and my little brother.

The first time in all that, that I was responsible for feeding myself was probably around about when we moved to Marsden, my mum did her own thing and all of us kids took care of ourselves. I was probably about 11 or so. My sister would make a four meal course and I would make another one, I usually made the desserts. Us kids just ate. Mum wasn't usually hungry – she was too stressed to eat, so sometimes she would but sometimes not.

Silke

Neither Silke's mother nor her father ever cooked. In these households, Silke typically ate only one meal a day, which either she or her sister prepared or it was take-away. When asked if that had always been her food intake pattern, Silke describes when she lived with her grandmother during her early primary school years. When asked to think of someone who she considered 'good with food', Silke thought of her Nanna straight away.

Well, I used to live up at Nanango. I don't know where my Mum was. Me and my sister stayed with her before my brother was born and we stayed up there for a very long time and went to school there. Nanna was really, really picky on the food. We had porridge for breakfast, we had this for lunch and we had this for dinner. It was all really good, healthy stuff. My Nanna, she's crazy. She grows her own vegetables. … She's not a part of our lives anymore apparently.

Silke

For young people who were homeless, their life-course and movements from their parental home were even more complex. Here Julia, who was 16 at the time of the interview, describes where she has lived over her life so far. Julia started being responsible for feeding herself at seven. She did not consider herself particularly good with food but was remarkable in how she organized her day-to-day eating to include food from each of the core food groups every day. Interview excerpts from Julia also appear in Component 2.3 where she demonstrates high level decision-making skills and adaptability to changing environments.

I was born in New Zealand and came to Australia at the start of 2008. I lived with my mother and then she – she had to go away to work and I lived with my aunty, I lived with my other aunty, stayed with my father, I came over to Perth when I was about six, I stayed here for about a year and then my mother took me back, lived with my uncle, my dad's brother, moved back in with my mum, I lived with my aunty again and then we moved over here. Now I live in Red Hill. We just got a place there yesterday actually. Before that I lived under a bridge for easy four months, and about two years ago before that, for about a year. Yeah. In between that I was – was with my mother actually. Just kind of sorted stuff out and then she went through a rough patch again and back out here and yeah. Now I have my own place. It's a motel. Yeah.

Julia

Here, Jewel, 20, interviewed at the Australian Red Cross Night Café, talks about where he has lived and its influence on his food intake. Jewel had a profound congenital physical disability requiring the use of a wheelchair. He was homeless.

I live in the city. I've lived there for nine months. I travel a lot. I normally don't stay in towns for more than a year – a year to two years, and then move. I was born in New Zealand. My mum's from over here. So I came over back and forth for years. And then when I turned 16, I just moved over here to live by myself. Moved over, stayed by myself. Lived with my dad for a bit. He put me back through school. When I was living with my mum, two little brothers, me, stepdad, mum, there were five of us. With my dad, it was on and off. At some point it was 12 people, some point it was four people, or two people. At one point, it was my dad, his wife, me, my brother, workmate, uncle, his wife, his two kids, uncle, his wife, his one kid in a five bedroom house. Whereas sometimes it could be just me and my dad.

I'm the type of person where I eat like once every two, three days. But it's been like that for about two or three years now. Before, I used to eat more than three meals a day constantly until I was about 17. I moved out on my own and to save money, I ate less. And my body got used to just eating less so I just kept going. I could either eat a lot of food but that I could be eating for a long time, or I could eat little bits here and there for a couple of days.

Jewel

Other disadvantaged young people had moved less often but leaving their parental home for the first time was usually abrupt and not their choice or a result of their planning.

Five women who had become mothers as teenagers participated in this study. For all of these women, this coincided with leaving their parental home. Here, Tina, the oldest mother, reflects on her living arrangements since becoming pregnant at 16. At the time of her interview, Tina worked full time, was studying and had her own business. Pregnant young women typically move through a series of family-like relationships. Their food literacy is particularly significant in that it potentially influences the subsequent generation.

> I currently live at Collingwood Park with my son. He's six. He's really cute. I've been living there four and a half years now. Before that I was living at Springfield with his father for three years. I grew up in The Gap. I moved here (Ipswich area) when I was about 13, and I was living in Bellbird Park. It was like my mum and dad, my family, and then I got kicked out of home, and I moved in with my friend and her family. From Bellbird Park I moved to Springfield with my friend and her family. And then I moved in with my surrogate grandfather – he was like my nan's boyfriend, but not really, in Goodna, and then from there I moved back in with my grandparents in The Gap, and from there I moved in with my friends in Redbank Plains, and from there I moved to Springfield, and from there I went to Collingwood Park.
>
> Tina

Interview excerpts from all of these young people appear in the descriptions of food literacy components in Chapter 3. They had all developed significant knowledge, skills and behaviours regarding food and eating at a younger age than the more advantaged participants. Those participants who were university graduates and whose parental home was in the same city typically were not responsible for feeding themselves until their early twenties when they got their first job and left home. Prior to this their involvement in meal preparation for more than one person was limited, and in the planning and purchasing of food almost non-existent.

Where young people learnt about food and from whom

Most participants learnt about food at home. Across all participant groups this was most often from a female household head. Among less disadvantaged participants, mothers were the main avenue for learning about food and the person participants identified as being 'good with food' (see Table 9.2). Participants that were more satisfied with how they used food tended to have this person in their life earlier and more consistently. It appeared as though when the adult carer in the household was constantly changing, the task of transferring domestic life skills, including feeding yourself, suffered.

Males still contributed to young people's relationship with food with several identifying fathers, stepfathers and male housemates as the main person from whom they learnt about food. When reflecting on their childhood, the large majority of participants did not consider that food work was necessarily a female role although most agreed that females more often did this work. Most identified males typically only taking on this role when the female head of the household was unable to or was not present. Several young people

Table 9.2 The person participants identified as being 'good with food' or the primary person they learnt about food from

Person	Recruitment site						Total
	Aust Red Cross Night Café	Albert Park Flexible Learning Centre	Kingston Flexible Learning Centre	Ipswich City Council	QUT School of business	Nutrition Australia QLD	
Family member:							
• Mother	0	4	1	2	6	1	14
• Grandmother	2	2	2	0	1	0	7
• Father	1	0	0	2	0	0	3
• Aunt	1	0	0	0	0	0	1
• Stepmother	0	1	0	0	0	0	1
• Stepfather	0	0	0	1	0	0	1
• Sister	0	0	0	0	1	0	1
Peer:							
• Housemate	0	1	0	1	1	0	3
• Boyfriend	0	2	0	0	0	0	2
• Girlfriend	1	0	0	0	0	0	1
• Personal Trainer	0	0	0	0	0	1	1
• Best Friend's Mother	0	0	1	0	0	0	1
• Youth Worker	0	1	0	0	0	0	1
No one identified	2	1	1	0	0	0	4
Total	7	12★	5	6	9★	2	41

Source: Young People Study Recruitment Site

Notes: ★some participants identified more than one person

talked about the impact of male celebrities in breaking down these stereotypes.

Despite specifically being asked about their involvement in cooking, food or health classes at school, very few young people identified these as being significant in the development of their food literacy. Cooking classes and demonstrations that took place in other settings, for example, youth shelters, seemed to be of interest to young people who already had a base level of skills and were interested in extending them, rather than those who were perhaps in greater need. Young people also learnt from peers, particularly boyfriends and girlfriends, housemates and older siblings. In identifying someone whom they considered to be 'good with food' all participants chose someone they knew personally rather than a celebrity.

Few young people followed recipes; rather, recipe books, television shows, celebrity chefs, magazines and their experiences of eating out were used as motivation and inspiration to try new foods, expand their repertoire, and experiment with ingredients. These strategies, however, were primarily used by those young people who already had experience with food rather than those who did not. Young people tended to talk about expanding their repertoire at calmer times in their lives rather than at key milestones. When first moving out of home, for example, young people tended to use convenience and take-away foods in the first instance. They then typically reached a point of needing to establish routines and budgets and then looked for recipes and other food choices that would help them to do that.

Most young people were content with their level of food knowledge. They were confident that they had all the knowledge and skills they needed to keep themselves fed and that they could access additional support or information to develop their skills and knowledge further over their life-course if they needed to. Young people eating a simple, limited and nutritionally inadequate diet were not interested in expanding their food intake beyond those foods they currently consumed. These young people may have identified that they had limited food literacy but did not consider this to be problematic or something that needed to be addressed.

It is unclear from the data whether different components of food literacy developed differently across the life-course, although this seems likely. There were a few participants who had rarely eaten commensally during their childhood and now found it difficult to do so as an adult; this impacted on their food intake and potentially, their ability to connect socially. Some young people had been thrust into being responsible for feeding themselves at quite a young age (that is, while still in their primary school years). This typically occurred in households where the responsible adult changed regularly or was absent. Those responsible for food provision for themselves and others at a young age tended to choose simple dishes that required simple preparation and assembly, for example, spaghetti Bolognese made by boiling a packet of pasta and opening a jar of sauce; or scrambling eggs and microwaving frozen vegetables. As young adults, these participants maintained this routine of preparing food this way and considered themselves competent providers of foods despite having a quite narrow repertoire of meals and limited skills in traditional cooking techniques.

Participants who were responsible for feeding themselves early also ate fewer meals and regularly missed meals. These participants talked about not taking any food to school rather than preparing anything. This habit developed over the years with many young people routinely eating only once a day. This was compounded by a lack of access to and affordability of food. These participants more often had to rely on foodservice options, for example, chips and soft drinks from a petrol station on the way home from school, which tended to be more expensive over time. Participants who had similarly poor access to affordable food but came from a home environment where food was prepared and shared, more often by a consistent adult carer, were more likely to have a healthier food intake, that is, they ate regularly and ate from the core food groups.

What does this mean for practice?

The people in this study describe their food literacy developing over time in response to individual, household, community and global changes in various aspects of their lives. They first looked to those around them, their peers and their household members, to support them in developing the knowledge, skills and behaviours to feed themselves. This began early in life. It follows then that child development theories may be more useful than learning theories in guiding practitioners. This is an important finding as food literacy is often described as something to be 'taught' resulting in an individual who is 'competent' or not (Glickman et al. 2012; Pendergast, Garvis & Kanasa 2011; Public Health Association of Australia 2009; Vandenbroeck, Goossens & Clemens 2007). The findings of this study, however, describe a continuously evolving relationship with food that is influenced by and responds to social, biological and environmental systems. In considering interventions to address food literacy, therefore, it follows that they would need to target not just individuals, but also households, communities and nations.

Home is clearly the primary setting for learning about food. Household members continue to be important over the life-course. Schools, cooking classes, mass media and food industry only had an influence when an initial interest in food had been developed in the childhood household. Bronfenbrenner's ecological model of human development describes the core central function of families in child development (Shaffer 2005). This microsystem extends as children get older to include peers, schools and neighbourhoods. His model extends to describe an exosystem of health services, social welfare services, workplaces, the mass media and a macrosystem of broader cultural attitudes and ideologies, each with a gradually weakening but significant influence on development. This model is useful in describing the findings of this study. When the initial interest in food was not established in the home, the importance of these other settings increased. However, only social learning approaches appeared to be effective (Bandura 1977). For example, in the welfare services settings, group cooking classes were not attractive to people who were not already engaged with food; however, these participants spoke about learning from individual caseworkers or peers at the service.

A second element of Brofenbrenner's model is the influence each of these systems has on each other. Close values and relationships between them optimize development. Conceptualizing food literacy as existing at individual, household, community, population and national levels helps to acknowledge that efforts and activity are needed at each level to effectively develop food literacy. For example, if a household is interested in food preparation, the child may engage more in cooking classes at school. Bronfenbrenner's model includes a temporal dimension which highlights the changes in the strength of influence of the systems over time. In this study, young people who could identify someone from whom they learnt about food early in their lives demonstrated more components of food literacy.

There was a broad range of ages at which participants in this study had been responsible for their food. Being responsible for food early was more likely if you were living in disadvantage and much more likely if you were female. Young people in this study, however, did not consider food work to be the role of one gender only. This is consistent with other Australian studies of food provisioning (Lupton 2000). However, as exemplified in this study, food work is usually done by women (Australian Bureau of Statistics 2008). It follows therefore that if the origins of food literacy are in the childhood home, these gendered roles will remain. Participants spoke about the role of celebrities in challenging these stereotypes, but these are likely to predominantly capture the attention of those already engaged in food. Additionally, celebrities are more likely to represent special occasion, rather than every-day, food provisioning. Schools play a role in universally developing food literacy and addressing gendered norms.

Disadvantage impacted on the development of food literacy in a range of ways: young people were responsible for food earlier; they were more likely to be responsible for multiple household members; they were less likely to have lived with a parent or learnt about food from them; and their poverty meant they were less able to experiment with food. Each of these factors worked in various ways to both enhance and inhibit the development of food literacy. Participants described different responses to what could be considered similar experiences. For example, some participants described having a mother who had never cooked as motivation for learning to prepare food, others cited this as the reason they never learnt. Knowledge is considered a determinant of attitudes and beliefs, but in this study values and beliefs influenced the demonstration and acquisition of knowledge (Nutbeam & Harris 1999).

This research examined the nature and source of 'food expertise'. It contrasted the views of national food experts against those for whom they write policies, develop interventions, practise, measure and judge behaviour. Many of the disadvantaged young people in this study had been responsible for food since they were in primary school. They considered themselves experts. They could feed themselves and others in very resource restricted circumstances. This often did not include the use of core foods, cooking from scratch or multiple courses, all of which are outcomes of current interventions and measures (Department of Health 2011; Government of South Australia July 2009; Larson et al. 2006; Queensland Health 2011). Practitioners must acknowledge these significant skills and experience and critically appraise the need for their extension. Across all levels of disadvantage, participants ate within a standard repertoire of foods. Practitioners should begin their activity within this repertoire. Vygotsky describes the role of the practitioner in scaffolding the learner to extend from what they can do on their own to what they need help to do (Berk 1995). Bandura describes self-efficacy as coming from the mastering of skills developed through opportunities to experiment and practise new skills (Bandura 1977). Education, welfare and health services can provide the opportunity to experiment when the resources of the individual or household make this difficult.

Leaving home did not appear to be a key transition point for diet quality, although it may be important in expressing one's food identity. Young people who enjoyed family foods and mealtimes continued these habits when living independently. Others chose to distance themselves from the food of their parental home. Neither of these approaches appeared to be associated with diet quality. A study of 18–25 year olds in Liverpool found the quality of the diets of people living independently was more likely to be 'good' when compared those living in their parental home. Diet quality was better the longer the person had been living away from home (Beasley, Hackett & Maxwell 2004). This is consistent with the findings of this study in which participants described establishing routines about food and eating some time after first moving into a new household. A study of over 18,000 adolescents aged 11–21 (mean 16 years) examined parental influence on food intake (Videon & Manning 2003). Neither adolescent autonomy, parental control, nor the presence of a parent when the child left or arrived home from school were associated with healthier food intake. The greatest influence came from the number of meals eaten in the presence of a parent. The significance increased with the frequency of meals consumed together. This highlights the complexity of parental influence.

Prior to this study, nutrition practitioners had anecdotally identified that food literacy appeared to be of greater interest to clients at key life transition points, including leaving the parental home. Literature regarding the existence or importance of key transition points to food choice is mixed (Riddell et al. 2011; Wills 2005; Zhang et al. 2012). The findings of this study indicate that there are few standard transition points across all population groups. Moreover, the significance of transition points varied considerably, and in this sense, their importance in shaping identity did also. For young people who are already socially excluded, mainstream transition points such as completing school, getting their first job and leaving the parental home for the first time have little relevance. This is consistent with the youth literature (Wyn & White 1997). Interventions which target these times, therefore, are likely to further marginalize these groups. For example, interventions which focus only on the conventional school setting may miss some of the most vulnerable groups.

It is unclear whether transition points are significant for populations not experiencing disadvantage. Some transitions, such as finishing school, were more consistently experienced, i.e. people were 17 years old, living at home and it happened at the end of the year with their peers. However, they did not necessarily pair with other milestones such as living independently or earning an income which are likely to be more important in the development of food literacy. It may be that practitioners who have anecdotally observed key transitions are identifying individuals who are ready for action in a phase of behaviour change, rather than a transition milestone that could be more universally applied (Prochaska, DiClemente & Norcross 1992). Learning about food and developing a relationship with it appear to continually happen over a lifetime. Participants identified multiple influences and key points in the development of their relationship with food.

Conclusions

Theories of learning appeared inadequate in describing the complexity of how food literacy develops. Models of child social development were more relevant. This is perhaps because learning about food does not have an endpoint, rather it develops over a lifetime. Being 'good with food', too, is not simply about knowledge and skills but also about a social relationship because it is part of our day-to-day lives.

Brofenbrenner's model of child development is widely used in policy and practice (Australian Institute of Family Studies 2009). This model describes various determinants of child development, and their levels of influence. The influence of these levels grows stronger the closer they are to the centre of the circle. The model is useful in describing who is involved in the development of our relationship with food and what might happen if there is a breakdown in one of these levels. Learning theories, then, are useful to describe how this relationship might develop, what factors will support and inhibit it, while taxonomies of learning help to organize what elements need to be part of this development.

Perhaps the most important finding of this study, however, is the significance of social, rather than educational, systems in the development of food literacy. In particular, the results challenge mainstream thinking about the role of traditional family structures in the development of food literacy. It is critical that practitioners acknowledge and consider this when planning their work.

References

Australian Bureau of Statistics 2008, *4153.0 How Australians Use Their Time, 2006*, Australian Bureau of Statistics, viewed 30 September 2010, <http://www.abs.gov.au/AUSSTATS/ abs@.nsf/Latestproducts/4153.0Main%20Features12006?opendocument&tabname= Summary&prodno=4153.0&issue=2006&num=&view=>.

Australian Institute of Family Studies 2009, *Key Research Questions*, Commonwealth Department of Families, Housing, Community Services and Indigenous Affairs, viewed 13 March 2013, <http://www.growingupinaustralia.gov.au/pubs/reports/krq2009/keyresearchquestions.html>.

Bandura, A. 1977, *Social Learning Theory*, Prentice-Hall, Englewood Cliffs, New Jersey.

Beasley, L.J., Hackett, A.F. & Maxwell, S.M. 2004, 'The dietary and health behaviour of young people aged 18–25 years living independently or in the family home in Liverpool, UK', *International Journal of Consumer Studies*, vol. 28, no. 4, pp. 355–363.

Berk, L.E. 1995, *Scaffolding Children's Learning: Vygotsky and Early Childhood Education*, National Association for the Education of Young Children, Washington, DC.

Department of Health 2011, *Expression of Interest DOHEO106/10: Development and Delivery of Healthy Promotion Campaigns and Programs in Western Australia*, Government of Western Australia, Perth.

Glickman, D., Parker, L., Sim, L.J., Del Valle Cook, H. & Miller, E.A. (eds) 2012, *Accelerating Progress in Obesity Prevention: Solving the Weight of the Nation*, National Academies Press, Washington DC, viewed 10 December 2015, <http://www.nap.edu/openbook.php?record_id=13275>.

Government of South Australia 2009, *Part B: Bid Rules: Requirements and Specifications*, Government of South Australia, Adelaide.

Larson, N.I., Perry, C.L., Story, M. & Neumark-Sztainer, D. 2006, 'Food preparation by young adults is associated with better diet quality', *Journal of the American Dietetic Association*, vol. 106, no. 12, pp. 2001–2007.

Lupton, D. 2000, 'The heart of the meal: Food preferences and habits among rural Australian couples', *Sociology of Health and Illness*, vol. 22, no. 1, pp. 94–109.

Nutbeam, D. & Harris, E. 1999, *Theory in a Nutshell: A Practical Guide to Health Promotion Theories*, 2nd edn, McGraw-Hill, Australia.

Pendergast, D., Garvis, S. & Kanasa, H. 2011, 'Insight from the public on home economics and formal food literacy', *Family and Consumer Sciences Research Journal*, vol. 39, no. 4, pp. 415–430.

Pink, B. 2008, 'Socio-Economic Indexes for Areas (SEIFA) – Technical Paper', Australian Bureau of Statistics, Canberra, viewed 10 December 2015, <http://www.abs.gov.au/AUSSTATS/abs@.nsf/DetailsPage/2039.0.55.0012006?OpenDocument>.

Prochaska, J.O., DiClemente, C.C. & Norcross, J.C. 1992, 'In search of how people change: Applications to addictive behaviors', *American Psychologist*, vol. 47, no. 9, pp. 1102–1114.

Public Health Association of Australia 2009, *A Future for Food: Addressing Public Health, Sustainability and Equity from Paddock to Plate*, Public Health Association of Australia, Deakin.

Queensland Health 2011, *Request for Offer: CSU201011014 Engagement of a Service Provider to Undertake a Healthy Lifestyle and Food Literacy Pilot Program*, Queensland Government, Brisbane.

Riddell, L.J., Ang, B., Keast, R.S.J. & Hunter, W. 2011, 'Impact of living arrangements and nationality on food habits and nutrient intakes in young adults', *Appetite*, vol. 56, no. 3, pp. 726–731.

Shaffer, D.R. 2005, *Social and Personality Development*, 5 edn, Wadsworth, Belmont, CA.

Vandenbroeck, P., Goossens, J. & Clemens, M. 2007, *Foresight: Tackling Obesities: Future Choices – Obesity System Atlas*, Government Office for Science, London, viewed 12 December 2012, <http://www.bis.gov.uk/assets/foresight/docs/obesity/11.pdf>.

Videon, T.M. & Manning, C.K. 2003, 'Influences on adolescent eating patterns: The importance of family meals', *Journal of Adolescent Health*, vol. 32, no. 5, pp. 365–373.

Wills, W.J. 2005, 'Food and eating practices during the transition from secondary school to new social contexts', *Journal of Youth Studies*, vol. 8, no. 1, pp. 97–110.

Wyn, J. & White, R. 1997, *Rethinking Youth*, Allen & Unwin, Sydney, Australia.

Zhang, Y., Tan, H., Dai, X., Huang, H. & He, G. 2012, 'Dietary patterns are associated with weight gain in newlyweds: Findings from a cross-sectional study in Shanghai, China', *Public Health Nutrition*, vol. 15, no. 5, pp. 876–884.

10 Developing food literacy through the education sector

A focus on home economics

Sandra Fordyce-Voorham and
Theresa Wai Ling Lai-Yeung

Introduction

Food literacy includes the knowledge, skills and behaviours young people use to plan, manage, select, prepare and eat foods to meet their needs. As described in the previous chapter, food literacy typically develops in the home; but, schools have an important role because they are a setting that allows programmes to reach and influence a large number of people. This is particularly important when home environments do not support healthy eating. Food and nutrition is typically included in school curricula around the world, but the extent to which hands-on food skills are present varies. Hands-on programmes are more likely to be present in middle school years rather than for younger children. In secondary schools, food literacy is generally developed through hands-on practical skills programmes, usually in Home Economics classes. A well-designed healthy eating skills-based programme needs to include a range of declarative (knowledge) and procedural (hands-on) skills that will enable young people to develop the food skills they need to be able to live healthy independent lives. This chapter outlines and explains these essential skills and how they can be incorporated strategically and easily into a school programme. Suggestions are made on how these food skills could be measured. A tool for measuring these skills, in the form of a food literacy skills checklist, is outlined for teachers and facilitators of such programmes.

This chapter aims to describe food literacy in an educational context by firstly reviewing current definitions and how they apply in an educational setting. Next, an overview of relevant models with particular attention to those applicable in an educational setting is presented. Finally, a sample of a generic food literacy measure and checklist based on and underpinned by a model (the Food Literacy Model) is described. The Food Literacy Measure and Food Literacy Checklist include sample activities designed for teachers to use in upper primary and junior secondary schools. Further, a sample of a pre- and post-evaluation series of questions based on the the Food Literacy Model is provided.

Definitions of food literacy

The term 'food literacy' has received burgeoning interest amongst health professionals in recent years as described in Chapter 2. This has been signalled as an area relevant to home economics education (Smith 2009). Among the various definitions, the one most aligned to home economics education is that of Slater (2013). She describes a three layered outline of declarative skills:

- functional food literacy (assessing, understanding and evaluating information);
- interactive food literacy (decision making, goal setting and practices to enhance nutritional health and well-being); and
- critical food literacy (respecting family, cultural and religious food beliefs, understanding the wider context of food production and nutritional health and advocating for personal, family and community changes to enhance nutritional health).

This definition is revisited later in the chapter and contextualized in the description of the Food Literacy Model.

A professional association for home economics teachers, Home Economics Victoria, has described food literacy as 'the knowledge, skills and the capacity to source, prepare, cook and share food in a sustainable manner to promote a healthy and balanced lifestyle. Food literacy is also about individuals understanding the role that food plays in communities and cultures' (Home Economics Victoria 2013).

The use of the term in schools has been a recent phenomenon. Most schools use the term 'food literacy' loosely to include any programme that includes nutritional knowledge and hands-on food preparation and cooking (Pendergast & Dewhurst 2012; Smith 2009). Due to time constraints imposed by crowded school curricula (Fordyce-Voorham 2014; Smith 2009), food literacy in schools has mostly focused on the procedural (hands-on) more than the declarative skills. Based on this definition, skill-based cooking programmes in schools need to do more than focus on the 'hands-on' procedural or cooking skills (Colatruglio & Slater 2014). However, with competing curriculum demands and time constraints, designers of these programmes (usually teachers) need to plan strategically to encompass other components of food literacy, for example the cultural and social significance of cooking, eating and feeding, and the health and social benefits of preparing and sharing food with others.

The role of schools in developing food literacy

Various reviews have failed to conclusively support food literacy programmes in schools as programmes tend to be short term and poorly and inconsistently evaluated (Brooks & Begley 2013; Contento, Randell & Basch 2002; Crawford &

Worsley 2004; Food Standards Agency 2005; Smith & de Zwart 2010; Wu, Seeley & Caraher 2008). Longer-term, embedded programmes tend to operate in secondary schools and are undertaken in home economics classes (Carleton et al. 1991; Klepp & Wilhelmsen 1993; Rescinow et al. 1999; Wu, Seeley & Caraher 2008). As the most likely specialist teachers to teach food literacy programmes at least in secondary schools, home economics teachers are given the important role of teaching young people the nutritional knowledge and the culinary skills they need to ameliorate the effects of these poor dietary habits on their health, especially as they move from childhood into adolescence (Lichtenstein & Ludwig 2010). Home economics teachers have a significant role in young people's lifelong learning about nutrition and healthy eating behaviour (Contento 2008; Home Economics Institute of Australia 1997; Klepp & Wilhelmsen 1993; Nowak & Buttner 2002; Pendergast & Dewhurst 2012; Slater 2013; Worsley & Crawford 2005).

An international investigation of 1,188 home economics teachers from 36 different countries reported on respondents' views of the role of Home Economics in developing food literacy (Pendergast & Dewhurst 2012). Respondents were provided with the following definition of food literacy as 'the capacity of an individual to obtain, interpret and understand basic nutrition information and services as well as the competence to use that information and available services that are health enhancing'. From a list of 18 elements derived from a posed question, '*How might you define food literacy education?*', respondents listed skill acquisition (food preparation and cooking activities, safe and hygienic practices, nutrition acquisition and application, consumer budgeting and costing) as priority activities and foci for food literacy education in schools.

As described in Chapter 6, food choice and behaviour are determined not only by physiological factors to satisfy hunger and nourish the body, but also by a range of interlocking factors including psychological, environmental, sociological and economic factors (Hjelmar 2011; Nestle et al. 2009; Salmon, Campbell & Crawford 2006; Steenhuis, Waterlander & De Mul 2011; Vartanian, Herman & Wansink 2008). Health practitioners have attempted to develop a more holistic approach to nutrition education which integrates theories and practices to empower young people with the skills that lead them to life-long healthy eating. The emergence of the term 'food literacy' in recent years is an attempt to acknowledge this. In addressing food literacy, a school programme, therefore, needs to include more than the 'hands-on' food preparation skills to prepare young people for life. Food literacy in schools needs to encompass themes such as environmental sustainability (for example, minimizing food waste) and the development of students' critical thinking skills in order to help them manage as successful consumers in the market place. Teachers are challenged to incorporate these ideas in the classroom and develop food education programmes (Pendergast & Dewhurst 2012; Smith 2009). The European Food Framework is one such example (see http://www.europea nfoodframework.eu/).

A whole school approach

Schools are increasingly recognized as a source of transference of skills and changing health behaviours of young people (Colatruglio & Slater 2014; Mikkelsen 2014). In a world where parents lack time (Lai-Yeung 2015), skills or the inclination to teach their children how to plan, prepare and cook meals, home economics teachers are in a unique position to design and teach students these food skills. Since home economics teachers work exclusively in schools they understand young people and their world. They have the nutritional background and pedagogical expertise to design skill-based healthy eating programmes that are sequential and match the age with the developmental needs and skill levels of their students. These are both integral to the design of successful healthy eating programmes (Backman et al. 2002; Colatruglio & Slater 2014; Pendergast & Dewhurst 2012).

In a whole school approach to healthy eating, teachers work collaboratively with key stakeholders including school managers, food suppliers (including canteen managers), parents, students and the wider community beyond the school gate. The example whole school approach developed by Home Economics Victoria (Home Economics Victoria 2013) built on existing capabilities of secondary schools to address food literacy and healthy eating.

Box 10.1 Four components embedded into the teacher guidelines of a whole school approach to a food literacy project

Source: Home Economics Victoria 2013

1   Food literacy knowledge

- Embed topics such as nutrition, food models, food systems and health eating across the curriculum
- Develop partnerships with local food producers and suppliers
- Contribute to the local food system
- Promote the relationship between health and food within the school
- Encourage and support students in advocating for making healthy food accessible and affordable.

2   Food literacy skills

- Embed topics such as budgeting, practical healthy cooking skills, recipe modification, seasonality
- Provide students with opportunities to learn and use practical cooking skills outside of the curriculum
- Create learning activities and tasks (e.g. students devise an advertisement for healthy foods)
- Provide students with opportunities to plan, shop and prepare healthy menus
- Motivate students to advocate about healthy eating and food literacy to the school community

3 Food literacy skills to be able to source (resources)

- Embed topics such as budgeting, shopping, excursions, food system mapping, etc.
- Establish partnerships with others in the community (e.g. through joining local food networks)
- Provide students with opportunities to engage in the local food system
- Provide students with a range of cultural food experiences
- Create local food challenges
- Provide students with the skills and opportunity to grow their own produce
- Provide healthy choices in the school canteen

4 Food sustainability (reduce food waste)

- Embed topics such as food hygiene, food storage, food security, portion sizing across curriculum areas
- Provide students with opportunities to plan, budget and shop for school activities
- Establish relationships with food relief organizations and provide students with opportunities to become involved
- Develop or utilize a school paddock to plate programme
- Consider portion sizing with all school food services
- Start a compost programme

Before the broader goals of school and community can be addressed, teachers need to help their students identify their own values of health and use of discretionary time as factors that might contribute to their eating behaviours. An overly narrowed approach that focuses solely on the benefits of healthy eating linked to chronic disease is considered to be too long-term for students, and young people generally (Fordyce-Voorham 2014). Instead a more balanced programme that focuses on healthy eating for the purposes of wellbeing and stamina to manage sporting and daily activities, and that takes into account the social and cultural benefits of sharing food amongst peers, augurs well for a food literacy programme that young people would find more attractive. The merits of such a programme underpin the concept of healthy eating as not only having physical health benefits but also cultural and social benefits that come from the enjoyment of preparing, cooking and sharing food with others.

Teachers then need to consider these factors in their teaching practices, as well as teaching the declarative (planning) and procedural (hands-on) or practical skills the students need to make healthy meals for themselves and others, so that they are less reliant on external food suppliers. Within the process of meal-making, declarative skills are the precursory skills required by individuals to make and evaluate decisions about meal planning, food shopping and meal preparation. These are considered to be fundamental components of teaching food literacy to students. The procedural skills, equally important, are the 'hands-on' skills required by individuals to prepare and cook meals and clean up after the meal is prepared.

Curriculum-based declarative and procedural skills

Food skills may be defined as 'the process of purchasing, preparing and cooking food materials (ingredients) using available resources to produce well-balanced and tasty meals appropriate to the age and needs of the individuals consuming them' (Fordyce-Voorham 2009: 17). Short (2007), for example, has used the term 'cooking skills' to describe the process of meal-making. More recently, Vanderkooy (2009: 22) modified Short's description to define food skills at an individual and household level as 'a complex, interrelated, person-centred set of skills, necessary to provide and prepare, safe, nutritious and culturally-acceptable meals for all members of one's household'.

The declarative skills described as the precursory decision-making knowledge and information required by an individual to make a meal is summarized in Table 10.1. Table 10.2 further shows the procedural shopping and task skills required to store, prepare and cook food and clean up after the meal. These align well with the components of food literacy described in Chapter 3 and detail their potential application and inclusion in the classroom. In addition to the content of skills taught, teachers can support their students' skill acquisition by:

- providing students with opportunities to practise and repeat tasks to develop confidence, especially those with special needs;
- allowing students to work individually to develop independence when preparing food;
- allowing students to work in teams to encourage co-operation and scheduling skills;
- encouraging students to take risks to try unfamiliar food and trial new food tasks;
- exposing students to positive real and simulated independent living experiences;
- allowing students the trial and error process of creating recipe variations to improvise and problem solve; and
- reminding students to be aware of eco-friendly practices in the food preparation and consumption processes.

These directional guidelines support the aims of food literacy in school programmes and empower young people to protect their diet quality through change; they support dietary resilience over time as young people develop the knowledge, skills and behaviours to plan, manage, select, prepare and eat foods to meet their needs and determine their intake.

The first stage of designing meals requires the food preparer to think about how best to meet the specific needs of the people consuming those meals. This

Table 10.1 Declarative food skills

Meal-making	Consumer	Nutritional health	Equipment	Cookery methods	Hygiene and safety	Use of terminology
Plan a variety of appetising meals that meet the dietary and sensory requirements of household members.	Recognize and purchase quality and value-for-money food produce through personal or on-line shopping.	Know the importance of eating a healthy meal in relation to meeting daily activity requirements.	How to use a cook's knife confidently, safely and skilfully.	Know the basic traditional and modern methods of cookery and how they affect the nutritional value, energy use, preparation and cooking time of foods and product outcome.	How and where to store food.	Follow instructions to deconstruct and accurately follow recipes and produce successful meals and food products.
Accurately calculate food amounts based on portion size and appetite demands of household members to reduce food wastage and plate waste.	Purchase appropriate quantities of food to match personal demands and reduce plate waste. Negotiate food purchases with food vendors.	Know the importance of enjoying and consuming a wide variety of nutrient dense food.	How to choose, use, clean, maintain and store essential items used in the kitchen.		Know the longevity of fresh food produce.	Understand descriptive and generic instructions.
Match allocated food budget with recommendations made in healthy eating guidelines.	Know how to store, prepare and cook food post-purchase.	How to select nutrient dense food in relation to vegetarian and healthier alternatives and portion size.	How to select alternative items of equipment in situations where the most appropriate item of equipment is not available.	How to match food products with appropriate cookery methods to achieve the best product outcome and value for money.	How to safely defrost frozen food.	Understand complex health terms and health promotional terms.
Allocate time in advance to write a shopping list.	Make 'food miles' and ethical purchase decisions.		How to adapt different items of equipment for different cooking or preparation purposes.		How to clean and use purposefully designed equipment and safe food handling techniques to prevent cross-contamination of raw and cooked food.	
Know how to stock a pantry and refrigerator with perishable and non-perishable items consumed on a regular basis.	Consider food packaging and the environment. Consider food processing on cost and nutritional value of raw food.		How to operate small and large kitchen appliances.		How to clean equipment, appliances, cooking and eating utensils.	
			How to evaluate appliances' purchase value in terms of frequency and versatility of use.		How long to cook 'at risk' fresh food (fish, meat, poultry and dried soaked beans) to reduce food poisoning risk.	
			How to use a microwave oven as a cooking as well as a re-heating or defrosting appliance.			

Table 10.2 Procedural food skills

Consumer	Seasonal produce	Food exposure	Use information sources	Hygiene and safety	Meal skills	Trouble-shooting
Interpret and act upon food labelling. Evaluate basic and optional equipment items for meal-making. Compare fresh, frozen, canned and processed foods when purchasing for recipe suitability. Budget, manage and make good food choices around money. Make informed and shared decisions to plan, prepare and cook quick, healthy meals and snacks instead of buying take-away dishes or pre-prepared food.	Select fruits and vegetables in season when cheaper, tastier, more nutritious and readily available. Know fruits and vegetables in season when selecting recipes. Evaluate and purchase food produce that is value for money, fresh, seasonal and ripe.	Experience a variety of foods from different cultures. Support and encourage new food experiences, particularly at a young age. Acknowledge importance of family, friends, school and community groups for broadening food preferences, fostering positive food interest and experiences.	Point of sale food sources, e.g. recipe cards and magazines, informed personnel who assist with produce selection. Cook books provide step–by–step and pictorial instructions to construct recipes; shopping information and terminology to assist with recipe construction. Internet provides international food recipe and multiple recipe ideas for one or more ingredients; access to food products not locally available through on-line shopping services; a source of food and nutrition information for some people.	Use cooking appliances and equipment safely and skilfully to prepare food efficiently and appropriately. Prepare for food preparation tasks. Apply first aid when necessary. Store, freeze and defrost food to avoid cross-contamination, microbial spoilage and rodent infestation. Evaluate food product labelling information and act upon if and how that food should be used, stored or discarded.	Prepare fresh food when constructing meals. Use flavouring ingredients and seasonings to enhance food and create flavoursome meals. Accurately weigh and measure ingredients. Use and adapt basic food proces-sing 'universal' skills to extend culinary repertoire. Deconstruct and organize a recipe into small tasks when constructing meals. Select temperature and adjust timing to control the cooking process.	Know that successful food product outcomes depend on careful reading and following of recipe instructions. Know why food product outcomes were not successful. How to rectify unsuccessful food product outcomes.

Consumer	Seasonal produce	Food exposure	Use information sources	Hygiene and safety	Meal skills	Trouble-shooting
Adjust serving sizes and purchase precise amounts of food that meet the appetite and budgetary requirements of household members. Economize: buy and cook in bulk when food produce is cheaper and store for later use. Recognize and purchase cheaper but equally nutritious food alternatives.			Television provides inspirational and fun ideas to motivate individuals to cook, particularly if programmes have matching cookbooks or DVDs. Advertising about food products and health education to assist individuals with purchase decisions.	Manage the physical environment of a kitchen: keep it clean, hygienic and safe for users.	Sequence cooking processes so that all meal components are optimally cooked and ready for service at the same time. Assess, tailor and match food preparation tasks with product outcomes so that food is attractively presented and looks appetizing. Manage and perform cleaning tasks.	

may mean them drawing upon their own food experiences, consulting their own 'food experts' (friends and parents, for example), recipe books, food magazines, television cooking shows and recipe websites to begin the creative process of solving the problem of 'what shall we have for dinner tonight?' To assist with this process, any of the online food resources that include built-in elements, such as shopping lists of ingredients, make it easier for food preparers to complete the next stage of the process – the planning. The planning step of food literacy is a crucial one which requires quite high level skills. Arguably, this step is more complex than the assembling, construction, preparing and cooking of the meal itself. There is no shortage of television 'infotainment' programmes which demonstrate how to cook meals; however, viewing such programmes does not always transfer to individuals, specifically young people, planning and cooking more meals (Goodchild 2012).

Meal planning requires a review of the human and material resources available: the time required to review the stock in the pantry and the refrigerator, put together a shopping list and then shop for the ingredients to construct the meal. Planning also includes the preparer's ability to read, understand and act upon food labels, know seasonal variations of fresh food and how to prepare a budget to purchase those ingredients. The material resources include the money available to buy those ingredients, and the tools and equipment and the costs of the energy (gas or electricity) required to make the meal.

Arguably, the most important skill of all is the food preparer's self-analysis of the procedural skills required to prepare and cook the meal. Here the food preparer needs to appraise whether they have those skills. As listed in Tables 10.1 and 10.2, a summary of declarative skills and procedural skills has been derived from data collected from 51 food experts in a recent study (Fordyce-Voorham 2010). The goal of any food skills programme is to develop people's (specifically young people's) food skills so that they can produce a tasty, healthy and well-balanced meal on the majority of eating occasions, one which meets their appetite, nutritional and situational needs. However, skill-based programmes in schools need to be underpinned pedagogically with a food literacy base and supported with a model on which teachers can plan and develop their programmes. The next section examines such relevant food literacy models and how they may be used by educators.

Using models to conceptualize food literacy development in schools

Conceptualizing declarative and procedural skills

Described below is a model based on the components of the Food-related Lifestyle Model (Grunert, Brunso & Bisp 1993) and Eating Competence Model (Satter 2007). The Food-related Lifestyle Model has direct relevance to educators. Application of this model to the development of food literacy programmes would indicate that teachers need to teach students the self-efficacy skills; how to plan and make meals that will help them to meet the health and wellbeing goals that are reflective of the values held by each individual. They need to provide opportunities for their students to practise and apply practical food preparation and cooking skills and allow them to choose and make food they enjoy eating.

This concept of 'enjoying food' simply for its intrinsic value underpins the principles of the Satter model (Satter 2008), which postulates that young people can be encouraged to become 'competent eaters' through awareness of intuitive eating capabilities and exposure to a wide variety of foods, including 'unhealthy' food. Based on the Food-related Lifestyle Model (Grunert, Brunso & Bisp 1993) and components of the Eating Competence Model (Satter 2007), an adaptation that incorporates the procedural and declarative skills is shown in a proposed model (Figure 10.1).

The *values* described in the Food-related Lifestyle Model are more broadly described here as *motivational factors* such as the desire for nutritional health that may prompt a particular *behaviour* such as an individual choosing food low in fat or purchasing fresh seasonal vegetables instead of the pre-prepared variety. They also encompass the *eating attitudes* (EA) outlined in the Satter model that include parental influences on children's eating behaviour determined by their own attitudes and beliefs about food (Satter 2008).

The *higher order attributes* featured in the Food-related Lifestyle Model (Grunert, Brunso & Bisp 1993) serve as modifying influences to the food choices made by individuals, but also incorporate components of the *eating attitudes* (Satter 2007), which depend on an individual's positive attitude towards foods when it is offered in a supportive and harmonious environment (in school and at home). *Usage situations*, a component used in both models, describe the circumstances that may influence or modify typical food selection or eating behaviours. For example, the main food preparer still values their family's nutritional health when they forgo cooking a meal from 'scratch' on those

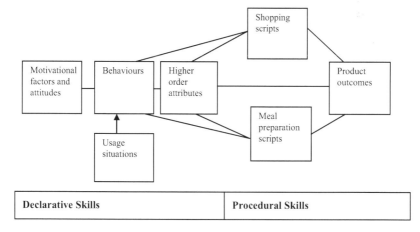

Figure 10.1 A proposed model depicting declarative and procedural food skills in context

occasions when convenience overrides health: for example, when the family eats purchased hot meat pies as a quick lunchtime meal before they leave to watch a football game on a winter's day. These decisions are precursors that are the declarative or person-centred skills which precede the procedural or task-centred actions of shopping for preparing and actually cooking (or re-heating) the food itself.

Using a health literacy model to conceptualize food literacy

A food literacy model based on Green's health literacy model (Green 1999, 2012) is described by Renwick (2013; see Table 10.3) and framed as a proposal

Table 10.3 Conceptualizing critical food literacy

Literacy		Possible questions or considerations about our food supply
Operational	Turning it 'on' Knowing what to do to make it 'work'	• Are a variety of foods available? • How can food life be extended through storage and preservation techniques? • Where does our food come from?
Cultural	Using 'it' to do something meaningful and effective	• What foods do we eat at home? • Is it reflective of a particular cuisine or family tradition? • Is the consumption dependent upon specific resources such as food knowledge, preparation skills or tools? • Where does the food come from? • What informs the purchasing of bought food, e.g. brand loyalty, where the food is sourced from, marketed or seasonality? • What particular foods might be grown or processed within the home?
Critical	Social practices and their meaning systems are: • Partial and selective • Shaped by power relations	• Do ethics inform our concerns about the production of food and therefore our choices? • How do our food purchasing choices impact on Australian food producers? • How does an available food in the supermarket vary between socio-economic areas and why do the same items differ in cost between areas? • What are the impacts of food choices on i) my personal health? ii) families in food producing communities? iii) the environment, e.g. being carbon neutral or food miles?

Source: Renwick 2013

specifically aimed at teachers to engage in critical pedagogy to develop their students' knowledge, research and analytical skills, as well as their own. She outlines various health models largely aimed at health professionals before arguing the case for a health literacy model that allows teachers to cultivate an environment where students engage actively, rather than passively, in their own learning. Teachers are shown how they can start students with a familiar base before stimulating them to move beyond into their own community and world. Together teachers and their students adopt a broader world view based on the freedom to become critical and reflective thinkers. In an example of the globalization of food supply, Renwick (2013) adapts Green's 3D literacy model and outlines how critical food literacy in three scaffolded level dimensions (operational, cultural and critical) could be conceptualized.

Bringing these models together

The proposed Food Literacy Model presented in Figure 10.2 brings a series of concepts from Green, Renwick and Bronfenbrenner together to describe the development of food literacy through schools. It consists of three levels comprising basic, intermediate and advanced food literacy skills. Each level is matched with Bronfenbrenner's theory of ecological systems (Bronfenbrenner 1979; Paquette & Ryan 2001).

Basic level

The basic level is described as the operational dimension (Renwick 2013). The tasks performed at this level focus on the individual and their interactions with food. The operational dimension aligns with the functional food literacy and the interactive food literacy described by Slater (2013). Examples include an individual's food likes and dislikes, access to different varieties (fresh and processed) and amount of food, basic knowledge of the origins of food ('paddock to plate'), and the chemical (nutritional) and sensory (aesthetic) properties of food in relation to their health.

Intermediate level

The intermediate level is described as the cultural dimension (Renwick 2013). The food tasks performed at this level involve the individual interacting with people (family, teachers, students and local shopping vendors) in their near environment (micro-meso system). The cultural dimension aligns with critical food literacy described by Slater (2013). Examples include family food likes and dislikes, food decisions ('gate-keeping' of food – who and what influences the food planned, purchased, stored, prepared and consumed in the home and school), availability of and access to food in the home (farmyard, backyard and balcony gardens and domestic food production of eggs and preservation of home-grown fruits, nuts and vegetables) and community (supermarkets, strip

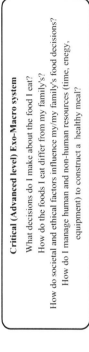

Critical (Advanced level) Exo-Macro system

What decisions do I make about the food I eat?

How do the foods I eat differ from my family's?

How do societal and ethical factors influence my/my family's food decisions?

How do I manage human and non-human resources (time, enegy, equipment) to construct a healthy meal?

Cultural (Intermediate level) Micro-Meso system

What does my family like to eat? Why do they eat those foods?

What foods are available to me/my family?

How does my family's food change over time?

How does my family meal plan, buy, store, prepare and cook food?

Operational (Basic level) Individual

What do I like to eat?

What foods are good for me? Available to me?

Where does my food come from?

How do I meal plan, buy, store, prepare and cook my food?

Figure 10.2 A proposed model for food literacy in schools

Source: An adaptation from Green's 3D (Green 1999) literacy model and Renwick's model (Renwick 2013). The proposed model for food literacy integrates concepts based on Bronfenbrenner 1979, Paquette & Ryan 2001, Green 1999 and Renwick 2013

shopping, fresh food vendors such as butchers, greengrocers, bakeries, roadside stalls and farmers' markets).

Advanced level

The advanced level is described as the critical dimension (Renwick 2013). The food tasks performed at this level involve the individual interacting with the social environment (media, culture, society, technology) and making ethical decisions about food (exo-macro system). This concept of a food literate individual operating as a citizen able to make ethical and responsible food decisions is described by Schnögl et al. (2006) and includes critical food literacy described by Slater (2013). Examples include social (including television, digital and print media, marketing activities and technology), ethical, sustainability considerations and cultural factors influencing and modifying individual and family food decisions and choices.

Each level operates independently or inter-relates as indicated by the two-way directional arrows. An individual can access and return to any level without the need to progress from the basic through to the intermediate and advanced levels of food literacy skills

Table 10.4 provides a sample range of activities for each of the three levels (basic, intermediate and advanced). Whilst the activities target upper primary and junior secondary school students aged between 9 and 14 years of age, the activities can be used by teachers at their own discretion to accommodate mixed age groups or capability level of students in the same classroom. In those schools where hands-on food preparation and cooking skills are not offered, the Food Literacy Model offers some practical ideas of how food literacy can be implemented into a classroom without access to a kitchen facility.

Table 10.5 provides teachers with a template they could use to evaluate student's learning achievements.

Conclusions

Home economics teachers possess pedagogical expertise as well as nutritional background in designing effective food literacy programmes to address the students' needs. Yet teachers may often focus on what they want to achieve in order to fit in demands such as limited time allocation in the timetable and integration of subject programmes in the school based curriculum. There is a need for a model on which to base their teaching programme so that they can flexibly tailor-make a specific scheme of work which conforms to the limitations and requirements of the school, caters to the needs of the students, and encompasses the cultural and social significance of cooking and eating, and the health and social benefits of preparing and sharing food with others. The Food Literacy Model (Figure 10.2) incorporates declarative and procedural skills from a broader and a more critical perspective, making available a guide and a reference for teachers to integrate declarative food skills as well as the procedural skills in any skill-based curriculum.

Table 10.4 An example of food literacy measure for upper primary and junior secondary students (based on the Food Literacy Model)

Basic	Intermediate	Advanced
I know what foods are good for me	My family chooses good food	I can recognize good food advertised or shown on television
Activity 1 What's for lunch? Over one school week, students *match* the contents of their lunchbox with the Guidelines. *Make suggestions* for improving the sensory and chemical properties of the food.	**Activity 1 What's for dinner?** Over one week, students *write down* what they eat for their evening meal. *Evaluate* each meal with the Guidelines. *Justify* reasons which account for variations in the family meals (family likes and dislikes, traditional/ indigenous foods, dietary modifications such as vegetarianism). *Make suggestions* for improving the sensory and chemical properties of the food presented. Does it take into account family members' likes and dislikes? Resource availability (for example, amount of money allocated to food, food availability, seasonal variation), health and dietary requirements?	**Activity 1 Watch a TV cooking food show** *Choose* a cooking food show on television and *evaluate* the meals constructed by the presenters. *Match* these with the Guidelines. *Make suggestions* for improving the sensory and chemical properties of the food presented. **Activity 2 Food ad watch survey** Over two evenings (4–6pm or 6–8pm) in one school week, students record the type of food advertised in their nominated time slot. Students create a table which names and describes the food advertised, the frequency of the advertisement in the time slots. At school, students *collate* the results, *create* a histogram and *make observations*. *Evaluate* the results making comparisons with the recommendations made in the Guidelines. *Provide* reasons for the frequency of recommended and limited foods and outline the impacts the messages conveyed have on health.
I can plan a week's meals that I like to eat and match with the Guidelines.	I can plan a week's meals that my family likes to eat, match with the Guidelines and consider my family's resources (time, energy, skills and money), dietary and cultural food decisions.	I can plan a week's meals that my family likes to eat, match with the Guidelines and consider my family's ethical food decisions.

Basic	Intermediate	Advanced
Activity 1 Recipe challenge Students conduct a 'Think, Pair and Share' *Think* – Students investigate and evaluate recipes from the internet, cookbooks, family recipes, supermarket magazines and plan one week's evening meals that they would like to eat and match with the Guidelines. Students *pair up* with a friend and swap two recipes that they would like to try. Students *justify* their two selected recipes. *Celebrate* and *share* a bank of recipes and *create* a class cookbook. **Optional activity** – Students *choose* a 'Recipe of the Week' from the class cookbook. Students *make* a shopping list and *arrange to go shopping* with their parents to buy the ingredients (online or in person), *discuss* transport home and storage of the food, *select* and safely *use* appropriate tools, utensils and equipment, prepare ingredients ('*mise-en-place*') and *cook* the meal. Students *evaluate* the sensory (appearance, texture, aroma, taste) and chemical properties of the meal. Students and parents *evaluate* the pre- and post-meal cleaning up. Suggestion: *create* an 'Evaluation of my selected meal' table and *record* the outcomes of each of the steps. *Include* a parent comment box. *Share* and *celebrate* student achievements.	**Activity 1 Family meal investigation** Students conduct a *Vox Populi* survey 'Investigation of my family meals'. **Step 1: Student brainstorm** Teacher or facilitator encourages students to *brainstorm* survey questions. Ask students to *reflect* on the meals their family ate last week (use findings from previous activity) and *give* reasons and *predict* why they think their family chose those meals. Examples of 'brainstorming questions' could include: Why did my family choose those meals? Who chooses those meals? How are those meals prepared? What factors influence meal selection? **Step 2: Parent survey** Students *compare their predictions* with their parents in a survey. **Step 3: Vox populi results and class evaluation** *Create* a class 'mind map' that *pools* students' survey results. The mind map will include factors such as resource availability (time, money, skills, energy), likes and dislikes, who's home to eat the meals, dietary requirements of family members.	**Activity 1 Food ethics** Teacher or facilitator conducts a *Vox Populi* survey on food ethics. *Conduct* a debate on contemporary topics, e.g. 'Caged eggs should be banned'/'Imported food should be restricted so that consumers buy local food products'. **Practical activity for home and family involvement** Students *trial* a meat free Monday. *Pool* results and *plan* an inter-class Meatless Monday challenge. **Activity 2 Plate waste survey** Class or school activity: over one week, each class collects and measures the lunchbox food and packaging waste produced by that class. *Plan* a reduce, recycle and reuse campaign and register the school for Nutrition Australia's Nude Food Day.

Table 10.5 Template for a student evaluation

Part A (Basic) Now that I have completed this programme...	Agree	Neutral	Disagree
Q 1	I have a better understanding of what fruits and vegetables are in season and how to prepare and cook them.			
Q 2	I am more likely to try a new food.			
Q 3	I have more confidence to prepare and cook new and familiar recipes.			
Q 4	I have a better understanding of where fresh food comes from and how I can buy it.			
Q 5	I have a better understanding of the food I need to eat to keep me healthy.			
Q 6	I have a better understanding of how I can make food look and taste better.			
Q 7	I have a better understanding of judging how much food to make to avoid food waste.			
Part B (Intermediate) Now that I have completed this programme...	**Agree**	**Neutral**	**Disagree**
Q 8	I have a better understanding of why I choose to eat particular foods.			
Q 9	I have a better understanding of why my family chooses to eat particular foods.			
Q 10	I have a better understanding of how the media (television, print and internet) influences people's food choices.			
Q 11	I feel more confident that I can contribute to the way my family decides what to eat.			
Q 12	I feel more confident that I can buy sufficient food that satisfies my family's appetite without food wastage.			
Q 13	I feel more confident that I can prepare and cook a healthy meal for my family.			
Part C (Advanced) Now that I have completed this programme...	**Agree**	**Neutral**	**Disagree**
Q 14	I can justify my decisions for eating the foods I do.			
Q 15	I am more aware of safety precautions, heat control and food hygiene during food preparation.			
Q 16	I feel more competent in integrating tasks in order to finish work efficiently within a time limit.			

Q 17	I have more confidence in judging the information about food presented in the media (television, print and internet).
Q 18	I have more confidence in making ethical decisions about the foods I eat.
Q 19	I can identify factors that might influence why people in different countries eat different foods to me.
Q 20	I feel that I could present a case for an ethical decision about food (for example, banning caged eggs or eating one meatless meal a week).
Q 21	I have the skills to evaluate my own and other's eating, shopping and sustainability practices (for example, acting on food conservation measures to prevent food wastage).
Q 22	I think the best part of the programme is:
Q 23	Because:
Q 24	I think the part which is least useful to me is:
Q 25	Because:
Q 26	Other comments:

References

Backman, D., Haddad, E., Lee, J., Johnston, P. & Hodgkin, G. 2002, 'Psychosocial predictors of healthful dietary behaviour in adolescents', *Journal of Nutrition Education and Behaviour*, vol. 34, pp. 184–193.

Bronfenbrenner, U. 1979, *The Ecology of Human Development: Experiments by Nature and Design*, Harvard University Press, Cambridge, MA.

Brooks, N. & Begley, A. 2013, 'Adolescent food literacy programmes: A review of the literature', *Nutrition and Dietetics*, vol. 71, no. 3, pp. 155–171.

Carleton, R., Sennett, L., Gans, K., Levin, S., Lefebre, C. & Lasater, T. 1991, 'The Pawtucket Heart Health Program. Influencing adolescent eating patterns', *Annals of the New York Academy of Sciences*, vol. 623, pp. 322–326.

Colatruglio, S. & Slater, J. 2014, 'Food literacy: Bridging the gap between food, nutrition and well-being', in Deer, F., Falkenberg, T., McMillan, B. & Sims, L. (eds), *Sustainable Well-being: Concepts, Issues, and Educational Practices*, ESWB Press, Winnipeg, pp. 37–55.

Contento, I.R. 2008, 'Nutrition education: linking research, theory, and practice', *Asia Pacific Journal of Clinical Nutrition*, vol. 17, no. 1, pp. 176–179.

Contento, I.R., Randell, J.S. & Basch, C.E. 2002, 'Review and analysis of evaluation measures used in nutrition education intervention research', *Journal of Nutrition Education and Behaviour*, vol. 34, no. 1, pp. 2–25.

Crawford, D. & Worsley, A. 2004, *Review of Children's Healthy Eating Interventions*, Deakin University, Deakin.

Food Standards Agency 2005, 'Dietary change: The evidence base and future research needs', Seminar, 20 January 2005.

Fordyce-Voorham, S. 2009, 'Essential food skills required in a skill-based healthy eating programme', paper presented to Daring to Dream: Preferred Futures through Home Economics, Darwin, Australia.

Fordyce-Voorham, S. 2010, 'Identification of food skills for healthful eating programmes in secondary schools', *Journal of Nutrition Education and Behaviour*, vol. 43, no. 2, pp. 116–122.

Fordyce-Voorham, S. 2014, 'Food skills in secondary schools', Doctor of Philosophy thesis, University of Wollongong.

Goodchild, R. 2012, 'The "reality" of the Australian "Junior Masterchef" television series for preadolescents and their parents', Bachelor of Psychology (Honours in Psychology) thesis, Murdoch University.

Green, B. 1999, 'The new literacy challenge', *Literacy Learning: Secondary Thoughts*, vol. 7, no. 1, pp. 36–46.

Green, B. 2012, 'Subject-specific literacy and school learning: A revised account', in Green, B. & Beavis, C. (eds), *Literacy in 3D: An Integrated Perspective in Theory and Practice*, ACER Press, Camberwell, pp. 2–21.

Grunert, K.G., Brunso, K. & Bisp, S. 1993, 'Food-related lifestyle: Development of a cross-culturally valid instrument for market surveillance', MAPP Working Paper, no.12, Aarhus Business School, Denmark.

Hjelmar, U. 2011, 'Consumers' purchase of organic food products. A matter of convenience and reflexive practices', *Appetite*, vol. 56, no. 2, pp. 336–344.

Home Economics Institute of Australia 1997, 'Home Economics Education in Australia: Understanding Home Economics Education'.

Home Economics Victoria 2013, *Healthy Eating and Food Literacy in Secondary Schools*, Home Economics Victoria, Mount Waverley, viewed 10 May 2015, http://www.homeeconomics.com.au/projects/hefl.aspx.

Klepp, K.I. & Wilhelmsen, B.U. 1993, 'Nutrition education in junior high schools: incorporating behaviour change strategies in home economics classes', *Health Education Research*, vol. 8, no. 4, pp. 547–554.

Lai-Yeung, T.W.L. 2015, 'Hong Kong parents' perceptions of the transference of food preparation skills', *International Journal of Consumer Studies*, vol. 39, no. 2, pp. 117–124.

Lichtenstein, A.H. & Ludwig, D.S. 2010, 'Bring back home economics education', *Journal of the American Medical Association*, vol. 303, no. 18, pp. 1857–1858.

Mikkelsen, B.E. 2014, 'School – a multitude of opportunities for promoting healthier eating', *Public Health Nutrition*, vol. 17, no. 6, pp. 1191–1194.

Nestle, M., Wing, R., Birch, L., Disogra, L., Drewnowski, A., Middleton, S., Sigman-Grant, M.. & Sobal, J. 2009, 'Behavioral and social influences on food choice', *Nutrition Reviews*, vol. 56, no. 5, pp. 50–64.

Nowak, M. & Buttner, P. 2002, 'Adolescents food-related beliefs and behaviours: A cross-sectional study', *Nutrition and Dietetics*, vol. 59, no. 4, pp. 244–252.

Paquette, D. & Ryan, J. 2001, 'Bronfenbrenner's Ecological Systems Theory', viewed 3 January 2008, http://pt3.nl.edu/paquetteryanwebquest.pdf.

Pendergast, D. & Dewhurst, Y. 2012, 'Home Economics and food literacy: An international investigation', *International Journal of Home Economics*, vol. 5, no. 2, pp. 245–263.

Renwick, K. 2013, 'Food literacy as a form of critical pedagogy: Implications for curriculum development and pedagogical engagement for Australia's diverse student population', *Victorian Journal of Home Economics*, vol. 52, no. 2, pp. 6–17.

Rescinow, K., Lazarus, A., Davis, M.S., Wang, D.T., Lyn, R., Kotler, H. & Hall, M. 2000, 'Go girls!: Development of a community-based nutrition and physical activity programme for overweight African-American adolescent females', *Health Education and Behavior*, vol. 27, no. 5, pp. 616–631.

Salmon, J., Campbell, K.J. & Crawford, D.A. 2006, 'Television viewing habits associated with obesity risk factors: A survey of Melbourne schoolchildren', *Medical Journal of Australia*, vol. 184, no. 2, p. 64.

Satter, E. 2007, 'Eating competence: Nutrition education with the Satter Eating Competence Model', *Journal of Nutrition Education and Behavior*, vol. 39, no. 5, pp. S189–S194.

Satter, E.M. 2008, 'Nutrition education in schools (Appendix H)', in *Secrets of Feeding a Healthy Family*, Kelcy Press, Madison, WI.

Schnögl, S., Zehetgruber, R., Danninger, S., Setzwein, M., Wenk, R., Freudenberg, M., Muller, C. & Groeneveld, M. 2006, *Savoury Dishes for Adult Education and Counselling*, BEST Institute, Vienna.

Short, F. 2007, 'Food and foodways – connecting people and places', paper presented at European Cultural Studies Conference, Norrkoping, Sweden.

Slater, J. 2013, 'Is cooking dead? The state of Home Economics Food and Nutrition education in a Canadian province', *International Journal of Consumer Studies*, vol. 37, no. 6, pp. 617–624.

Smith, G. & de Zwart, M. 2010, *Home Economics: A Contextual Study of the Subject and Home Economics Teacher Evaluation*, Teachers of Home Economics Specialists Association (THESA), British Columbia.

Smith, M.G. 2009, 'Food or nutrition literacy? What concept should guide home economics education?', *International Journal of Home Economics*, vol. 2, no. 1, pp. 48–64.

Steenhuis, I.H.M., Waterlander, W.E. & De Mul, A. 2011, 'Consumer food choices: The role of price and pricing strategies', *Public Health Nutrition*, vol. 14, no. 12, pp. 2220–2226.

Vanderkooy, P. 2009, 'What are food skills and who has them?', paper presented to the Ontario Public Health Convention, 6 April 2009.

Vartanian, L.R., Herman, C.P. & Wansink, B. 2008, 'Are we aware of the external factors that influence our food intake?', *Health Psychology*, vol. 27, no. 5, pp. 533–538.

Worsley, T. & Crawford, D. 2005, *Promoting Healthy Eating for Children - A Planning Guide for Practitioners*, Government Department of Human Services, Victoria.

Wu, M., Seeley, A. & Caraher, M. 2008, *A Movable Feast*, Centre for Food Policy, City University, London.

11 Developing food literacy through the health sector

Andrea Begley

Introduction

The perception that food literacy skills are declining and being devalued has translated into concern that people are no longer cooking with healthy raw ingredients or cooking at home and that this is having a substantial impact on dietary intakes and health outcomes (Begley & Gallegos 2010; Engler-Stringer 2010; Jaffe & Gertler 2006). The concern around decline and devaluing of food literacy, particularly expressed as cooking, is paralleled by the evidence that the overall dietary intakes in countries such as Australia are less than ideal, particularly in low socio-economic groups (Backholer et al. 2015). The rise in obesity is portrayed as an outcome of this concern with declining and/or devaluing of food literacy (Alkerwi, Crichton & Hebert 2014; Dixon, Hinde & Banwell 2006). Yet the evidence for food literacy skills and their relationship to health is scant.

Public health nutrition aims to promote and maintain the nutrition-related health and wellbeing of the population. Public health nutrition policy and practice has always referenced the need for some form of nutrition education and/or food skills as part of multilevel interventions to achieve dietary recommendations. As an example, when Australia's Food and Nutrition Policy (FNP) was launched in 1992, there was reference to the need to improve individual knowledge and skills. The recognition and targeting of the nutrition gatekeeper was highlighted as one method to achieve this. The policy stated: 'The role of many women as "gatekeepers" of their family's health requires special attention. Women in poverty … may need improved food skills to obtain good nutrition from foods which they can afford' (Commonwealth Department of Health, Housing and Community Services 1992: 5).

There is now increasing reference to this concept of food literacy in policy and a reframing of nutrition education as food literacy in programme delivery. The health sector may be increasingly taking up the food literacy space vacated by governments which no longer mandate home economics as a source of these skills (Caraher 2012). For countries like Australia it would appear that food literacy programmes are being funded as a panacea for a range of public health nutrition issues such as increasing obesity, chronic disease and food insecurity, with the assumption that a lack of practical knowledge and skills is the main contributing factor. The complexity of issues contributing to the increase in obesity and food insecurity results in what Lang and Rayner (2007) refer to as policy cacophony, whereby policy makers are faced with competing diagnoses of the problems.

The focus on food literacy programmes by governments fits a neo-liberalistic response to shift the responsibility for health to the individual level by focusing on what individuals need to be doing, without including a similar response at a structural level. The focus on personal skills is an easy and potentially cheaper solution for governments, but this does not address changing food systems with increasing convenience and cheap foods with variable nutrition qualities. Food literacy may be incorporated into broader programme delivery such as social marketing campaigns to increase fruits and vegetable consumption.

It is important that policy and practice are evidence based. Currently there is a need to establish criteria to guide policy and funding decisions by governments for investing in food literacy programmes. It is not possible to always implement randomized controlled trials and previously the findings from reviews have led to a false inference that there is an absence of sufficient evidence to guide appropriate action or define best practices (King et al. 2011). In tight fiscal environments policy options need to demonstrate best practice principles.

Best practice criteria for food literacy programmes

Best practice has come to mean taking account of 'best available evidence' for interventions. Best practice is a management idea which asserts that there is a programme that is more effective at improving, in this case, food literacy than another programme (Nutbeam 1996). In the context of population health, a best practice would enhance the diet quality and the health status of individuals and communities (King et al. 2011). On this basis, best practice in food literacy programmes should be understood as resulting from the efficacious content of the intervention itself and the integrity and quality of the process that delivers that intervention. Table 11.1 describes three principles which can be used to judge the quality of interventions (Baker, Auld & MacKinnon 2014; King et al. 2011; Nutbeam 1996).

Food literacy programmes are at their core nutrition education programmes. Nutrition education has been defined as 'any combination of educational

Table 11.1 Best practice food literacy programme principles

What?	Demonstrated effectiveness (dietary behaviour change), efficacy (efficient delivery and cost-effective delivery)
How?	Use of appropriate well-documented public health nutrition programme planning, implementation and evaluation research and methods
Why?	Suitability given the available evidence and particular context for programme delivery

strategies, accompanied by environmental supports, designed to facilitate voluntary adoption of food choices and other food- and nutrition-related behaviours conducive to health and well-being' (Contento et al. 1995: 279). Nutrition education is delivered through multiple venues and involves activities at the individual and community levels and support at policy levels. Food literacy programmes appear to have evolved as experiential practice forms of nutrition education that move away from reliance on nutrition knowledge transmission. Part of the increasing interest in food literacy programmes is their evolution as a form of nutrition education as driven by a need to consider specific target groups. Food literacy programmes such as cooking skill interventions appeal to practitioners who are working with lower literacy and numeracy populations such as socio-economically disadvantaged and indigenous groups (Cooper & Begley 2011).

The principles described in Table 11.1 can be used to judge food literacy interventions. The first of these would be demonstrating programme management principles for nutrition education as described by Contento and colleagues (Contento et al. 1995; Contento 2008a, b; Contento, Randell & Basch 2002). When undertaken by the health sector, food literacy programmes should importantly demonstrate a positive change in dietary behaviour. Secondly, past nutrition education reviews have highlighted the importance of behaviour change theoretical applications and consideration of andragogical and pedagogical learning principles depending on the target population (Baker, Auld & MacKinnon 2014; Contento et al. 1995). Thirdly, programmes should contain sufficient content and contextualization of food literacy domain applications and should be based around current dietary recommendations such as evidence based dietary guidelines.

Best practice programme management

There are very few programmes that meet all the known criteria to be labelled as best practice food literacy programmes. The next sections will discuss what is known and provide other examples of programmes that meet some of the elements. This discussion will provide directions for moving forward to develop best practice food literacy programmes.

Dietary behaviour change

A best practice food literacy programme must be able to demonstrate an impact evaluation showing a positive change in knowledge, skills, and ultimately dietary behaviour. Evaluating behaviour changes as a result of the intervention is an important outcome (Contento, Randell & Basch 2002). Typically this would be measured with a valid and reliable dietary assessment tool such as a food frequency questionnaire or 24 hour recall. Community programmes may use an adapted tool such as a brief food frequency questionnaire to reduce respondent burden and cost involved with complex evaluation.

A major limitation to date is that published food literacy programmes do not always report on dietary behaviour changes. Those that do show mixed results (Bisset et al. 2008; Hyland et al. 2006; Levy & Auld 2004; Stead et al. 2004; Tessaro et al. 2006, 2007; Wrieden et al. 2007; Wu, Seeley & Caraher 2008). There is some change in attitudes and knowledge; however, dietary behaviour is rarely a specified objective or measured outcome (Brooks & Begley 2013; Levy & Auld 2004; Reicks et al. 2014).

Consistent results have, however, come from the Expanded Food and Nutrition Education Program (EFNEP). This government funded programme aims to improve the nutritional knowledge, skills, behaviours and attitudes necessary for low income families in order to improve diet quality (Burney & Haughton 2002). In 2012, 130,485 adults attended the EFNEP, 85% of whom had incomes below the poverty line and 75% from ethnic minorities (National Data Report 2012). At this time, 95% of adults participating in the EFNEP have improved their diet including consumption of an additional cup of fruit and vegetables.

In addition to the 24 hour diet recall, the EFNEP also uses the EFNEP behaviour checklist. Both tools are implemented pre- and post-intervention to measure programme impact. The EFNEP behaviour checklist is a ten item checklist developed over five years to become a practical, valid and reliable measure (Baral et al. 2013; Bradford et al. 2010). Questions included in the checklist relate to food and nutrition practices and behaviours (Murphy et al. 2001; Wardlaw & Baker 2012). Specifically the checklist measures four constructs: food resource management practices, nutritional practices, food safety practices and food security. The programme demonstrates improvement in food resource management practices and in 2012 the EFNEP reported that 90% of adults improved their nutrition practices, 85% their food resource management practices, and 66% their food safety practices (Lohse et al. 2015; National Data Report 2012).

A major consideration of food literacy is how else these programmes can achieve health outcomes. There is the potential social benefit from the group processes being used and the value in sharing food which may in turn affect mental health. The need to cook healthy food is not always the main reason practitioners used such programmes, as those reported in indigenous populations demonstrated their use as an engagement strategy which relates to social inclusion (Abbott et al. 2010). Some process evaluation demonstrates that the social aspects of such programmes may be an important impact to evaluate. Recent evidence from Jamie's Ministry of Food in Australia demonstrated improvements in social interactions in the home (Herbert et al. 2014).

Economic effectiveness

A cost–benefit analysis measures the cost of achieving specific dietary or health outcomes. The EFNEP is the only programme to demonstrate cost–benefit analysis and is seen as a good use of US government dollars (Schuster et al. 2003). Other attempts with the EFNEP have estimated cost–benefit ratio based on potential prevention of diet-related chronic diseases and conditions (Dollahite, Kenkel & Thompson 2008; Rajgopal et al. 2002).

Given the level of funding the EFNEP receives, the cost-effectiveness of the programme has also been investigated. The cost–benefit of the programme looks at the total cost of the programme in relation to overall outcomes. US $1.1 million was spent on the EFNEP per year per state/territory (2000–2006), an average of $520 per participant (Baral et al. 2013). Outcomes were looked at in terms of food resource management practices, nutritional practices and food safety practices. All but three states were deemed cost-effective when looking at the cost per quality adjusted life years, providing support to continue funding the ongoing programme (Baral et al. 2013). EFNEP's impact on quality of life for participants and educators has found improvements in both groups, in different domains. The study used the Quality of Life (QOL) Profile, tested for reliability and validity (Auld et al. 2013).

Formative research

Programmes should follow a planning, implementation and evaluation cycle that informs their future development. Formative research is necessary for an intervention to be appropriately tailored to the target audience. This involves collecting information and data to assist the development and implementation of programmes and resources. It is important that communities and stakeholders be engaged in informing the intervention. Formative research methods include focus groups, interviews and surveys. There is little published on the formative evaluation and consultation with target group and stakeholders for food literacy programmes but when conducted it is more likely to lead to positive results (Condrasky et al. 2010; Thomas & Irwin 2012; Thompson et al. 2011).

Capacity building

Capacity building is an established effective component of public health practice. Capacity building can be defined as the process by which various levels (individuals, groups, organizations, workforce, systems, state, ecosystem) are developed to perform effectively, efficiently and in a sustainable manner (Baillie et al. 2009). The tenets of partnerships, intervention management, workforce development and community development are critical determinants of capacity, supported by leadership, resourcing and intelligence (Baillie et al. 2009).

One way that food literacy programmes contribute to capacity building is through the use of peer educators; they may be general community members or facilitators sharing specific characteristics with the programme's intended target group. A number of programmes have described the peer nutrition educators as 'local community members with an interest in nutrition' (Anderson, Mullan & Thomson 2012; Caraher & Richards 2007; Community Foodies 2010;

Dick & Telfer 2010; Food Fairness Illawarra 2012; Glasson et al. 2012; Ness, Elliott & Wilbur 1992; Sanders 2006). In contrast, some peer educators were specifically selected with a view to reaching a specific target group, such as university students (Garcia, Henry & Zok 2000), primary or secondary school students (Foodbank for New York City 2013; Story et al. 2002), people from specific culturally and linguistically diverse groups (Herrmann, Williams & Hunt 2001; Taylor et al. 2000), older adults (Hyland et al. 2006; Lynde 1992), or parents (Marshak, De Silva & Silberstein 1998; Tasmanian Government 2014; Wong & Keller 2010). A high degree of similarity between peer educators and the target group is suggested to bring both benefits, in terms of empathy and understanding of the audience, and challenges, in terms of peer educators facing similar life crises to their participants, potentially resulting in higher educator turnover (Anliker et al. 1999). Paraprofessionals are employed as front-line Community Nutrition Educators (CNEs) for the EFNEP. These CNEs are local residents from the target population and are hired on the basis that their life experiences will improve rapport with the programme audience (Auld et al. 2013; Dickin, Dollahite & Habicht 2005).

Few programmes have extensively evaluated the effectiveness of peer nutrition educator training, programme delivery and outcome measures in programme participants, with most programmes focusing on evaluating only one or two of these elements. The importance of providing peer educators with training, support and monitoring in collecting detailed and accurate evaluation data is suggested to be of key importance (Anliker et al. 1999). Training effectiveness has largely been evaluated through the use of pre- and post-training questionnaires and qualitative interviews with peer educators. Evaluation has focused on change in peer nutrition educator knowledge as a result of training, and self-reported confidence of educators in performing nutrition-related behaviours and disseminating nutrition information or delivering nutrition education sessions.

With respect to changes in dietary behaviours, Dickin, Dollahite and Habicht (2005) demonstrated a significant increase in the magnitude of participant behaviour change following the provision of training to paraprofessional staff facilitators. Glasson et al. (2012) reported significant increases in fruit and vegetable servings among parents who attended a nutrition education session facilitated by community members. A number of other programmes have reported positive changes in participant knowledge, attitudes and skills (Cason 2001; Christofferson et al. 2012; Marshak, De Silva & Silberstein 1998; Taylor et al. 2000).

Programme duration, intensity and reach

A programme must be of sufficient duration and intensity to support behaviour change. Depending on the objectives sought, longer more intensive programmes are required compared to a one-off session. A review of nutrition education programmes found that between 15 and 50 hours might be needed to change attitudes and behaviours (Contento et al. 1995). Reviews of cooking programme duration find programmes consisting of one session to two-year programmes. This variation in duration makes it difficult to determine sufficient or minimum duration and intensity required. The varying durations are often the result of different aims and incorporation of food literacy domains (Hersch et al. 2014). There appears to be a general consensus that six to eight sessions lasting for at least two hours is a common delivery format to achieve dietary behaviour change (Auld et al. 2014; Flynn, Reinert & Schiff 2013; May et al. 2014). A review of school based cooking programmes with additional food literacy components found that most commonly programmes consisted of 10–15 hours of cooking classes in 5–10 sessions of 1–2 hours each (Caraher & Seeley 2010; Chen et al. 2014; Markow, Coveney & Booth 2012; Seeley, Wu & Caraher 2010). Food literacy programmes are therefore intensive to deliver given the number of sessions and potential numbers of people able to attend at any one time. The reach of a programme is an important consideration for funders as the cost of the programme usually means it has limited reach.

Fidelity

Fidelity describes the ability to deliver consistent programme content across settings and facilitators. Fidelity of implementation needs to be measured so that its impact on evaluation can be assessed. For example, FOODcents is a budgeting, food label and cooking programme outsourced by the Department of Health in Western Australia to three organizations. This challenges programme fidelity as described in a recent evaluation of the programme (Pettigrew et al. 2015).

There are numerous types of fidelity considerations for food literacy programmes. These include adherence to an intervention design; consistent exposure or dose; quality of delivery by the facilitator; and facilitation strategies such as the provision of manuals, guidelines, training, monitoring and feedback. Also important for fidelity is documenting programme differentiation which relates to identifying unique features of different components or programmes, and identifying what programmes components are essential, and without which the programme will not have its intended effect. Well-managed programmes are essential, as EFNEP research has found (Dickin, Dollahite & Habicht 2005), and it is important to publish details of training, for instance in the development of training manuals (Condrasky et al. 2013; Saunders et al. 2014; Whiteley & Matwiejczyk 2015). Programme developers and evaluators should balance fidelity with adaptability, and consider contextual factors such as the food environment.

Through process evaluation, interventions are able to monitor and document the reach and fidelity of the programme (Cates et al. 2014; Saunders et al. 2014). Fidelity can be assessed through observations or interviews with educators of the programme to ensure that all necessary components of the intended programme are being delivered (Cates et al. 2014).

Best practice theory and learning principles

Behaviour change models

Programmes must acknowledge the application of one or more theoretical behaviour change frameworks or models. Dietary behaviour change is the goal of food literacy programmes conducted in the health sector. Programmes that only disseminate food literacy information are unlikely to be effective. Food literacy programmes must build self-efficacy, confidence, self-motivation and participant's perceived control over their eating (Lytle 2005; Michie et al. 2009). Therefore it is important that programmes include some form of intention formation activity, specific goal setting, providing feedback on food literacy skill development and experiences and enabling review of behavioural goals (Achterberg & Miller 2004). Learning outcomes for each session would then be expected to reflect the translation of behavioural theory, and learning activities would be developed to achieve these outcomes (Achterberg & Miller 2004).

There has been limited research conducted regarding the most effective method of nutrition education for low income groups (Ball et al. 2013). However, it is recognized that programmes with a behavioural theory basis are more effective than information or knowledge based nutrition interventions (Contento et al. 1995). The Social Cognitive Theory (Ball et al. 2013; Condrasky et al. 2010; Cullen et al. 2010; Hoover, Martin & Litchfield 2009; Mitchell, Ash & McClelland 2006), Theory of Planned Behaviour (Carson & Hedl 1998) and the Trans-theoretical Model (Chung & Hoerr 2007; Pulver 2008; Strolla, Gans & Risica 2006) are examples of theories that have been used in programme development. Behaviour change theories are applied to food literacy programmes to provide guidance for programme content and predict outcomes.

Learning theory principles

Best practice programmes consider the application of andragogy and/or pedagogy (adult and child) learning principles in their programme design. It is important that adults can self-assess and individualize their dietary goals. Goal setting is the most common strategy implemented in adult nutrition education interventions to facilitate behaviour change. A number of programmes targeting low literacy/limited resources groups have incorporated goal setting, including the EFNEP and Supplemental Nutrition Assistance Programmes (Ball et al. 2013; Cullen et al. 2010; Derrickson et al. 2003). Goal attainment has been linked to positive food choice behaviour outcomes amongst this target group. Goals such as eating more fruit and vegetables can be achieved by developing self-efficacy in participants for planning fruit and vegetable consumption (Cullen et al. 2010).

Nelson, Corbin and Nickols-Richardson (2013) propose Kolb's Cycle of Experiential Learning as a framework for considering the importance of experiential learning for food literacy development. The authors use this cycle as a model for what they refer to as culinary skills education in schools for adolescents. Kolb's cycle suggests that there are four stages in learning which follow from each other and all this may happen instantly or over days, weeks or months, depending on the topic, and there may be skills development within different stages at the same time. Applying Kolb's cycle to food literacy development in recognizing these stages then raises the question as to how much experiential learning adults need in and between food literacy programmes to have a positive impact on dietary behaviour change.

For low literacy and low income groups traditional methods of learning that require high literacy levels and extensive vocabulary are not suitable (Albright et al. 1997). Experiential education as opposed to didactic or lecture interventions is preferable (Vineyard, Franck & Burney 2010). This may include cooking or food preparation, shopping tours, and other hands-on activities, such as measuring out the sugar content of sugary drinks.

Promising practices in food literacy programmes

In addition to considering best practices there is also a need in the area of food literacy programmes to consider promising or what are also described as emerging practices (Government of Canada 2010a; Washington State Department of Health 2009). The criteria for considering an emerging or promising practice for the purposes of this chapter are listed in Table 11.2.

Many food literacy programmes have a number of characteristics in line with best practice programmes; however, a food literacy programme might only be considered a promising practice if, for instance, there has been limited impact evaluation to prove its effectiveness or the programme only focuses on one aspect of food literacy such as cooking.

Table 11.2 Promising practices for food literacy programmes

Evaluation data	Programme has an evaluation plan in place to measure programme impact, but it may not yet have evaluation data available to demonstrate the effectiveness of positive outcomes, or has some quantitative and qualitative data showing positive outcomes, but does not yet have enough research or replication to support generalizable positive public health outcomes.
Food literacy domains	Programme only focuses on one or more food literacy domains, e.g. cooking, but not all.
Best practice characteristics	Programme incorporates characteristics and patterns of other best practice programmes by continually incorporating lessons learned, feedback, and analysis to lead toward improvement or positive outcomes.
Contextual considerations	Programme is based on guidelines that will lead to effective public health outcomes because it considers the contextual factors impacting on food literacy.

A programme might be considered a promising practice if it addresses contextual factors known to affect food literacy. Food literacy development and application is context dependent. A person cannot become food literate in a vacuum and food choices have been conceptualized as a function of circumstances (Bisogni et al. 2005). The Australian research described in Chapters 3 and 4 of this book identified a number of contextual factors that influence the ability of food literacy to influence diet quality.

Canadian research recognized similar factors in an ecological framework that emphasizes the societal determinants – socio-cultural and learning environments, living supports, and food and cooking facilities – that facilitate and enable food literacy for individuals. Participants in the Canadian research demonstrated differences in use of food literacy skills on a daily basis dependent on psycho-social, environmental and financial circumstances (Desjardins et al. 2013). Table 11.3 contains a description of how people's personal contexts

Table 11.3 Food literacy contextual factors and types of programmes to suit them

Contexts	Factors	Barriers	Types of food literacy programmes
Social and psychological environment	Food experiences, normalization of skills, emotional support	Social isolation, lack of role models for healthy food preparation, weight concerns, depression, stress, lack of self-esteem	Community kitchens Lay advisor-/peer educator-led programmes School kitchen gardens Family meal programmes
Learning environment	Literacy, numeracy, experiential learning, engagement	High literacy and numeracy requirements; food literacy programmes are absent, are poorly taught, or are not geared to needs or interests	Cooking classes Supermarket tours
Food, food preparation facilities and food environments	Food availability, meal provision and cooking facilities	Poor housing with limited cooking and food storage facilities; lack of utensils and ingredients for home cooking; and poor access to healthy food	Farmers' markets Cooking classes Recipe books
Living conditions	Income, employment and housing	Low income, unemployment and household food insecurity	Community kitchens Food vouchers Meal programmes for homeless or those in transition

Source: Desjardins et al. 2013

provide barriers to food literacy development and use of these skills. Consideration of the factors and barriers for each context then becomes a basis for selecting programmes.

Cooking skill interventions

Cooking skill interventions (CSIs) are promising food literacy programmes because their explicit intention is primarily to support one food literacy domain. Whilst the programmes may incorporate aspects of other domains, for example food selection, it is not always clear from programme descriptions. These programmes also have the potential to assist learners in intervening in broader physical and social environments to address barriers to improved food choices and cooking practices.

There have been a number of reviews of cooking class type programmes in the peer and grey literature. There have been reviews in the UK (Rees et al. 2012), Scotland (Community Food and Health 2012), Ireland (Mac Con Iomaire & Lydon 2011) and Canada (Government of Canada 2010a, 2010b; The Conference Board of Canada 2013) in the past few years, and systematic reviews on adults, adolescents and school children aged 5–12 (Hersch et al. 2014; Reicks et al. 2014). All demonstrate large activity in these types of programmes but numerous issues in study design and lack of high quality evaluation which limit development of best practice examples.

The UK review found that the usual delivery of classes was programmes offered to existing community groups rather than advertised to individuals. They were usually conducted in a variety of community settings such as all-purpose centres through to venues with purpose built kitchens. The cooking programmes were delivered in three ways: firstly they could be tailored to specific needs of people with illness, ethnic backgrounds or life stages, secondly they recruited from the general community who then were able to teach others in a train the trainer model, and lastly they were initiated by research teams for evaluation purposes.

There are only two systematic reviews of cooking programmes to date: the systematic review of effectiveness and appropriateness of interventions to introduce 16 years+ adults to home cooking in the UK (Rees et al. 2012) and the review of cooking programmes from a range of countries (Reicks et al. 2014). Interventions generally included practical cooking skills with some elements of food safety and hygiene, and shopping on a budget. The evidence of programme duration indicates that participants needed more intensive delivery than a one-off 'cook and taste' session to encourage the development of skills. Participants need opportunities for experiential/hands-on learning (ranging from taste testing to demonstrations to cooking and food preparation skills) to promote and build self-confidence and self-efficacy through skill development. Supportive learning environments, including a social support component and regular positive reinforcement, are also important and enable participants to set goals (May et al. 2014). Usually a theoretical basis or at least some defendable assumptions were lacking.

In these reviews only a few studies were found that included a comparison control group. At this point in time the lack of high quality food literacy programme evaluations demonstrating dietary behaviour change is disappointing. Issues with evaluation, included recruiting a control group and attrition before research completed. The UK review made a number of recommendations, primarily about evaluation, including the need to build rigorous evaluation into the provision of home cooking programmes before commencing. Evaluations need to be of a sufficient size, with robust designs that can provide reliable evidence about impact. Researchers must ensure that sufficient resources and feasibility testing are built into the recruitment stages of evaluation. There is a need for validated yet simple to administer evaluation tools that can be used and analysed by the diverse range of professionals and non-professionals delivering food literacy programmes (McClone, Dallison & Caraher 2005).

Conclusions

Food literacy programmes are a key policy strategy for addressing a range of health issues; however, a major limitation to date is the lack of programme evaluation demonstrating consistent impact on dietary behaviour change and health outcomes. Many programmes insufficiently demonstrate a range of best practice criteria. There is certainly a need for research on effective programme designs.

More broadly, there are the other impacts on food literacy that also need consideration. Food literacy has not instigated serious programme delivery and policy debate over its importance in today's society. Despite evidence that nutrition problems require large scale system changes, government responses continue to place the responsibility on individuals. CSIs have been designed to focus on individual practices to provide the knowledge and skills for people to select and cook healthier foods and to resist food industry developments in fast foods, quick-serve and convenience foods. These approaches assume people just need more knowledge or skills to fill some presumed 'deficit' that contributes to poor dietary behaviours. This ignores social structure variables that are not within an individual's decision-making capability. Whilst food literacy programmes are embedded in the 'developing personal skills' individualism of public health nutrition programme delivery, cooking and eating are highly social activities and therefore we need to consider social processes and social relationships.

There is clearly a challenge to the use of best practice food literacy programmes when considering just a health focus. Initiatives are required to change cultural attitudes to food literacy. Food literacy programmes have the potential to build capacity for individuals, agencies, organizations and communities by connecting all participants into community endeavours that support healthy eating.

References

Abbott, P., Davison, J., Moore, L. & Rubinstein, R. 2010, 'Barriers and enhancers to dietary behaviour change for Aboriginal people attending a diabetes cooking course', *Health Promotion Journal of Australia*, vol. 21, no. 1, pp. 33–38.

Achterberg, C. & Miller, C. 2004, 'Is one theory better than another in nutrition education? A viewpoint: more is better', *Journal of Nutrition Education and Behavior*, vol. 36, no. 1, pp. 40–42.

Albright, C.L., Bruce, B., Howard-Pitney, B., Winkleby, M.A. & Fortmann, S.P. 1997, 'Development of a curriculum to lower dietary fat intake in a multiethnic population with low literacy skills', *Journal of Nutrition Education*, vol. 29, no. 4, pp. 215–223.

Alkerwi, A., Crichton, G.E. & Hebert, J.R. 2014, 'Consumption of ready-made meals and increased risk of obesity: findings from the Observation of Cardiovascular Risk Factors in Luxembourg (ORISCAV-LUX) study', *British Journal of Nutrition*, pp. 1–8.

Anderson, I., Mullan, C. & Thomson, K. 2012, *Cooking with the Community in 5 Easy Steps*, Fife Community Food Project, viewed 20 December 2015, <http://www.communityfoodandhealth.org.uk/wp-content/uploads/2012/05/cooking-in-the-community.pdf>.

Anliker, J., Damron, D., Ballesteros, M., Feldman, R., Langenberg, P. & Havas, S. 1999, 'Using peer educators in nutrition intervention research: Lessons learned from the Maryland WIC 5 A Day Promotion Programme', *Journal of Nutrition Education*, vol. 31, no. 6, pp. 347–354.

Auld, G., Baker, S., Bauer, L., Koszewski, W., Procter, S.B. & Steger, M.F. 2013, 'EFNEP's impact on the quality of life of its participants and educators', *Journal of Nutrition Education and Behavior*, vol. 45, no. 6, pp. 482–489.

Auld, G., Baker, S., Conway, L., Dollahite, J., Lambea, M.C. & McGirr, K. 2014, 'Outcome effectiveness of the widely adopted EFNEP curriculum Eating Smart Being Active', *Journal of Nutrition Education and Behavior*, vol. 47, no. 1, pp. 19–27.

Backholer, K., Spencer, E., Gearon, E., Magliano, D.J., McNaughton, S.A., Shaw, J.E. & Peeters, A. 2015, 'The association between socio-economic position and diet quality in Australian adults', *Public Health Nutrition*, pp. 1–9.

Baillie, E., Bjarnholt, C., Gruber, M. & Hughes, R. 2009, 'A capacity-building conceptual framework for public health nutrition practice', *Public Health Nutrition*, vol. 12, no. 8, pp. 1031–1038.

Baker, S., Auld, G. & MacKinnon, C. 2014, *Best Practices in Nutrition Education for Low-Income Audiences*, Department of Food Science and Human Nutrition Colorado State University supported by the National Institute of Food and Agriculture (NIFA), USDA, through Award 2012-48757-20337, viewed 20 December 2015, <http://snap.nal.usda.gov/snap/CSUBestPractices.pdf>.

Ball, K., McNaughton, S.A., Le, H., Andrianopoulos, N., Inglis, V., McNeilly, B., Lichomets, I., Granados, A. & Crawford, D. 2013, 'ShopSmart 4 Health – protocol of a skills-based randomised controlled trial promoting fruit and vegetable consumption among socioeconomically disadvantaged women', *BMC Public Health*, vol. 13, p. 466.

Baral, R., Davis, G.C., Blake, S., You, W. & Serrano, E. 2013, 'Using national data to estimate average cost effectiveness of EFNEP outcomes by state/territory', *Journal of Nutrition Education and Behavior*, vol. 45, no. 2, pp. 183–187.

Begley, A. & Gallegos, D. 2010, 'What's cooking for dietetics? A review of the literature', *Nutrition & Dietetics*, vol. 67, no. 1, pp. 26–30.

Bisogni, C., Jastran, M., Shen, L. & Devine, C. 2005, 'A biographical study of food choice capacity: Standards, circumstances, and food management skills', *Journal of Nutrition Education and Behavior*, vol. 37, no. 6, pp. 284–291.

Bisset, S., Potvin, L., Daniel, M. & Paquette, M. 2008, 'Assessing the impact of the primary school-based nutrition intervention Petits cuistots-parents en réseaux', *Canadian Journal of Public Health*, vol. 99, no. 2, pp. 107–113.

Bradford, T., Serrano, E.L., Cox, R.H. & Lambur, M. 2010, 'Development and testing of a nutrition, food safety, and physical activity checklist for EFNEP and FSNE adult programmes', *Journal of Nutrition Education and Behavior*, vol. 42, no. 2, pp. 123–130.

Brooks, N. & Begley, A. 2013, 'Adolescent food literacy programmes: A review of the literature', *Nutrition & Dietetics*, vol. 71, no. 3, pp. 158–171.

Burney, J. & Haughton, B. 2002, 'EFNEP: A nutrition education programme that demonstrates cost–benefit', *Journal of the Academy of Nutrition and Dietetics*, vol. 102, no. 1, pp. 39–45.

Canada, Go 2010, *Improving Cooking and Food Preparation Skills: A synthesis of the Evidence to Inform Program and Policy Development*, Health Canada, Canada, viewed 20 December 2015, <http://www.hc-sc.gc.ca/fn-an/nutrition/child-enfant/cfps-acc-synthes-eng.php>.

Caraher, M. 2012, 'Cooking in crisis: lessons learned from UK', paper presented to Dublin Gastronomy Symposium, Dublin, viewed 20 December 2015, <http://arrow.dit.ie/dgs/2012/june512/6/>.

Caraher, M. & Richards, L. 2007, *An Evaluation of the Community Nutrition Assistant Training Programme Camden*, City University, London, viewed February 27 2014, <http://openaccess.city.ac.uk/488/2/Camden%20CNA%20Evaluation%23D20C0.doc.pdf>.

Caraher, M. & Seeley, A. 2010, 'Cooking in schools: Lessons from the UK', *J HEIA*, vol. 17, no. 1, pp. 2–9.

Carson, J. & Hedl, J. 1998, 'Smart shoppers tours: Outcome evaluation', *Journal of Nutrition Education*, vol. 30, pp. 323–331.

Cason, K.L. 2001, 'Evaluation of a preschool nutrition education programme based on the theory of multiple intelligences', *Journal of Nutrition Education*, vol. 33, no. 3, pp. 161–164.

Chen, Q., Goto, K., Wolff, C., Bianco-Simeral, S., Gruneisen, K. & Gray, K. 2014, 'Cooking up diversity: Impact of a multi-component, multi-cultural, experiential intervention on food and cooking behaviors among elementary-school students from low-income ethnically diverse families', *Appetite*, vol. 80, pp. 114–122.

Christofferson, D., Christensen, N., LeBlanc, H. & Bunch, M. 2012, 'Developing an online certification programme for nutrition education assistants', *Journal of Nutrition Education and Behavior*, vol. 44, no. 5, pp. 407–414.

Chung, S.J. & Hoerr, S.L. 2007, 'Evaluation of a theory-based community intervention to increase fruit and vegetable intakes of women with limited incomes', *Nutrition Research and Practice*, vol. 1, no. 1, pp. 46–51.

Commonwealth Department of Health, Housing and Community Services 1992, *Food and Nutrition Policy*, Australian Government Publishing Service, Canberra.

Community Food and Health 2012a, 'What's cooking in Scotland? Part One How Scotland's community food initiatives are addressing the challenges of setting up cookery courses within low-income communities', Community Food and Health, Scotland, viewed 20 December 2015, <http://www.communityfoodandhealth.org.uk/wp-content/uploads/2012/05/cfhs-whats-cooking-part-one3.pdf>.

Community Food and Health 2012b, 'What's cooking in Scotland? Part Two How community food initiatives are finding out about the impact of cookery courses', Community Food and Health, Scotland, viewed 20 December 2015, <http://www.communityfood andhealth.org.uk/wp-content/uploads/2012/10/cfhs-whats-cooking-in-scotland-part2. pdf>.

Community Foodies 2010, *Community Foodies*, viewed 27 February 2014, <http://www.communityfoodies.com/>.

Condrasky, M.D., Baruth, M., Wilcox, S., Carter, C. & Jordan, J. 2013, 'Cooking training for Faith, Activity and Nutrition project with AME churches in SC', *Evaluation and Programme Planning*, vol. 37, pp. 43–49.

Condrasky, M.D., Griffin, S.G., Catalano, P.M. & Clark, C. 2010, 'A formative evaluation of the Cooking with a Chef program', *Journal of Extension*, vol. 48, no. 2, p. 2FEA1.

Contento, I.R. 2008a, 'Nutrition education: Linking research, theory and practice', *Asia Pacific Journal of Clinical Nutrition*, vol. 17, no. 1, pp. 176–179.

Contento, I.R. 2008b, 'Review of nutrition education research in the *Journal of Nutrition Education and Behavior*, 1998 to 2007', *Journal of Nutrition Education and Behavior*, vol. 40, no. 6, pp. 331–340.

Contento, I.R., Balch, G.I., Bronner, Y.L., Lytle, L., Maloney, S., Olson, C. & Swadener, S. 1995, 'The effectiveness of nutrition education and implications for nutrition education policy, programs, and research: A review of research', *Journal of Nutrition Education*, vol. 27, no. 6, pp. 277–418.

Contento, I.R., Randell, J.S. & Basch, C.E. 2002, 'Review and analysis of evaluation measures used in nutrition education intervention research', *Journal of Nutrition Education and Behavior*, vol. 34, no. 1, pp. 2–25.

Cooper, S. & Begley, A. 2011, 'WA health practitioners and cooking: How well do they mix?', *Nutrition & Dietetics*, vol. 68, no. 1, pp. 65–69.

Cullen, K.W., Thompson, D.I., Scott, A.R., Lara-Smalling, A., Watson, K.B. & Konzelmann, K. 2010, 'The impact of goal attainment on behavioral and mediating variables among low income women participating in an Expanded Food and Nutrition Education Programme intervention study', *Appetite*, vol. 55, no. 2, pp. 305–310.

Derrickson, J., Buchanan, C., Asing, K. & Okuma, A. 2003, 'Lessons learned from the "Spend Less. Eat Well. Feel Better" Programme Efficacy Trial', *Journal of Nutrition Education and Behavior*, vol. 35, no. 1, pp. 30–36.

Desjardins, E., Davidson, L., Samra, R., MacDonald, A., Dunbar, J., Thomas, H., Munoz, M., King, B., Maxwell, T., Wong-McGraw, P. & Shukla, R. 2013, '"Making something out of nothing." Food literacy among youth, young pregnant women and young parents who are at risk for poor health', Food Secure Canada, viewed 20 December 2015, <http://foodsecurecanada.org/resources-news/resources-research/making-something-out-nothing-food-literacy-among-youth-young>.

Dick, G. & Telfer, A. 2010, *Healthy Cooking in the Community: A Comprehensive Manual for the Delivery of Practical Cooking Sessions to Encourage Healthier Eating*, Department of Nutrition and Dietetics, NHS Ayrshire and Arran, viewed 20 December 2015, <http://www.communityfoodandhealth.org.uk/wp-content/uploads/2010/08/healthy cookinginthecommunitynhsayrarran-1430.pdf>.

Dickin, K.L., Dollahite, J.S. & Habicht, J.-P. 2005, 'Nutrition behavior change among EFNEP participants is higher at sites that are well managed and whose front-line nutrition educators value the program', *Journal of Nutrition*, vol. 135, no. 9, pp. 2199–2205.

Dixon, J., Hinde, S. & Banwell, C. 2006, 'Obesity, convenience and "phood"', *British Food Journal*, vol. 108, no. 8, pp. 613–615.

Dollahite, J., Kenkel, D. & Thompson, C.S. 2008, 'An economic evaluation of the expanded food and nutrition education programme', *Journal of Nutrition Education and Behavior*, vol. 40, no. 3, pp. 134–143.

Engler-Stringer, R. 2010, 'Food, cooking skills and health: A literature review', *Canadian Journal of Dietetic Practice and Research*, vol. 71, no. 3, pp. 141–145.

Flynn, M.M., Reinert, S. & Schiff, A.R. 2013, 'A six-week cooking program of plant-based recipes improves food security, body weight, and food purchases for food pantry clients', *Journal of Hunger & Environmental Nutrition*, vol. 8, no. 1, pp. 73–84.

Food Fairness Illawarra 2012, *Stir It Up!*, viewed 27 February 2014, <http://foodfairnessillawarra.org.au/projects-stories/stir-it-up/>.

Foodbank for New York City 2013, *EATWISE CookShop for Teens*, viewed 27 February 2014, <http://eatwiseteens.org/learn/about/>.

Garcia, A.C., Henry, C.J. & Zok, A. 2000, 'Peer education in nutrition for students: Part I program development and process evaluation', *Foodservice Research International*, vol. 12, no. 3, pp. 163–173.

Glasson, C., Chapman, K., Gander, K., Wilson, T. & James, E. 2012, 'The efficacy of a brief, peer-led nutrition education intervention in increasing fruit and vegetable consumption: a wait-list, community-based randomised controlled trial', *Public Health Nutrition*, vol. 15, no. 7, pp. 1318–1326.

Government of Canada 2010a, *Improving Cooking and Food Preparation Skills: A Profile of Promising Practices in Canada and Abroad*, Health Canada, viewed 20 December 2015, <http://www.hc-sc.gc.ca/fn-an/nutrition/child-enfant/cfps-acc-profil-apercu-eng.php>.

Government of Canada 2010b, *Improving Cooking and Food Preparation Skills: A synthesis of the Evidence to Inform Program and Policy Development* Health Canada, viewed 20 December 2015, <http://www.hc-sc.gc.ca/fn-an/nutrition/child-enfant/cfps-acc-synthes-eng.php>.

Herbert, J., Flego, A., Gibbs, L., Waters, E., Swinburn, B., Reynolds, J. & Moodie, M. 2014, 'Wider impacts of a 10-week community cooking skills programme – Jamie's Ministry of Food, Australia', *BMC Public Health*, vol. 14, p. 1161.

Herrmann, J., Williams, G. & Hunt, D. 2001, 'Effect of nutrition education by para-professionals on dietary intake, maternal weight gain, and infant birth weight in pregnant Native American and Caucasian adolescents', *Journal of Extension*, vol. 39, no. 1.

Hersch, D., Perdue, L., Ambroz, T. & Boucher, J. 2014, 'The impact of cooking classes on food-related preferences, attitudes and behaviours of school-aged children: A systematic review of the evidence 2003–2014', *Preventing Chronic Disease*, vol. 11, no. E193.

Hoover, J.R., Martin, P.A. & Litchfield, R.E. 2009, 'Qualitative tools to examine EFNEP curriculum delivery', *Journal of Extension*, vol. 47, no. 3, p. 3FEA.

Hyland, R., Wood, C., Adamson, A., Mathers, J., Hill, M., Seal, C. & Moynihan, P. 2006, 'Peer educator's perceptions of training for and implementing a community-based nutrition intervention for older adults', *Journal of Nutrition for the Elderly*, vol. 25, no. 3–4, pp. 147–171.

Jaffe, J. & Gertler, M. 2006, 'Victual vicissitudes: consumer deskilling and the (gendered) transformation of food systems', *Agriculture and Human Values*, vol. 23, pp. 143–162.

King, L., Gill, T., Allender, S. & Swinburn, B. 2011, 'Best practice principles for community-based obesity prevention: Development, content and application', *Obesity Reviews*, vol. 12, no. 5, pp. 329–338.

Lang, T. & Rayner, G. 2007, 'Overcoming policy cacophony on obesity: An ecological public health framework for policymakers', *Obesity Reviews*, vol. 8, pp. 165–181.

Levy, J. & Auld, G. 2004, 'Cooking classes outperform cooking demonstrations for college sophomores', *Journal of Nutrition Education and Behavior*, vol. 36, no. 4, pp. 197–203.

Lohse, B., Beleu, R., Smith, S., Wamboldt, P. & Cunningham-Sabo, L. 2015, 'About eating: An online programme with evidence of increased food resource management skills for low income women', *Journal of Nutrition Education and Behavior*, vol. 47, no. 3, pp. 265–272.

Lynde, B.D. 1992, 'Nutrition promotion for mature adults: A case study in peer education', *Journal of Nutrition for the Elderly*, vol. 11, no. 3, pp. 19–31.

Lytle, L.A. 2005, 'Nutrition education, behavioral theories, and the scientific method: Another viewpoint', *Journal of Nutrition Education and Behavior*, vol. 37, no. 2, pp. 90–93.

Mac Con Iomaire, M. & Lydon, J. 2011, 'The current state of cooking in Ireland: The relationship between cooking skills and food choice', paper presented to Tourism and Hospitality Research in Ireland Conference, Athlone Institute of Technology, 14–15 June.

Markow, K., Coveney, J. & Booth, S. 2012, 'Enhancing food literacy through school-based cooking programmes: What's working and what's not?', *J HEIA*, vol. 19, no. 2, pp. 2–11.

Marshak, H.H., De Silva, P. & Silberstein, J. 1998, 'Evaluation of a peer-taught nutrition education programme for low-income parents', *Journal of Nutrition Education*, vol. 30, no. 5, pp. 314–322.

May, J., Brady, A., Van Offelen, S. & Johnson, B. 2014, 'Simply Good Cooking: Online curriculum for the Interactive SNAP-Ed classroom', *Journal of Nutrition Education and Behavior*, vol. 46, no. 1, pp. 85–87.

McClone, P., Dallison, J. & Caraher, M. 2005, *Evaluation Resources for Community Food Projects*, National Health Service, London.

Michie, S., Abraham, C., Whittington, C. & McAteer, J. 2009, 'Effective techniques in healthy eating and physical activity interventions: A meta-regression', *Health Psychology*, vol. 28, no. 6, pp. 690–701.

Mitchell, R.E., Ash, S.L. & McClelland, J.W. 2006, 'Nutrition education among low-income older adults: A randomized intervention trial in congregate nutrition sites', *Health Education & Behavior*, vol. 33, no. 3, pp. 374–392.

Murphy, S.P., Kaiser, L.L., Townsend, M.S. & Allen, L.H. 2001, 'Evaluation of validity of items for a food behavior checklist', *Journal of the American Dietetic Association*, vol. 101, no. 7, pp. 751–761.

National Data Report 2012, *The Expanded Food and Nutrition Education Programme (EFNEP)*, United States Department of Agriculture, Washington, DC.

Nelson, S., Corbin, M. & Nickols-Richardson, S. 2013, 'A call for culinary skills education in childhood obesity-prevention interventions: Current status and peer influences', *Journal of the Academy of Nutrition & Dietetics*, vol. 113, no. 8, pp. 1031–1036.

Ness, K., Elliott, P. & Wilbur, V. 1992, 'A peer educator nutrition programme for seniors in a community-development context', *Journal of Nutrition Education*, vol. 24, no. 2, pp. 91–94.

Nutbeam, D. 1996, 'Achieving "best practice" in health promotion: Improving the fit between research and practice', *Health Education Research*, vol. 11, no. 3, pp. 317–326.

Pettigrew, S., Moore, S., Pratt, I.S. & Jongenelis, M. 2015, 'Evaluation outcomes of a long-running adult nutrition education programme', *Public Health Nutrition*, May, pp. 1–10.

Pulver, M.J. 2008, 'Behavior change among Hawaii Expanded Food and Nutrition Education Program (EFNEP) participants: Effects of ethnicity and the paraprofessional', *Journal of Nutrition Education and Behavior*, vol. 40, no. 4, pp. S24–S25.

Rajgopal, R., Cox, R.H., Lambur, M. & Lewis, E.C. 2002, 'Cost-benefit analysis indicates the positive economic benefits of the Expanded Food and Nutrition Education Programme related to chronic disease prevention', *Journal of Nutrition Education and Behavior*, vol. 34, no. 1, pp. 26–37.

Rees, R., Hinds, K., Dickson, K., O'Mara Eves, A. & Thomas, J. 2012, 'Communities that cook: A systematic review of the effectiveness and appropriateness of interventions to introduce adults to home cooking', Research Unit, Institute of Education, University of London, viewed 20 December 2015, <https://eppi.ioe.ac.uk/cms/Default.aspx?tabid=3322>.

Reicks, M., Trofholz, A.C., Stang, J.S. & Laska, M.N. 2014, 'Impact of cooking and home food preparation interventions among adults: Outcomes and implications for future programmes', *Journal of Nutrition Education and Behavior*, vol. 46, pp. 259–276.

Sanders, L. 2006, 'Community Foodies: Community peer educators working to foster community knowledge and skills about food and nutrition', paper presented at ISEqH 4th Biennial International Conference, Adelaide, Australia.

Saunders, R., Wilcox, S., Baruth, M. & Dowda, M. 2014, 'Process evaluation methods, implementation fidelity results and relationship to physical activity and healthy eating in the Faith, Activity and Nutrition (FAN) study', *Evaluation and Program Planning*, vol. 43, pp. 93–102.

Schuster, E., Zimmerman, Z.L., Engle, M., Smiley, J., Syversen, E. & Murray, J. 2003, 'Investing in Oregon's expanded food and nutrition education programme (EFNEP): Documenting costs and benefits', *Journal of Nutrition Education and Behavior*, vol. 35, no. 4, pp. 200–206.

Seeley, A., Wu, M. & Caraher, M. 2010, 'Should we teach cooking in schools? A systematic review of the literature of school-based cooking interventions', *J HEIA*, vol. 17, no. 1, pp. 10–18.

Stead, M., Caraher, M., Wrieden, W., Longbottom, P., Valentine, K. & Anderson, A. 2004, 'Confident, fearful and hopeless cooks. Findings from the development of a food-skills initiative', *British Food Journal*, vol. 106, no. 4, pp. 274–287.

Story, M., Lytle, L.A., Birnbaum, A.S. & Perry, C.L. 2002, 'Peer-led, school-based nutrition education for young adolescents: Feasibility and process evaluation of the TEENS', *Journal of School Health*, vol. 72, no. 3, pp. 121–127.

Strolla, L.O., Gans, K.M. & Risica, P.M. 2006, 'Using qualitative and quantitative formative research to develop tailored nutrition intervention materials for a diverse low-income audience', *Health Education Research*, vol. 21, no. 4, pp. 465–476.

Tasmanian Government 2014, 'Family Food Patch', viewed 27 February 2014, <http://www.familyfoodpatch.org.au/index.html#welcome>.

Taylor, T., Serrano, E., Anderson, J. & Kendall, P. 2000, 'Knowledge, skills, and behavior improvements on peer educators and low-income Hispanic participants after a stage of change-based bilingual nutrition education program', *Journal of Community Health*, vol. 25, no. 3, pp. 241–262.

Tessaro, I., Rye, S., Parker, L., Mangone, C. & McCrone, S. 2007, 'Effectiveness of a nutrition intervention with rural low-income women', *American Journal of Health Behavior*, vol. 31, no. 1, pp. 35–43.

Tessaro, I., Rye, S., Parker, L., Transgrund, K., Mangone, C., McCrone, S. & Leslie, N. 2006, 'Cookin' up Health: Developing a nutrition intervention for a rural Appalachian population', *Health Promotion Practice*, vol. 7, no. 2, pp. 252–257.

The Conference Board of Canada 2013, *What's to Eat: Improving Food Literacy in Canada*, Canada, viewed 20 December 2015, <http://www.conferenceboard.ca/e-library/a bstract.aspx?did=5727>

Thomas, H. & Irwin, J. 2012, 'Cook It Up! Formative evaluation of a community-based cooking programme for at-risk youth in London, Ontario', *International Journal of Home Economics*, vol. 5, no. 1, pp. 64–83.

Thompson, D., Cullen, K.W., Reed, D.B., Konzelmann, K. & Smalling, A.L. 2011, 'Formative assessment in the development of an obesity prevention component for the expanded food and nutrition education programme in Texas', *Family Community Health*, vol. 34, no. 1, pp. 61–71.

Vineyard, M., Franck, K. & Burney, J. 2010, *Comparative Evaluation of Interactive, Facilitated-discussion and Indirect Nutriton Education Methods for SNAP-Ed Clients*, University of Tennessee Extension, Family and Consumer Services, Tennessee.

Wardlaw, M. & Baker, S. 2012, 'Long-term evaluation of EFNEP and SNAP-Ed', Forum for Family and Consumer Issues, viewed 20 December 2015, <https://ncsu. edu/ffci/publications/2012/v17-n2-2012-summer-fall/wardlaw-baker.php>.

Washington State Department of Health 2009, 'Promising practices in nutrition education: Choosing the right nutrition education curriculum for your program', viewed 20 December 2015, <http://www.doh.wa.gov/portals/1/Documents/Pubs/345-250-PromisingPracticesNutritionEducation.pdf>.

Whiteley, C. & Matwiejczyk, L. 2015, 'Preschool programme improves young children's food literacy and attitudes to vegetables', *Journal of Nutrition Education and Behavior*, vol. 47, no. 4, pp. 397–398.

Wong, S.S. & Keller, S.D. 2010, 'A pilot study of paraprofessional peer teaching by teen moms in a teen parenting nutrition education program', *FASEB Journal*, vol. 24, viewed 20 December 2015, <http://www.fasebj.org/cgi/content/meeting_abstract/24/1_MeetingAbstracts/940.10>.

Wrieden, W., Anderson, A., Longbottom, P., Valentine, K., Stead, M., Caraher, M., Lang, T., Gray, B. & Dowler, E. 2007, 'The impact of a community-based food skills intervention on cooking confidence, food preparation methods and dietary choices: An exploratory trial', *Public Health Nutrition*, vol. 10, no. 2, pp. 203–211.

Wu, M., Seeley, A. & Caraher, M. 2008, *A Moveable Feast. Evidence for School Based Cooking Interventions to Improve Children's Food Behaviours and Diets*, Centre for Food Policy, City University, London.

12 Developing food literacy through food production

Heather Yeatman

Introduction

Food production and consumption have underpinned and defined societies through the ages. Transitioning from a hunter-gatherer existence to farming and agriculture resulted in communities developing different identities depending on the plant and animal sources available to them and their environment and climate. Communities' food production, storage and preparation practices developed in response to their environments depending on whether they had harsh food production environments or lived in locations with favourable conditions that enabled food to be produced and accessed year round. Trade and transport of food between communities and from different regions of the world further enabled the development of cultural food practices, from basic salting of food for preservation, to spicing of foods to signify status in a community. Development of different techniques to store foods safely was critically important, including fermentation of foods (for example making yoghurts and cheeses in Europe and Middle Eastern countries and soya sauce and tofu in Asia). Environmental disasters such as floods, droughts and earthquakes, along with man-made challenges during periods of conflict, also acted to shape the culinary characteristics of communities. Values relating to food and its production and preparation were embedded in individuals and communities to underpin and help ensure their food cultures and ultimately their survival.

These early relationships with food production and preparation remain part of our current food preferences and practices but may be less acknowledged and valued. However, recognition of the knowledge, skills and valuing of food production, preparation and storage may be experiencing a renaissance (Tarcher 2005). Greater contemporary recognition has developed of the importance of food preparation and nutrition in individual and community health. The importance of sustainable food production practices and water availability to the viability of communities and the world more generally is also being acknowledged. Global human population projections of up to an additional 2.5 billion people by 2050 and the balance (54% in 2014 rising to 66% by 2050) of the population living in urban areas (United Nations 2015) has directed decision makers' and communities' attention to our food system and its viability.

The importance of sustainable food production practices and water availability issues has refocused attention on the need for people to be literate in food supply matters and able to make informed decisions in terms of their own food choices and the short and long term consequences of these. Greater food literacy of food production also enables people to participate in discussion and debates on policy developments and decisions that have impacts on the food supply more broadly.

We learn much about our food and develop our food skills through our lived experiences – in the home and in our communities. Traditionally agriculture has been part of everyone's life, as people lived on farms, lived in rural communities, or food production was co-located with cities. Having experience with food production ensured that people developed literacies and confidence not only with supplying food for themselves, but also how to prepare and safely store a wide range of foods that were seasonally available.

This chapter has a particular focus on how food literacy is developed through experiences with food production in different settings (agriculture, urban food production and home and school gardens). Some work has explored the development of agricultural or environmental food literacies in the agricultural sector but less research has explored the links between food literacies and urban, community or home gardens. It would be expected that community and cultural food practices could be developed through lived experiences, thus embedding food literacy, appreciation and enjoyment within people's everyday lives. However, little work has been reported on the development of food literacies and food production in a systematic manner. It will be concluded that reconnecting communities with food production should be encouraged and examined for its potential to contribute to the development of food literacies.

Aspects of knowledge

Consideration of food literacy and food production processes requires reflection on different aspects of knowledge. Yang's (2003) work on the epistemology of knowledge identifies three facets: explicit, implicit and emancipatory. Explicit knowledge refers to content areas, for example knowledge of food production processes, animal husbandry, enrichment of soil and the effects of weather and climate conditions. Implicit knowledge is more skill related, such as undertaking farming, vegetable growing or fishing. Emancipatory aspects of knowledge relate to values, an increasingly important consideration in relation to different types of food production techniques (for example organic or intensive farming), animal welfare issues, food sovereignty considerations and legitimacy of power and ownership of food production. This framework has recently been developed by Sanaz Sadegholvad in her studies to elucidate what young adults need to know about the food system and nutrition (University of Wollongong, unpublished). It will provide a framework for considering food literacy in relation to food production.

Food literacy and agriculture

Food system literacy is increasingly recognized as important to underpin informed food choices and health outcomes. Knowing how food is produced, the processes involved and the seasonality of food may all be important to underpin healthy and sustainable food choices (Story et al. 2007) at the individual level, and important to inform food system policy making at the population level. Food system decisions are critically important to enable the provision of a sustainable and healthy food supply at a time of diminishing resources and rapid expansion of the world's populations.

With the increasing urbanization of the world's population and with fewer people directly involved in agriculture, judgements about agricultural and food system issues and policies are increasingly being made by people with limited knowledge of and experience with the sector. This is particularly the case in Australia, where only a quarter of the population live outside the major cities, agricultural land is relatively cheap and food purchases are very much driven by cost at point of sale rather than food system considerations (Britnell 2011).

The globalization of food systems, rise in technologies, international trade pressures and impacts of environmental and manmade disasters on food production add to the complexities of food systems (Kovar & Ball 2013). Being 'knowledgeable' about food systems, being able to participate in related discussions or even making informed food selections based on food system considerations such as minimizing environmental impacts or maximizing nutritional quality, thus become challenging for all but a very small number. So what then could be considered the basic elements of food system or agri-food literacy?

Agri-food literacy

Literacies deemed relevant to an issue are shaped by particular perspectives. As outlined in the first chapter, components of food literacy related to food production encompassed environmental sustainability, food security, active citizenship and informed consumerism, as well as nutrition outcomes. However, others have approached food production literacies from different perspectives, particularly those of agriculture and environment.

The need for agricultural literacy is based on the imperative for societies to have viable food production systems to feed current and future populations and agricultural endeavours and competence underpin the important area of trade in food commodities. There is also support for agricultural literacies from food manufacturing industry sectors, for which agricultural literacies and viable agricultural production help to ensure supply of components for their food processing or food retail interests. Urban-based communities may be less engaged in agricultural pursuits and thus less mindful of the need to support development of agricultural literacy.

In the area of agricultural literacy, Frick, Kahler and Miller (1991) established eleven agricultural subject areas needed to achieve such literacy. The eleven areas were 1) relationship with the environment, 2) agricultural processing, 3) public policies, 4) relationship with natural resources, 5) animal products, 6) societal significance, 7) plant products, 8) economic impact, 9) agriculture marketing, 10) distribution and 11) global significance. These literacy areas are primarily explicit knowledge areas related to food production and the implicit knowledge needed for agricultural endeavour. Emancipatory knowledge, that based more on values, has a lower emphasis within the agricultural literacies literature, perhaps reflecting their more (agricultural) science based origins. However, lack of emphasis on societal and cultural values related to agriculture and farming may limit the valuing of and support for these endeavours within society.

Environmental literacies

Food production increasingly is affected by other imperatives, notably environmental influences and the need for environmental literacies. Recognition of the importance of environmental education emerged in the mid 1970s, when the UNESCO-UNEP identified that the goal of environmental education is:

> To develop a world population that is aware of, and concerned about, the environment and its associated problems, and which has the knowledge, skills, attitudes, motivations and commitment to work individually and collectively toward solutions of current problems and the prevention of new ones.
>
> (UNESCO 1976: 2)

The UNEP (United Nations Environment Programme) has continued to be active in its support for environmental concerns being factored into food security debates. Sustainable food production and consumption relies on individual consumers changing their food consumption habits. In turn, this requires supportive measures such as public engagement on the issue and consumer education to support sustainable dietary guidelines (UNEP 2012).

While there are components of environmental literacy that relate to explicit and implicit knowledge, compared with agricultural literacy there is a greater component of values based or emancipatory knowledge. The UNEP definition above and the work of public advocates for environmental literacy include literacy components relating to awareness, attitudes, motivations, commitments and actions. Thus the work on environmental literacy more strongly includes values based knowledge than does the field of agricultural literacy.

The goals of agricultural literacy and of environmental literacy do not necessarily align. Malalignment between agricultural and environmental perspectives can arise in countries such as Australia where the population is predominantly urban and more environmentally than agriculturally literate, and where wealth is high and food shortages are not common. In such circumstances positive attitudes to environmental sustainability and food are likely to be dominant compared with a focus on or imperative of feeding the expanding population of the world. For example, Thalbitzer (2010) described a situation in Denmark where the government agreed to return waterways back to their original condition based on environmental grounds but at the expense of agricultural interests which had farmed drained wetlands for over a hundred years. A proclaimed preference by consumers for organic produce may also reflect a desire for less industrialized agriculture and greater commitment to environmental principles. However, this has not been borne out in the research. Lockie et al. (2002) found that individualized concern for personal wellbeing (perceived healthiness) was a stronger driver for purchase of organic food as compared with environmental concerns regarding food production methods.

There are also a growing number of examples where environmental and agricultural outcomes align. The Carbon Farming Initiative in Australia established in 2011 encouraged carbon farming activities that reduced greenhouse gas (GHG) emissions on the land, such as planting and maintaining trees on farms or feeding cattle supplements to reduce methane production (Australian Farm Institute 2014). The United Nations (1992) and signatory governments clearly identified the need to link sustainability and agriculture in the Agenda 21 document, Chapter 14, when they identified that the major objective is to increase food production in a sustainable way and enhance food security. More recently, the Post-2015 Development Agenda in its Goal 2 identified the need for sustainable agriculture and its link to ending hunger and achieving food security and improved nutrition (United Nations 2015).

Agri-food literacy and society

A third dimension not so commonly considered a component of agri-food literacy is its role in social order and the maintenance of culture and tradition. The production of food has traditionally been a component of what defines a community or population. This is still very apparent in many traditional and indigenous communities and is stronger in some developed countries (such as France) than in other countries where urban-based concerns are more pervasive. With less focus on agriculture as a social enterprise and one that underpins the social integrity of a community, those communities become more vulnerable to city-based concerns.

A common social issue relating to food is price. There is a tension in many countries between the affordability of food and the financial viability of farming to produce that food. High food prices can lead to social unrest, as was witnessed in 2008 when rapidly rising food prices led to civil unrest, riots, looting and some deaths (Schneider 2008). In these circumstances policy settings that encourage low food prices can become dominant, but as a consequence farmers can be penalized and achieve little return for their efforts. This can occur in a less dramatic manner through supermarket competition, such as occurs in Australia. Supermarkets Coles and Woolworths have been heavily criticized for their low payments to farmers in order to maintain low cost marketing strategies to their customers (Port Curtis Milk Suppliers Co-operative Association 2014).

Thus public engagement in policy debates around food price mechanisms requires only understanding of the need for food to be affordable to low income earners. However, knowledge of the impacts on farmers is also required, so that farmers can remain viable in their food production. Otherwise farmers will seek other agricultural pursuits, such as production of biofuels, or other mechanisms to achieve financial gain, such as sub-division of their land for housing. The net result is that food availability will decline and there will be greater dependency on imported, often processed, foods.

Agri-food literacies that enable people to assess the relative costs and benefits of food prices thus are important. An examination of the motivation of 300 people attending farmers markets in Canada did reveal some understanding of social value, as depicted by the desire to support the local community and the importance of the quality of the product, above price or convenience (Dodds et al. 2014). Wilkins et al. (2002) explored the links between local and seasonal foods and community economic growth, environmental sustainability, human nutrition and food markets or businesses. They concluded that exploring the public's perceptions of terms such as 'local' and 'seasonal' helped to expand food and agriculture system education (Wilkins, Bowditch & Sobal 2002).

A second example of a potential clash between agriculture and social values is the increasing focus in more affluent, educated and urbanized communities on considering the impacts of agricultural practices on animal welfare. Lack of knowledge and in some cases assumptions about animal husbandry practices have led to public outrage when selective footage and reporting of poor animal handling practices have been highly publicized (Bryant 2011). This is an area where concerns may be considered selective, or focused on issues that might be more emotionally appealing. For example, people have a greater affinity with the circumstances of animals with which they are familiar, such as chickens, and may demand and attempt to select food in good faith to support what they believe to be better animal husbandry practice, such as choosing eggs that are 'free range' (Harper & Makatouni 2002). People are less engaged in questions about animal versus plant food sources in a healthy and sustainable diet or the impacts on fish stock sustainability and fish welfare of wild fish capture to appease culinary preferences (Vanhonacker, Berbeke & Sioen 2006).

Agri-food literacy and power

A fourth dimension to agri-food literacy is the issue of power over food production, or food sovereignty. Weiler et al. (2014) argue that a food sovereignty approach moves considerations away from a more simplistic approach of developing individuals' food literacy in terms of food knowledge and cooking skills that result in their becoming rational economic actors responsible for their own health. They argue that a food sovereignty approach encompasses a broader vision of communities' power over food system resources and their abilities to engage with the system on their own terms. It has a particular focus on equalizing power in the food system. Agri-food literacies within such a frame would focus on the political, economic and social power within the food system, mechanisms to address barriers preventing access by communities to socially created solutions to the imbalances of power, democratic participation and equalizing access to material well-being (Weiler et al. 2014). Within this context, individual implicit and explicit food knowledge such as cooking and gardening skills need to be complemented by more emancipatory knowledge of ecological considerations, rights-based perspectives of food production and capacities for collective decision-making and action.

There has been some work to identify the extent to which people are knowledgeable about agri-food systems. Studies of knowledge of agriculture have generally found low levels of agricultural literacy amongst both students (Pense & Leising 2004) and teachers (Terry, Herring & Larke 1992). Harmon and Maretzki (2006) undertook a more broadly based food system survey of students to determine their knowledge, attitudes and experiences. Participants were found to be least knowledgeable about food system sectors, sustainability and agriculture; more knowledgeable about nutrition and food origins; and most knowledgeable about food safety, local foods and hunger. The students' attitudes favoured local food systems, but these attitudes were not supported by their behaviours. The authors found that food system knowledge and attitudes supportive of sustaining the local food system were positively associated with participation in youth clubs, gardening and food related activities at home and negatively associated with television viewing (Harmon & Maretzki 2006). Attempts to increase agricultural literacy also have been found to be inter-mittent (Jepsen, Pastor & Elliot 2007) or exclusionary of older audiences who are directly involved in policy decisions relating to the food system (Igo & Frick 1999). For the agri-food system to be sustainable and successful in meeting the growing demands of the world's expanding population, an agri-food literate society is required. As Livingstone and Smith (2010: 1) concluded in their review of agricultural education:

> There are clear challenges for agriculture in a world with a looming food security crisis, a changing climate, a need to adapt to changing technology, and political discourse that embraces the need to be more green as well as the need to be mindful of the way we undertake animal production processes and outputs. These are not just challenges for agriculture. They are challenges for humanity if we wish to live in a stable world that has a hope of adequately feeding its growing population. This is the same world, which at least in Australia, is seeing a decline in the number of providers of agricultural edu-cation and training, and the number of individual participant learners. In here lie the threats and the opportunities for agricultural education and training.

Overall there is an absence of systematic research of agri-food system literacies, more encompassing than agricultural or environmental literacies alone. The limited research on levels of agricultural literacy has reported low levels of literacy. Thus there is little evidence available to support claims of links between such literacies and outcomes such as improved agri-food systems, greater food security, more healthy or sustainable food choice behaviours or better nutrition.

Urban food production and food literacy

The dominance of urban living around the world has created significant challenges to food production. The continually enlarging cityscapes and sprawling suburban areas encroach on prime agricultural land, with less and poorer lands available for future farming. At the same time the rapidly growing populations require feeding and management of their food and other wastes, which creates environmental challenges. Not only are urban dwellers increasing in number, their food selection preferences place different pressures on food production, with higher demand for meat, fruit and vegetables compared with rural dwellers who eat more cereals, tubers and roots.

The growing divide between the urban dwelling population and the agri-food system that sustains them requires consideration of alternative or at least complementary food production systems. Urban food production is increasingly considered as a viable option to produce food in a sustainable manner. Not only is it deemed to be a location to promote communities' literacies in relation to sustainable production of healthy food that is accessible and affordable, it is also viewed as a mechanism to improve local food security and employment. Urban food production is of increasing importance in agri-food system and urban planning considerations.

Urban agriculture

Urban food production is not new, as human settlements first developed in conjunction with the food production practices that sustained them. Modern industrially based cities initially were no exception. Atkins provides an interesting account of the food sources of London and Paris in the mid-1850s. Then as now, changes in the food systems reflected the technological developments of the time. For example, while initially food was being grown within a walking radius of the city or town, the introduction of railways enabled food to be rapidly transported into the city from more distant localities, much like the rapid transport of food via air travel today. Social changes of the times also impacted on aspects of the cities' food systems. The influx of migrants into London in the 1850s led to an expansion of mobile street vendors while at the same period of time the increased population density of Paris gave rise to food shops and cafes and the expulsion of dairies and fresh meat butchery practices to outside the city (Atkins 2007). Later, around the turn of the nineteenth century, the Garden City Movement in the United Kingdom enjoyed a short-lived popularity and also spread to North America (Buder 1990).

More recently a very wide range of urban-based food production initiatives have been developed, from small scale gardens on road verges and in planter boxes in shopping malls, through to employment schemes, institutionally based food gardens (e.g. in hospital grounds) and large scale economically driven food growing initiatives. Such endeavours aim to maximize food production in a small area for purposes beyond that for home consumption or educational purposes, and may also include farms supplying urban farmers markets, community supported agriculture, and family farms located in metropolitan greenbelts (Golden 2013).

There have been a number of reasons why urban agriculture and community gardens have gained in both urgency and popularity in the past few decades. In 2008 during the time of the global financial crisis, urban and peri-urban agriculture was identified as a strategy to alleviate urban food insecurity and build cities that were more resilient to crisis (Food and Agriculture Organization 2008). However, for this to be successful and sustainable in the longer term will require a paradigm shift in urban design policy and planning that is 'more focussed on urban food security, improved environmental management and enhanced rural-urban linkages' (Food and Agriculture Organization 2008: 3).

Other drivers include concerns about the environmental footprint of food production, issues of food sovereignty and communities wishing to reclaim power in the agri-food system (Grayson, Richards & Rose 2013), concerns about the increasingly processed nature of foods and associated health concerns, recognition of urban agriculture as an avenue of employment for youth and new migrants (Moustier & Danso 2006), addressing food insecurity within urban areas (Karanja & Njenga 2011) and also the increasing recognition of the role that food production can play in people's lives (Mansfield & Kelly 2013). A recent review by Warren, Hawkesworth and Knai (2015) of the impacts of urban agriculture found some associations with increased dietary diversity and food consumption but variable outcomes in relation to improving food security. Unfortunately evidence of the benefits of urban agriculture initiatives is limited due to scarce studies and poor research designs.

This array of issues with potential to be linked with urban agriculture thus makes it challenging to identify specific food literacies pertaining to or arising from these initiatives. Some view urban agriculture as an opportunity to increase implicit and explicit knowledge of food production, seasonality, food safety measures or basic familiarity with primary food products for households and generations unfamiliar with the production of food, especially when specifically linked with onsite education programmes (Travaline & Hunold 2010). Some of these inferred food knowledge areas are deemed to translate into viable employment skills (Meenar & Hoover 2011). There are also many claims about emancipatory knowledge related to urban agriculture, for example that engagement in local food production or markets will assist in reclaiming power within the agri-food system through influencing planning and retail policies or greater understanding of ecological citizenship (Travaline & Hunold 2010).

However, there are also those who have more cautious views of the value of urban agriculture. One more cynical perspective by Hallsworth and Wong

(2013) attributed the expansion of urban agriculture to political popularism rather than to real gains in availability or affordability of fresh foods for city dwellers. These concerns were echoed by Meenar and Hoover (2012) who also raised limitations of urban agriculture to address the food security and social equity goals often claimed by proponents. While acknowledging the important role of urban agriculture in relation to community food security, particularly in disadvantaged communities, they identified several areas of concern, such as inaccessibility of project information, social exclusion, inequitable food distribution and limited economic contributions in poor neighbourhoods.

In conclusion, there is some limited research evidence in relation to links between urban agriculture and the development of food system or nutrition literacy. There is clear evidence that urban agriculture can play an important social role within communities and is positively valued. Confirming its potential beyond the aesthetic or emotional appeal to also being a functional and core component of urban living is still to be achieved.

Community gardens

Community gardens could be considered a sub-group of urban food production mainly characterized by being managed by a group of people from the local community. They can be considered in a variety of forms. As larger initiatives, they could be similar to urban agriculture, with greater land areas involved and the aim of producing food for local communities. The victory gardens during war times are one example, where local municipalities converted public lands to food production locations tended on a voluntary basis by local residents (Armstrong 2000), with reportedly close to 40% of fresh vegetables consumed in the USA during the Second World War being produced in community gardens (Murphy cited in Armstrong 2000). Smaller scale community gardens have become increasingly common in more recent years, with local residents reclaiming vacant lands or rooftop spaces for gardening.

The incentives for smaller scale community gardens have been cited as numerous, including reconnecting with the land, promoting green space, increasing social connectedness and consumption of locally produced foods. Community gardeners themselves perceive numerous health benefits, including improved nutrition, increased physical activity and improved mental health. Community gardens are also seen to promote social health and community cohesion. These reported benefits are claimed despite limited understanding of gardening by the community members, insecurity of access to locations for the gardens, resistance by government officials, inconsistent access to resources and sometimes concerns about soil contamination (Wakefield et al. 2007).

Some studies report improved health behaviours related to community gardening, while others identify lack of strong supporting research evidence. A review of the impacts of community gardens by McCormack et al. (2010) found few well designed research studies (those incorporating control groups) utilizing valid and reliable dietary assessment methods to evaluate the influence of community gardens on nutrition-related outcomes. However, more recently Litt et al. (2011) found that community garden participation was significantly associated with (self-reported) fruit and vegetable intake. Barnidge et al. (2013) using both intercept and population-based surveys also found that participation in a community garden was associated with higher self-reported fruit and vegetable consumption. However, while these studies have found promising results in relation to food behaviours, albeit self-reported, the extent to which community gardens may impact on participants' food literacy skills is yet to be fully explored.

Home gardens/school food gardens

Home gardens have been a tradition in many areas of the world, in affluent households (the landed gentry and churches could afford property and produce their own foods) through to small scale subsistence farmers, whose home garden produce sustained them during times of hardship or between seasons.

Home gardening refers to 'the cultivation of a small portion of land which may be around the household or within walking distance from the family home' (Odebode 2006: 48). Home gardens in developed countries are usually small areas for production of food for personal or family use. However, globally, home gardens serve many purposes, for example for production of indigenous medicines, to provide fuel (manure from cattle) or to produce food for the local market to supplement the household's income. The potential benefits of home gardening are thus multiple, including improved nutrition and food security, and social, economic or environmental impacts (Landon-Lane 2004). These benefits can be especially great for women-headed households (Odebode 2006). Home gardens in developed countries have recently received greater media attention, driven by celebrity chefs and cooking competitions more than by considerations of population based benefits or benefits to vulnerable communities.

The benefits of home gardening, especially in relation to food literacy, nutrition and health outcomes, have not been well researched. There is some support for the health benefits of participation in gardening (Schmutz et al. 2014) but the sustainability of home gardens has been questioned, as has been their potential longer term economic benefits or empowerment opportunities (Langellotto 2014). However, the potential benefits of home gardens in conflict or post-conflict communities have received heightened attention with the increase in civic unrest in many countries. For viable models of home gardening that may provide economic or nutritional value, structural support such as access to new technologies, extension and advisory services, and women empowerment strategies are required.

School food gardens have also been recorded for many decades. More recently they have been established in response to community and government concerns about food security in poor neighbourhoods, lack of children's food knowledge and the rising rates of obesity of children and adults.

The school food garden may take many forms. At one level it may be a focus of a particular teacher, enthused to encourage students to understand where their food comes from or to support organic or permaculture gardening principles. Food gardens in schools also may be much grander affairs, adopted by the whole school community and closely linked with the school's curriculum. When integrated across the whole school there is some evidence that participation in school food gardens can improve children's fruit and vegetable consumption (Christian et al. 2014). One example of an integrated approach to the school food gardens is the Stephanie Alexander Kitchen Garden Program. Initiated in the state of Victoria, Australia, this school food garden is closely linked with a kitchen in which to prepare the foods grown in the garden. Links across the curriculum are encouraged, with mathematics being taught through adjusting recipes or measuring garden plots, and science and sustainability taught in the gardens.

School food gardens have undergone several evaluations, indicating positive changes in students' knowledge of growing foods, their confidence and skills in preparing foods and their enjoyment of eating foods that they had grown and prepared (Yeatman et al. 2013). These evaluations primarily have been based on qualitative reporting, with as yet limited quantitative evidence (Gibbs et al. 2013; Hutchinson et al. 2015). However, these evaluations do provide some support to the improvement of food literacy through participation in school food gardening, especially if the gardening initiatives are part of wider food-based education programmes and experiences in schools.

Conclusions

Food production is no longer a daily part of the majority of people's lives. One consequence of this is that opportunities to benefit and learn from engaging in food production activities have been diminished or lost altogether. While the economic and political benefits to society of having people concentrated in urban areas are great, some essential elements of living, such as knowledge and understanding related to the fundamental act of eating to maintain health and well-being or the essential roles that food plays in society, culture and economics, have been significantly diminished.

Understanding the role that being engaged or associated with food production has in developing food literacies and influencing healthy eating behaviours is not yet well researched. There has been some limited work in the area of agricultural literacies but this appears to be ineffectual. Development of environmental literacies has reported wider successes but these initiatives may not have positive outcomes for sustainable and sufficient food production.

Recent reports of evaluation of school garden initiatives may provide some important insights into the links between food production and development of food literacies. Greatest impacts have been reported when whole school approaches have been undertaken, embedding food production as a valued and core element of the school, integrated in wider school curricula and underpinned by the school's relationships with its community. This implies that a more systemic, institutional change is required to instil a valuing of food production and food literacies as core elements of children's education.

Incorporating values into the development of food literacies is consistent with Yang's epistemology of knowledge as comprising implicit, explicit and emancipatory knowledge areas. While food knowledge and skills are essential elements of food literacy, so too is the value that food has in our lives, including the many roles that it plays socially, culturally, economically and environmentally. Involvement with and understanding of food production processes and systems can assist people in recognizing the social and environmental impacts of their food choices. More broadly, such knowledge and understanding enable people to understand societal systems more broadly, as food systems are reflective of wider changes, locally and globally, affecting everyone's lives.

References

Armstrong, D. (2000) A survey of community gardens in upstate New York: Implications for health promotion and community development. *Health & Place* 6, 319–327.

Atkins, P.J. (2007) A tale of two cities: A comparison of food systems in London and Paris in the 1850s, in Lummel, P., Oddy, D.J. & Atkins, P.J. (eds) *Food in the City in Europe since the Late Eighteenth Century*. pp 25–38. Ashgate, England.

Australian Farm Institute (2014) *Carbon Farming Extension and Outreach: Case Studies for Farmers and Land Managers*, Australian Farm Institute, Surry Hills, Australia.

Barnidge, E., Hipp, P.R., Estlund, A., Duggan, K., Barnhart, K. & Brownson, R. (2013) Association between community garden participation and fruit and vegetable consumption in rural Missouri. *International Journal of Behavioral Nutrition and Physical Activity* 10, 128–136.

Britnell, R. (2011) *Agricultural Literacy – Farming Matters. A Report for Nuffield Australia*. Nuffield Australia Project No. 1102, Nuffierd Australia, New South Wales.

Bryant, N. (2011) *Australia Bans all Live Cattle Exports to Indonesia*. BBC, 8 June. Retrieved 6 August 2015 from http://www.bbc.com/news/world-asia-pacific- 13692211.

Buder, S. (1990) *Visionaries and Planners: The Garden City Movement and the Modern Community*. Oxford University Press, Oxford.

Christian, M., Evans, C., Nykjaer, C., Hancock, N. & Cade, J. (2014) Evaluation of the impact of a school gardening intervention on children's fruit and vegetable intake: A randomised controlled trial. *International Journal of Behavioural Nutrition and Activity* 11(19). Retrieved 3 September 2015 from http://www.ijbnpa.org/content/pdf/s12966-014-0099-7.pdf.

Dodds, R., Holmes, M., Arunsopha, V., Chin, N., Le, T., Maung, S. & Shum, M. (2014) Consumer choice and farmers' markets. *Journal of Agricultural and Environmental Ethics* 27, 397–416. DOI:10.1007/s10806-013-9469-4.

Food and Agriculture Organization (2008) *Food for the Cities*. Retrieved 6 August 2015 from http://www.fao.org/fcit/upa/en/.

Frick, M.J., Kahler, A.A. & Miller, W.W. (1991) A definition and the concepts of agricultural literacy. *Journal of Agricultural Education* 32(2), 49–57. DOI:10.5032/jae.1991.02049.

Gibbs, L., Staiger, P., Johnson, B., Block, K., Macfarlane, S., Gold, L., Kulas, J., Townsend, M., Long, C. & Ukoumunne, O. (2013) Expanding children's food experiences: The impact of a school-based kitchen garden program. *Journal of Nutrition Education and Behavior* 45(2), 137–146.

Golden, S. (2013) *Urban Agriculture Impacts: Social, Health and Economic: A Literature Review.* UC Sustainable Agriculture Research and Education Program, Agricultural Sustainability Institute at UC Davis. Retrieved 18 August 2015 from http://asi.ucdavis.edu/resources/publications/UA%20Lit%20Review-%20Golden%20Reduced%2011-15.pdf.

Grayson, R., Richards, C. & Rose, N. (2013) *The People's Food Plan. A Common-sense Approach to a Tasty, Resilient and Fair Food System for all Australians Policy Directions.* Australian Food Sovereignty Alliance. Retrieved 6 August 2015 from http://www.australianfoodsovereigntyalliance.org/wp-content/uploads/2012/10/PFP-policy-august13.pdf.

Hallsworth, A. & Wong, A. (2013) Urban gardening: A valuable activity, but... *Journal of Agriculture, Food Systems, and Community Development* 3(2), 11–14. Retrieved 20 December 2015 from http://dx.doi.org/10.5304/jafscd.2013.032.010.

Harmon, A.H. & Maretzki, A.N. (2006) A survey of food system knowledge, attitudes, and experiences among high school students. *Journal of Hunger & Environmental Nutrition* 1(1), 59–82. DOI: 10.1300/J477v01n01_05.

Harper, G.C. & Makatouni, A. (2002) Consumer perception of organic food production and farm animal welfare. *British Food Journal* 104, 287–299. DOI: org/10.1108/00070700210425723.

Hutchinson, J., Christian, M., Evans, C., Nykjaer, C., Hancock, N. & Cade, J. (2015) Evaluation of the impact of school gardening interventions on children's knowledge of and attitudes towards fruit and vegetables. A cluster randomised controlled trial. *Appetite* 91(2015), 405–414.

Igo, C. & Frick, M. (1999) A case study assessment of standard and benchmarks for implementing food and fibre systems literacy. *Proceedings of the 18th Annual Western Region Agricultural Education Research Meeting.* Retrieved 6 August 2015 from http://pubs.aged.tamu.edu/conferences/WRAERC1999/pdf/wr-1999-218.pdf.

Jepsen, H., Pastor, M. & Elliot, J. (2007) Agricultural perceptions of the participants of the Summer Agricultural Institute. *Proceedings of the 2007 Association for Career and Technical Education Research 41st Annual Research Conference.* Retrieved 6 August 2015 from http://www.agedweb.org/WRAEC/2006/documents/c3poster.pdf.

Karanja, N. & Njenga, M. (2011) Feeding the cities, Chapter 10 in *Worldwatch Institute, State of the World 2011: Innovations that Nourish the Planet.* Worldwatch Institute, Washington, DC.

Kovar, K. & Ball, A. (2013) Two decades of agricultural literacy research: A synthesis of the literature. *Journal of Agricultural Education* 54(1), 167–178. DOI: 10.5032/jae.2013.01167.

Landon-Lane, C. (2004) *Livelihoods Grow in Gardens.* Agricultural Support Systems Division, Food and Agriculture Organization of the United Nations, Rome. Retrieved 3 September 2015 from ftp://ftp.fao.org/docrep/fao/006/y5112e/y5112e00.pdf.

Langellotto, G.A. (2014) What are the economic costs and benefits of home vegetable gardens? *Journal of Extension* 52(2) article # 2RIB5. Retrieved 3 September 2015 from http://www.joe.org/joe/2014april/pdf/JOE_v52_2rb5.pdf.

Litt, J., Soobader, Mah-J., Turbin, M., Hale, J., Buchenau, M. & Marshall, J. (2011) The influence of social involvement, neighborhood aesthetics, and community garden participation on fruit and vegetable consumption. *American Journal of Public Health* 101, 1466–1473. DOI:10.2105/AJPH.2010.300111.

Livingstone, S. & Smith, P. (2010) Agricultural education and the challenges of now and the future, Industry Paper. Retrieved 20 December 2015 from http://www.marcusold ham.vic.edu.au/_literature_115161/Agricultural_Education_and_the_Challenges_of_ Now_and_the_Future_-_August_2010.

Lockie, S., Lyons, K., Lawrence, G. & Mummery, K. (2002) Eating green: Motivations behind organic food consumption in Australia. *Sociologia Ruralis* 42(1), 23–40. DOI: 10.1111/1467-9523.00200.

Mansfield, B. & Kelly, T. (2013) *What Feeds Us: Vancouver Food Strategy.* City of Vancouver. Retrieved 6 August 2015 from http://vancouver.ca/files/cov/vancouver-food-strategy-final.PDF.

McCormack, L.A., Laska, M.N., Larson, N. & Story, M. (2010) Review of the nutritional implications of farmers' markets and community gardens: A call for evaluation and research efforts. *Journal of the American Dietetic Association* 110, 399–408.

Meenar, M. & Hoover, B. (2011) *Food Insecurity and Spatial Inequality in Philadelphia's Lower-income Neighbourhoods: Analysing the Role of Community Gardens.* Centre for Sustainable Communities, Temple University. Retrieved 6 August 2015 from https:// phillyfoodjustice.files.wordpress.com/2011/10/meenar2011_philacommgarden_food insecurity.pdf.

Meenar, M. & Hoover, B. (2012) Community food security via urban agriculture: Understanding people, place, economy, and accessibility from a food justice perspective. *Journal of Agriculture, Food Systems, and Community Development* 3(1), 143–160. Retrieved 6 August 2015 from http://dx.doi.org/10.5304/jafscd.2012.031.013.

Moustier, P. & Danso, G. (2006) *Local Economic Development and Marketing of Urban Produced Food.* Resource Centres on Urban Agriculture & Food Security. Retrieved 8 August 2015 from http://www.ruaf.org/

Odebode, S.O. (2006) Assessment of home gardening as a potential source of household income in Adinyele local government area of Oyo state. *Nigerian Journal of Horticultural Science* 11(1), 47–55.

Pense, S.L. & Leising, J.G. (2004) An assessment of food and fiber systems knowledge in selected Oklahoma high schools. *Journal of Agricultural Education* 45(3), 86–96. DOI: 10.5032/jae2004.03086.

Port Curtis Milk Suppliers Co-operative Association (2014) A fair price for fresh QLD Milk – that's all we ask. Agricultural competitiveness white paper submission – IP286 Port Curtis Milk Suppliers Co-operative Association Limited. Retrieved 6 August 2015 from http://agwhitepaper.agriculture.gov.au.

Schmutz, U., Lennartsson, M., Williams, S., Devereaux, M. & Davies, G. (2014) *The Benefits of Gardening and Food Growing for Health and Wellbeing.* Garden Organic and Sustain. Retrieved 3 September 2015 from http://www.sustainweb.org/resources/ files/reports/GrowingHealth_BenefitsReport.pdf.

Schneider, M. (2008) We are hungry! A summary report of food riots, government responses, and states of democracy in 2008. Retrieved 6 August 2015 from http:// www.academia.edu/238430/.

Stephanie Alexander Kitchen Garden Foundation. Retrieved 3 September 2015 from http s://www.kitchengardenfoundation.org.au/.

Story, M., Kaphingst, K.M., Robertson-OBrien, R. & Glanz, K. (2007) Creating healthy food and eating environments: Policy and environmental approaches. *Annual Review of Public Health* 29, 253–272. DOI: 10.1146/annurev.publhealth.29.020907.090926.

Tarcher, J.P. (2005) *The Real Food Revival*, Penguin, New York.

Terry, R., Jr., Herring, D.R. & Larke, A., Jr. (1992) Assistance needed for elementary teachers in Texas to implement programs of agricultural literacy. *Journal of Agricultural Education*, 33(2), 51–60.

Thalbitzer, A.F., (2010) cited in Britnell, R. *Agricultural Literacy - Farming Matters. A Report for Nuffield Australia*. Nuffield Australia Project No 1102. Retrieved 6 August 2015 from http://www.nuffieldinternational.org/rep_pdf/1354671353Roma_Brit nell_final_report.pdf.

Travaline, K. & Hunold, C. (2010) Urban agriculture and ecological citizenship in Philadelphia. *Local Environment* 15(6), 581–590.

UNEP (2012) *Avoiding Future Famines: Strengthening the Ecological Foundation of Food Security through Sustainable Food Systems*. United Nations Environment Programme (UNEP), Nairobi, Kenya. Retrieved 6 August 2015 from http://www.unep.org/.

UNESCO (1976) The Belgrade Charter. A global framework for environmental education. *UNESCO-UNEP Environmental Education Newsletter* 1(1), 2. Retrieved 6 August 2015 from http://unesdoc.unesco.org/images/0015/001533/153391eb.pdf.

United Nations (1992) *Agenda 21. Sustainable Development*. United Nations Conference on Environment & Development, Rio de Janiero, Brazil, 3–14 June 1992.

United Nations (2015) Draft resolution submitted by the President of the General Assembly. Draft outcome document of the United Nations summit for the adoption of the post-2015 development agenda. General Assembly. Retrieved 2 September 2015 from http://www.un.org/ga/search/view_doc.asp?symbol=A/69/L.85&Lang=E.

Vanhonacker, F., Berbeke, W. & Sioen, I. (2006) Consumer perception about ethical and sustainability issues of fish, in Kaiser, M. & Lien, M. (eds) *Ethics and the Politics of Food*. Wageningen Academic Publisher, The Netherlands.

Wakefield, S., Yeudall, F., Taron, C., Reynolds, J. & Skinner, A. (2007) Growing urban health: Community gardening in South-East Toronto. *Health Promotion International* 22, 92–101.

Warren, E., Hawkesworth, S. & Knai, C. (2015) Investigating the association between urban agriculture and food security, dietary diversity, and nutritional status: A systematic literature review. *Food Policy* 53, 54–66.

Weiler, A., Hergesheimer, C., Brisbois, B., Wittman, H., Yassi, A. & Spiegel, J. (2014) Food sovereignty, food security and health equity: A meta-narrative mapping exercise. *Health Policy and Planning*, 1–15. DOI:10.1093/heapol/czu109.

Wilkins, J. L., Bowdish, E. & Sobal, J. (2002) Consumer perceptions of seasonal and local foods: A study in a US community. *Ecology of Food and Nutrition* 41, 415–439.

Yang, B. (2003) Toward a holistic theory of knowledge and adult learning. *Human Resource Development Review* 2(2), 106–129.

Yeatman, H., Quinsey, K., Dawber, J.P., Nielsen, W.S., Condon-Paoloni, D., Eckermann, S., Morris, D., Grootemaat, P.E. & Fildes, D.L. (2013) *Stephanie Alexander Kitchen Garden National Program Evaluation: Final Report*. Centre for Health Service Development, Australian Health Services Research Institute, University of Wollongong.

13 Measuring food literacy

Rebecca McKecknie

Introduction

A previous lack of understanding and formal definition of food literacy has resulted in significant variation in the methods of assessment used to evaluate food literacy programmes or to measure this phenomenon in scientific literature. Even with the development of a formal definition, the multidimensional and contextual nature of food literacy creates complexities in regards to its potential measurement. This chapter discusses the rationale behind the measurement of food literacy, the complexities associated with its measurement as well as limitations of and recommendations for current practice in the measurement and evaluation of food literacy programmes and research.

The importance of measuring food literacy

Why do we measure?

To measure is to 'ascertain the size, amount or degree of something' (typically using an instrument, device or measurement scale), and to 'assess the importance, effect or value' (*Oxford Dictionary of English* 2010). Measurement is an essential component across many disciplines (health-related and other), whether it be in practice, research or as an act of everyday living. Across all disciplines and levels of health specifically, decisions must be made about healthcare in order to justify actions, assess effectiveness of and improve services, maximize efficiencies and direct resources appropriately. Thus, the ability to measure and subsequently identify tangible values and the importance or effect of a determinant or outcome is required in order to make critical decisions regarding health-related issues and care (Streiner & Norman 2008).

The selection of an appropriate tool or device to measure a construct is based on the concepts of validity and reliability. Validity refers to the ability of a tool, device or scale to measure what it is intended to measure. Reliability refers to the ability of a device, tool or scale to measure in a consistent and reproducible fashion. Whilst seemingly simple in theory, there are in fact multiple procedures through which validity and reliability are assessed (McDowell 2006; Streiner &

Table 13.1 Processes for assessing/stages of testing for validity and reliability

Process of assessing/stage of testing for validity and reliability	Description
Validity	
Face validation	The degree to which, on face value, a scale appears to be measuring the desired concept
Content validation	The degree to which a scale measures all required underlying content domains, constructs or concepts, usually confirmed by expert review
Criterion/concurrent validation	The degree to which a scale is correlated with another measure of the same trait, ideally the gold standard (i.e. the degree to which a measure of food literacy correlates with another measure of food literacy)
Convergent validation	The degree to which a scale correlates with other factors known to be associated with the concept to be measured
Construct validation	The degree to which a scale measures the desired concept or construct
Reliability	
Test-retest/intra-rater reliability	The degree to which a scale will measure a concept consistently when repeated across two time points
Inter-rater reliability	The degree to which a scale will measure a concept consistently when measures are repeated by different interviewers/examiners
Internal consistency	The degree to which relevant items included in a scale are measuring the same concept

Norman 2008). Table 13.1 summarizes the various procedures for the assessment of validity and reliability of a health-related measurement scale. The ideal tool for measurement of any concept is both valid and reliable; that is, it is able to actually measure the intended concept in a consistent and reproducible fashion.

Should we measure food literacy?

Acknowledging the importance of food literacy to diet and health, various nutrition policies and interventions across countries internationally include a key focus on improving nutrition through enhanced food literacy (International Union of Nutrition Sciences 2005; Parliament of Australia 2009). However, there have been conflicting views as to the necessity for measuring food literacy; as food literacy is unanimously acknowledged as being an important and implicit component to diet and health, its measurement has been regarded as potentially redundant. However, in a climate of limited resources, practitioners and policy makers have a responsibility to ensure that the use of resources is transparent and directed to programmes and interventions that are creating effective outcomes amongst 'at need' groups. Evaluation of such programmes allows for judgement as to how they are planned and implemented, the performance of staff, improvements in the implementation and subsequent effectiveness of programmes, and to satisfy programme sponsors and stakeholders (Oshaug 1997).

It has been acknowledged that a marked gap exists in surveillance and intervention data surrounding food literacy programmes, which limits understanding of and potential to improve this important determinant of food and health (Government of Canada 2010). The previous lack of a formal definition for food literacy, and a limited understanding of its underlying domains and their association with nutrition, resulted in the use of varying terminology related to 'food knowledge', 'food skills' or 'food behaviours' being used in place of and interchangeably with 'food literacy' (Vidgen 2014). As such, the evaluation of interventions and strategies aimed at enhancing food literacy is often limited to only the process and impact of the nutrition intervention (i.e. with failure to assess the longer term outcome), and/or to only one component of food literacy, such as improvements in knowledge or food preparation skills (Byrd-Bredbenner 2004; Caraher et al. 1999; Devine, Farrell & Hartman 2005). Furthermore, there has been no apparent consistency or consensus regarding the tools that are used to evaluate aspects of food literacy, resulting in the use of varying evaluation tools and techniques across programmes, leaving limited opportunity for comparisons of programme implementation and effectiveness, or for the identification of specific limitations of programmes as to which domains of food literacy they are able and unable to address.

The limitations associated with evaluation mean that there is a lack of evidence regarding the effectiveness of food literacy programmes within their respective population subgroups. As such, the true efficacy, legitimacy and sustainability of previous and existing programmes remain unknown, limiting accountability and opportunities for improvement and tailoring of interventions and strategies (Vidgen 2014). With the large number of varying programmes designed to enhance food literacy, the ability to define and subsequently accurately measure food literacy is essential to assess effectiveness, for comparison of effectiveness across programmes and population sub-groups, to assess need and for justification of resource allocation. Accurate measurements will allow for better understanding of the concept of food literacy, and will assist public health officials, policy makers and service providers in assessing the changing needs of target populations and tailoring interventions to specifically meet the needs of these groups. Furthermore, the measurement of food literacy and subsequent evaluation of food literacy aligns with the best practice principles of food literacy programmes as outlined in Chapter 11.

Considerations for measuring food literacy

Broader considerations for measuring food literacy

Food literacy is a complex, multidimensional concept, with individual but inter-related domains consisting of food related knowledge and skills, and the behavioural responses to these, which combined define an individual or household's 'food literacy' (Vidgen 2014; Vidgen & Gallegos 2014). A comprehensive measure of food literacy should seek to assess the three characteristics (knowledge, skills and behaviours) across each identified domain.

As with many other health related concepts, food literacy is not able to be 'directly' measured (as is the case with characteristics such as weight and height). Instead, its measurement requires consensus as to the concepts underlying food literacy (as created in the work by Vidgen 2014) and the assembly of multiple indicators to reflect the combination of these concepts (McDowell 2006). To date, only one tool exists that specifically measures 'food literacy' as a concept with multiple underlying domains. This tool was developed and validated among a population of New Zealand school children aged nine to ten years (O'Sullivan 2015). Attempts to extend this tool for use to other populations have not been undertaken, so its validity and reliability outside of the specific population in which it was developed remain unknown. However, food and eating are essential to life; learning processes associated with these are ongoing and occur to varying degrees across the life course; and the settings in which this learning occurs vary, including informal settings such as the home, cooking shows on television and celebrity chefs, and planned educational programmes implemented through schools, formal cooking classes and demonstrations (Vidgen 2014). In addition, whilst food literacy is most often discussed as an individual characteristic, it may also change in response to changes at the global, national, community and household level (Vidgen & Gallegos 2014). As such, the concept of food literacy, and the concepts relevant to its measurement, may exist to varying degrees and importance across each of these and it is unlikely that one single measure of food literacy will be able to assess the full continuum. Instead, a range of measures addressing the various stages of the life course and levels at which food literacy is affected are likely to be required. In developing such measures, the use of pre-existing tools is desirable, due to potential savings in terms of time and cost, and such items are more likely to have undergone testing and have been identified as psychometrically valid. Alternatively, the creation of new items requires careful thought, and significant time commitments, as once finalized, statistical manipulation is not able to rectify the inaccuracies that may arise from poorly worded or ambiguous questions (Streiner & Norman 2008). Regardless, both the selection and/or development of items to create a tool to measure food literacy must be done within the context of some unique challenges.

Food literacy is a highly contextual phenomenon; the nature of each underlying domain and its importance relative to other domains varies according to context. As such, the identification or development of a valid and reliable measure of food literacy requires consideration as to how domains are contextually driven, and the implications that a change in one domain may have on other domains. Depending on the context and situation, one or more domains may not be relevant and therefore should not be measured. For example, an intervention may seek to specifically enhance knowledge and skills for reading labels – warranting measurement of the 'selection' domain, but not other domains of food literacy. To accommodate this, measures of food literacy would ideally allow for the measurement of each domain to 'stand alone' as well as be combined in an overall score. This in turn also poses unique challenges for the classification of food literacy 'status', and the identification of respective cut-off points. There are no acknowledged criteria for what constitutes 'good' or 'poor' levels of food literacy, and, as mentioned above, the importance and relevance of the different domains of food insecurity vary across population sub-groups, situations and stages of the life course (Vidgen 2014). As such, lower scores in one domain of food literacy may not necessarily reflect low food literacy within a particular context, making the potential scoring and subsequent categorization of responses to a measure particularly complex.

As the activities associated with cooking and eating are often activities of daily living embedded within unconscious practices, people may find it particularly difficult to verbalize factors or considerations associated with these (Dowler, Caraher & Lincoln 2007; Dowler et al. 2011), particularly in response to quantitative enquiry, as would most likely be the case in the development of a measurement scale. Thus the accuracy of a quantitative tool to assess food literacy may be limited. Furthermore, efforts at measuring food literacy may be impeded by response bias and differential responses to items. It is well known that questions relating to food and diet are prone to social desirability bias (Herbert et al. 1995); previous studies have identified that when asked about fruit and vegetable intake, respondents to questions tend to overestimate the amount of fruit and vegetables that they eat (Herbert et al. 2008). In the context of food literacy, questions pertaining to financial management and beliefs and behaviours pertaining to healthy eating may be more likely to elicit positive or affirmative responses, not necessarily because they are true, or a beneficial outcome has been achieved by a programme, but due to intentional manipulation of answers by respondents based on the desire to report what they believe will be appreciated or respected by the researcher (van de Mortel 2008). In order to truly and more accurately capture the essence and depth of food literacy, an approach incorporating mixed methods may be more appropriate in its measurement.

There is debate as to whether the assessment of food literacy should include knowledge, attitudes and skills specific to food, or whether these should be assessed as generic activities that complement daily living. For example, measures for budgeting and financial skills may not necessarily investigate financial skills and ability within the context of food or food literacy. Rather, many exist that assess general budgeting ability across a variety of activities or tasks (Cramer et al. 2004; Gundersen & Garasky 2012). It could be argued that the ability to manage finances as an activity of everyday life would translate to ability to adopt a food budgeting system. The use of generic scales or items in particular may address some of the complexities associated with measuring a concept as contextual as food literacy as their use may maximize the generalizability of results, allowing comparisons across a broader range of contexts and situations. Furthermore, as more generic or unrelated measures exist in the published literature, utilizing generic items may maximize chances of identifying suitable alternatives that have previously been validated. In addition, generic scales may provide the opportunity to truly assess the main effect of interventions, which may extend beyond the improvement of knowledge, attitudes and skills beyond the context of food and food literacy (i.e. such as the case of financial management and planning skills and abilities). However, the use of a generic scale may include items that are not conducive to measurement within the context of the construct being measured, effectively creating 'white noise' and more items than necessary for inclusion in a scale. In the context of tool development, items that are not conducive to measurement should be removed from a tool, and the aim is to create a scale that contains as few questions as possible (Streiner & Norman 2008).

Finally, given the varying contexts in which a tool to measure food literacy may be applied, considerations as to response options and categories, formatting and the mode of administration (i.e. face-to-face, interviewer administered, online, paper-based, etc.) are also warranted, and should focus on identifying the most appropriate for each relevant target group.

Considerations for measuring specific domains of food literacy

Planning and management

The concepts underlying planning and management include prioritizing money (budgeting) and time for food, planning food intake, and making feasible decisions which balance food need with available resources. Balancing food decisions based around need compared to resources often comprises consideration of how money is managed and spent, and budgeting is also considered an important component for the efficient planning of meals. As such, the concepts that make up this domain are inextricably linked and may be measured interchangeably or within the same tool.

A variety of strategies exists through which individuals and households manage finances; as such there is a limited understanding or consensus as to what concepts define the knowledge, skills and behaviours associated with budgeting and/or finances, and therefore limited consensus regarding how they can be measured (Huston 2010). Whilst opportunity exists to qualitatively investigate the variety of strategies and adoption of these across different contexts and situations, the assessment of budgeting and/or financial management via a simple or self-administered quantitative survey is more of a challenge (Dowler 1998). Budgeting strategies and balancing food decisions are context specific, and more common strategies rely on certain conditions, including easy access to adequate food retail and/or transport to access such facilities, which may fail to be acknowledged in a measurement context (Dowler 1998). In addition, the nature of the topic is often considered sensitive by those from whom data is collected, increasing the possibility of response bias as people become concerned about criticism or judgement of financial mismanagement or poor decision making (Dowler 1998); this risk may be particularly prevalent among lower income individuals or households.

Previous attempts have been made to measure food budgeting behaviours by assessing total dollar expenditure on food, and, in some instances, specific expenditure on fruits and vegetables and take-away or fast foods (Flego et al. 2013; Herbert et al. 2014). Whilst it has been identified that low-income households are able to accurately recall the amount of money spent on purchasing food (Dowler 1998), limited information is available as to whether this accuracy is maintained when asking about healthy foods specifically. A focus on healthy foods may predispose a budget recall question to response bias, with households potentially over-reporting healthy food expenditure. To address the potential issue of response bias associated with budget recall methods, evaluations of nutrition programmes in the USA have adopted objective measurement strategies by incorporating the provision of receipts for food purchasing (Burney 2002). Budgeting skills are also assessed in terms of confidence, investigating self-perceptions of confidence in being able to prepare meals that are low in price, or purchasing fruits and vegetables on an existing budget (Flego et al. 2013). Such measures rely on the informant being able to accurately report on their financial abilities, and as mentioned above, risk the participant intentionally inflating estimates of such capabilities due to perceived fear of judgement of financial mismanagement or poor decisions (Cramer et al. 2004).

Efforts to measure 'meal planning' have incorporated some of the budgeting measures identified above, as well as the use of shopping lists (as shopping lists have been identified as being associated with meal planning and the adoption of healthier eating habits, specifically an increased consumption of vegetables). The most common method of assessing use of a shopping list is to ask the participant the frequency with which one is utilized (to which responses may be either predetermined frequency categories, or a continuous response from the participant) (Burney 2002; Fruh et al. 2013). Investigations have also assessed the frequency of preplanning meals, including how frequently meals are planned prior to 9am each day, frequency with which menus are planned two to three days in advance and a week in advance (Fruh et al. 2013). The validity and reliability of these existing measures have not been identified, so it is unclear the extent to which these truly reflect meal planning practices. Furthermore, relying on the use of lists to assess the ability to plan meals may not accurately capture the true extent of a person's food literacy; it is possible that with enhancements/improvements across the other domains of food literacy, a person may have less use/requirement for a shopping list as their overall food literacy is enhanced.

The potential to assess balancing food need in relation to resources is complicated by individuals or households developing their own systems and beliefs around food preferences, need and therefore decisions. The combination of such factors is complex, highly individualized and context specific; as such, this component of food literacy may be particularly difficult to assess (Asp 1999). Due to the complexities associated with food-related decision making, this concept may be more appropriately investigated via qualitative methodologies, which would allow for the collection of rich, in-depth data in order to understand how individuals, families and households balance food need with available resources (Gillespie & Gillespie 2007). Previous efforts at capturing data pertaining to balancing food need in relation to resources has been limited to the factors or barriers influencing food decisions, failing to acknowledge how these decisions are balanced in the context of available resources (Furst et al. 1996).

Selection

Assessing the 'selection' domain requires investigations into food access, food shopping practices and understanding and utilizing food products.

Food access is characterized by a number of underlying components, including both aspects of physical and financial access to food. Measures to assess food access have traditionally incorporated environmental audits and mapping, including the collection of information regarding food retail outlets and their location. Such data provides opportunity to identify the potential food access available to residents in a particular area or region, but is unable to capture the combination of sources through which an individual or household might access food, or their understanding of the benefits or disadvantages associated with the sources that they may access. Some efforts to capture food shopping practices have been undertaken, in which individuals have been asked about the location of shopping and store type, and reasons for shopping at particular food retail outlets (Ayala et al. 2005). The reasons for shopping at a particular outlet are often investigated, and may provide insight into people's perceived benefits and thus decisions to shop in particular locations, but these methods fail to directly assess the knowledge of the advantages and disadvantages of accessing foods from a variety of sources. Such information may be particularly difficult to capture through quantitative investigation, as the perceived advantages and disadvantages of different food sources are likely to differ between individuals, situations, sociodemographic factors and geographic location; thus the use of qualitative inquiry may be more prudent for investigating the perceived benefits and disadvantages associated with relevant sources of food access.

Understanding and utilizing food products is often assessed via the ability to read labels, which is also a key skill in the ability to assess food quality. Food label use has been assessed in a variety of ways. Firstly, self-reported label reading habits, ease of reading labels, perceived accuracy and usefulness, and the influence of label reading on food selection have been assessed. However, the assessment of self-reported use and confidence in label reading does not necessarily translate to ability to read or interpret labels. Indeed, it has previously been found that although self-reported label use may be high among consumers, many users simply look at the nutrition information panel without further processing information to make a decision (Cowburn & Stockley 2005). As such, the reliance on self-reported frequency of label use is likely to artificially inflate indications of higher food literacy. Furthermore, the frequency with which labels may be read does not necessarily correlate with food literacy; that is, the reliance on the use of labels may decrease as one's food literacy is enhanced. Addressing these limitations, other measures have investigated knowledge of and ability to use food labels by providing brief tasks able to be answered via multiple-choice options (Cowburn & Stockley 2005). Of consideration, however, are the potential differential abilities of respondents to complete task related questions or assessment; older people were identified to perform less well on label reading tasks compared to their younger counterparts (Levy & Fein 1998). This may suggest the need for specifically tailored interventions to assist in skills development, and/or tailored assessment items that differ between groups to suit varying levels of comprehension.

Preparation

The measurement of food preparation, cooking skills or food safety skills is well suited to the use of practical activities for the assessment of knowledge, confidence and ability pertaining to these components. Such measures would provide objective means of assessing the knowledge that underpins these concepts, as well as the skills and confidence of the individual to undertake tasks associated with these. However, practical assessment of skills and ability is rarely adopted due to time constraints and limited practicality or appropriateness (Byrd-Bredbenner 2004; Caraher et al. 1999; Porter, Capra & Watson 1999); instead the assessment of concepts underpinning this domain mainly occurs through investigation of self-reported frequency or self-perceived confidence in preparing food (i.e. 'How often do you cook?' or 'How confident are you in preparing/stir frying/cooking, etc.?'), or in the self-reported use or perceived importance of food safety practices ('Do you wash your hands before preparing food?' or 'How important do you think it is to wash your hands before preparing food?'). The assessment of confidence or self-efficacy relating to food preparation skills is supported by the notion that not cooking is a result of a lack in confidence rather than a lack in skill (Lang & Caraher 2001). However, confidence in food preparation and cooking does not necessarily equate to these tasks being undertaken more often, therefore both should be measured (Crombie et al. 2009).

There are several limitations associated with the assessment of food and/or meal preparation. Firstly, within a constantly changing food system in which processed and convenience foods are ubiquitous, the notion of 'cooking' and food preparation skills becomes more difficult to deconstruct and understand. Efforts to capture food preparation skills often incorporate use of the terms 'basic' or 'pre-prepared' to distinguish between food types and level of skill in food preparation; however, it has been acknowledged that dichotomizing foods as such is simplistic, and fails to acknowledge that many foods in contemporary food systems could in fact be classified as both (e.g. tinned vegetables or dried pasta) (Engler-Stringer 2010). The concepts of food or meal preparation may also be understood or interpreted in different ways across varying contexts, including across cultures and generations, and the skills required for one to be 'food literate' also are likely to vary across contexts (Engler-Stringer 2010; Vidgen 2014). Furthermore, attempts to capture food preparation mainly consider the preparation of planned meals, often failing to account for snacking or grazing (Kristensen & Holm 2006). In addition, with technological advancements, the skills that are required to 'sufficiently' prepare and cook food continue to change over time. In assessing food preparation skills, it is also necessary to consider the relationships between planning and organizing foods intake (Domain 2 in the food literacy definition) and subsequent food preparation. This interplay may have implications on measurement and overall 'food literacy' (Engler-Stringer 2010; Vidgen 2014).

Finally, the reliance on self-reported use of or frequency of food safety practices is likely prone to social desirability bias, with respondents providing affirmative responses out of fear of judgement. This may be particularly true of post-intervention assessment and may result in overestimates of a programme's true effectiveness.

Eating

Understanding the important role of food for wellbeing and demonstrating awareness of the need to balance food intakes for health (including foods to include and exclude, serving sizes and proportions) represent 'traditional' food and nutrition knowledge based on dietary recommendations. Food and nutrition knowledge is widely assessed in practice and throughout academic literature, but its measurement is deceptively simple. Knowledge is influenced by many factors, including individual experiences and beliefs. The belief structure of an individual is of great importance to knowledge, as knowledge will only be adopted if one believes something to be true (as influenced by one's life experiences). With the establishment of the nutrition expert, nutrition pseudo-experts, gaining interest in nutrition, the ubiquity of nutrition information and misinformation widespread on social media, and the dynamic and changing nature of nutrition research, the experience of the individual is highly variable, and thus the acceptance of knowledge varies (Pollan 2008; Vidgen 2014), and there appears to be little consensus as to what constitutes important nutrition-related knowledge for food literacy (Worsley 2002).

Given the variations in dietary requirements based on individual characteristics, belief states, life experiences, disease states and stages of the life course, variations in recommendations across countries and the complexities of food needs and preferences that span across cultures, unsurprisingly there exist a vast number of approaches to assess 'nutrition knowledge', and these vary depending on the context in which data is being collected. In the context of food literacy, knowledge questions are not only an explicit component of the 'Eating' domain, but an implicit inclusion across the remaining three domains, with knowledge required to underpin the skills, attitudes, beliefs and behaviours associated with each component (Vidgen 2014). As such, measures that assess food related knowledge are required to capture a broad range of content, from knowledge regarding planning or budgeting techniques, to the use of food labels and appropriate use of cooking and preparation techniques, and 'knowledge' is the mostly widely addressed and measured component of food literacy. Adding to the complexity of capturing food and nutrition related knowledge are the differing degrees of development and importance and contribution to 'food literacy' across the life course. As such, the development of knowledge related questions to assess food literacy requires careful consideration of a multitude of factors, and measures are required to be unique to the context in which they are administered. This however is likely to create complexities in the comparing and contrasting of findings across various situations and settings. Opportunities to address these via the adoption of a framework underpinning food literacy programmes to assist in the development of similar/consistent goals and objectives and subsequently evaluation techniques are further discussed in the following section.

The majority of previous investigations into social eating have relied on self-reported frequency of social activities around meals, including frequency with which most people in a household consumed meals with each other eating at the dinner table and eating in front of the television (Herbert et al. 2014; Larson et al. 2013). These existing measures have been designed within the context of a traditional family unit, and as such it is unknown how these may be translated by people living alone, or in 'non-traditional' family situations. Furthermore, whilst focusing solely on eating together in the house and at the dinner table as the indicator for social eating, these measures fail to account for a multitude of other social eating situations, including dining out with others and attendance at other social events, which may be important considerations for some individuals, households or cultures.

Implications of measurement and recommendations for evaluation and monitoring of food literacy and interventions

A vast number of food literacy programmes exist, targeting various stages of the life course (including childhood, adolescence, adulthood, the elderly), general health, chronic conditions and varying combinations of the underlying domains of food literacy. The existence of so many programmes and target groups reinforces the highly complex, contextual nature of food literacy and its measurement.

A combination of the varying nature of the programmes and the food literacy domains they target, the respective target groups to which they are tailored, and varying use of terminology and understanding of 'food literacy' has resulted in the use of a multitude of different assessment techniques and tools for evaluation, making comparisons between programmes difficult. Whilst a number of programmes adopt scales previously developed and validated among similar populations, many developed unique measures that have been tailored to assess factors that relate to the specific content of the individual intervention itself (Abood, Black & Feral 2003; Devine, Farrell & Hartman 2005; Keller et al. 2004; Levy & Auld 2004; Rustad & Smith 2013). In these instances, the validation of scales is most often limited to face and content validation and confirmation of test-retest reliability and internal consistency among the sample in which the intervention was implemented (Abood, Black & Feral 2003; Greenwell & Sobal 2000; Levy & Auld 2004). As such, the evaluation of many programmes is limited by the use of measures for which the true validity of assessment scales, and therefore the accuracy of the findings, remains unknown. In part, this variation in assessment methods has likely been compounded by the previous lack of formal definition and consensus regarding the components that underpin food literacy, resulting in inconsistencies in the development of programme goals, objectives and strategies and subsequently in the selection of measurement scales for outcome, impact and process evaluation. The formal definition of food literacy developed by Vidgen (2014) now provides a potential framework to underpin the development, implementation and subsequent evaluation of food literacy programmes, which may provide an opportunity to streamline goals, objectives and strategies across various groups and populations and for the identification or development of valid scales that may be used more consistently for evaluation and monitoring purposes.

Few programmes have incorporated the use of objective or observational techniques for assessing the knowledge, attitude and belief changes associated with food literacy interventions, as these options are associated with higher cost and are limited in their practical application. Instead, items employed in the evaluation of most food literacy programmes mainly rely on self-report regarding knowledge, attitudes and beliefs. This form of subjective measurement is used for its simplicity, low cost and ability to provide qualitative detail beyond the information obtained through more objective measures. However, the use of subjective measurement is notoriously prone to response bias, with respondents overestimating affirmative or positive responses and underestimating negative ones. In addition, the lack of rigorous construct validation for a number of tools used in existing programme evaluations may make the generalization of findings to the broader target group and population inappropriate (McDowell 2006). Further efforts are required to rigorously validate existing and new scales to minimize potential bias and allow for the collection of data that may be confidently used to guide intervention and policy development for a broader population.

The majority of food literacy intervention evaluations assess food knowledge, food-related attitudes and self-efficacy. However, even within the assessment of similar components of food literacy there appear to be inconsistencies as to what constitutes characteristics such as knowledge, attitudes, belief and confidence/self-efficacy. For example, the question 'Do you know how to use a knife?' has been assessed as knowledge (Levy & Auld 2004); however, this question does not appropriately capture knowledge of using a knife, but rather one's confidence in doing so. Such inconsistencies, along with the limited validation undertaken for many newly developed tools, may explain some of the variation in the types of scales used for assessment. These inconsistences are further exacerbated by the use of a range of different response options for varying scales, ranging from oversimplified dichotomous outcomes (true or false for knowledge, yes or no for attitudes, beliefs and behaviours) through to the use of Likert scales (four and five point scales being the most common throughout the evaluation literature) to assess the spectrum of knowledge, attitudes and beliefs. As such, the comparison of evaluation outcomes between interventions is difficult, and the limited validation of many existing scales risks inaccurate measurement of the true effectiveness of these programmes or inefficiencies in being able to correlate changes in knowledge, attitudes and beliefs with the overall desired behavioural change. This in turn has significant implications for demonstrating programme effectiveness (Streiner & Norman 2008).

The progressive reviews by Contento and colleagues have identified the importance of demonstrating programme effectiveness through the assessment of dietary behaviour change as a key outcome of food literacy programmes (see Contento 2008a, b; Contento, Randell & Basch 2002; Contento et al. 1995). Consistent with this recommendation, and aligning with goal evaluation as a best practice principle, a majority of food literacy programmes incorporate measurements of dietary change (food or nutrient intakes), and to a lesser extent weight change or a change in other health indicators. However, there appears to be limited consensus on the use of these variables, with few evaluations investigating the associations between the components of food literacy and these health outcomes. Such information would provide valuable insight into the components of food literacy that facilitate the desired diet and health changes; this would allow for refinement and consensus about the domains and components that underpin food literacy, tailoring of interventions to enhance food literacy and consensus regarding its measurement.

Conclusions

Food literacy is an inherent component to healthy eating and health and well-being. Acknowledging this, a plethora of education programmes exist to enhance food literacy, but in the previous absence of a formal definition, the evaluation of these programmes has been limited in scope, assessing only one or two domains of food literacy using a variety of different tools. Whilst arguments exist as to whether food literacy needs to or should be measured, best practice dictates that the incorporation of principles of evaluation (and therefore measurement) is required, particularly in an environment of constrained resources in which the practitioner is responsible for ensuring the use of resources is directed towards programmes that are effective and tailored to groups most in need.

The contextual and varying nature of food literacy creates complexities for its measurement and as such it is unlikely that one measure could be used to investigate food literacy across a variety of populations and sub-groups. Rather, several scales may be required to accommodate the contextual nature of this issue. Currently, no existing measures assess all identified domains of food literacy. As such the measurement and evaluation of food literacy has relied on combining several individual scales, many of which have been developed in consideration of a unique population and food literacy programme and have not undergone rigorous validation studies. The recently developed formal definition of food literacy and identification of the underlying components may be used as a framework on which to base future food literacy programmes, providing opportunities for the identification of consistent goals, objectives and strategies and subsequently consistency in measurement across evaluation, monitoring and surveillance efforts.

References

Abood, D., Black, D. & Feral, D. 2003, 'Nutrition education worksite intervention for university staff: Application of the health belief model', *Journal of Nutrition Education & Behavior*, vol. 35, no. 5, pp. 260–267.

Asp, E. 1999, 'Factors affecting food decisions made by individual consumers', *Food Policy*, vol. 24, no. 2, pp. 287–294.

Ayala, G., Mueller, K., Lopez-Madurga, E., Campbell, N. & Elder, J. 2005, 'Restaurant and food shopping selections among Latino women in Southern California', *Journal of the American Dietetic Association*, vol. 105, no. 1, pp. 38–45.

Burney, J. 2002, 'EFNEP: A nutrition education program that demonstrates cost-benefit', *Journal of the American Dietetic Association*, vol. 102, no. 1, pp. 39–45.

Byrd-Bredbenner, C. 2004, 'Food preparation knowledge and attitudes of young adults: Implications for nutrition practice', *Topics in Clinical Nutrition*, vol. 19, no. 2, pp. 154–163.

Caraher, M., Dixon, P., Lang, T. & Carr-Hill, R. 1999, 'The state of cooking in England: The relationship of cooking skills to food choice', *British Food Journal*, vol. 101, no. 8, p. 590.

Contento, I.R. 2008a, 'Nutrition education: linking research, theory and practice', *Asia Pacific Journal of Clinical Nutrition*, vol. 17, no. 1, pp. 176–179.

Contento, I.R. 2008b, 'Review of nutrition education research in the *Journal of Nutrition Education and Behavior*, 1998 to 2007', *Journal of Nutrition Education and Behavior*, vol. 40, no. 6, pp. 331–340.

Contento, I.R., Balch, G.I., Bronner, Y.L., Lytle, L., Maloney, S., Olson, C. & Swadener, S. 1995, 'The effectiveness of nutrition education and implications for nutrition education policy, programs, and research: A review of research', *Journal of Nutrition Education*, vol. 27, no. 6, pp. 277–418.

Contento, I.R., Randell, J.S. & Basch, C.E. 2002, 'Review and analysis of evaluation measures used in nutrition education intervention research', *Journal of Nutrition Education & Behavior*, vol. 34, no. 1, pp. 2–25.

Cowburn, G. & Stockley, L. 2005, 'Consumer understanding and use of nutrition labelling: A systematic review', *Public Health Nutrition*, vol. 8, no. 1, pp. 21–28.

Cramer, K., Tuokko, H., Mateer, C. & Hultsch, D. 2004, 'Measuring awareness of financial skills: Reliability and validity of a new measure', *Aging & Mental Health*, vol. 8, no. 2, pp. 161–171.

Crombie, I., Kiezebrink, K., Irvine, L., Wrieden, W., Swanson, V., Power, K. & Slane, P. 2009, 'What maternal factors influence the diet of 2-year-old children living in deprived areas? A cross-sectional survey', *Public Health Nutrition*, vol. 12, no. 8, pp. 1254–1260.

Devine, C., Farrell, T. & Hartman, R. 2005, 'Sisters in health: Experiential program emphasizing interaction increases fruit and vegetable intake among low-income adults', *Journal of Nutrition Education & Behavior*, vol. 37, no. 5, pp. 265–270.

Dowler, E. 1998, 'Budgeting for food on a low income in the UK: The case of lone-parent families', *Food Policy*, vol. 22, no. 5, pp. 405–417.

Dowler, E., Caraher, M. & Lincoln, P. 2007, 'Inequalities in food and nutrition: Challenging "lifestyles"', in *Challenging Health Inequalities*, Policy Press, Bristol.

Dowler, E., Kneafsey, M., Lambie, H., Inman, A. & Collier, R. 2011, 'Thinking about "food security": Engaging with UK consumers', *Critical Public Health*, vol. 21, no. 4, pp. 403–416.

Engler-Stringer, R. 2010, 'Food, cooking skills, and health: A review', *Canadian Journal of Dietetic Practice & Research*, vol. 71, no. 1, pp. 141–145.

Flego, A., Herbert, J., Gibbs, L., Swinburn, B., Keating, C., Waters, E. & Moodie, M. 2013, 'Methods for the evaluation of the Jamie Oliver Ministry of Food program, Australia', *BMC Public Health*, vol. 13, no. 1, p. 411.

Fruh, S., Mulekar, M., Hall, H., Adams, J., Lemley, T., Evans, B. & Dierking, J. 2013, 'Meal-planning practices with individuals in health disparity zip codes', *Journal for Nurse Practitioners*, vol. 9, no. 6, pp. 344–349.

Furst, T., Connors, M., Bisogni, C., Sobal, J. & Falk, L. 1996, 'Food choice: A conceptual model of the process', *Appetite*, vol. 26, no. 3, pp. 247–265.

Gillespie, A. & Gillespie, G. 2007, 'Family food decision-making: An ecological systems framework', *Journal of Family & Consumer Sciences*, vol. 99, no. 2, pp. 22–28.

Government of Canada 2010, *Improving Cooking and Food Preparation Skills: A Synthesis of the Evidence to Inform Program and Policy Development*, Health Canada, Ottawa.

Greenwell, C. & Sobal, J. 2000, 'Food practices and nutrition knowledge after graduation from the Expanded Food and Nutrition Program (EFNEP)', *Journal of Nutrition Education*, vol. 32, no. 3, pp. 130–138.

Gundersen, C. & Garasky, S. 2012, 'Financial management skills are associated with food insecurity in a sample of households with children in the United States', *Journal of Nutrition*, vol. 142, pp. 1865–1870.

Herbert, J., Clemow, L., Pbert, L., Ockene, I. & Ockene, J. 1995, 'Social desirability bias in self-report may compromise the validity of dietary intake measures', *International Journal of Epidemiology*, vol. 24, no. 2, pp. 389–398.

Herbert, J., Flego, A., Gibbs, L., Waters, E., Swinburn, B., Reynolds, J. & Moodie, M. 2014, 'Wider impacts of a 10-week community cooking skills program – Jamie's Ministry of Food, Australia', *BMC Public Health*, vol. 14, p. 1161.

Herbert, J., Hurley, T., Peterson, K., Resnicow, K., Thompson, F., Yaroch, A., Ehiers, M., Midthune, D., Williams, G., Greene, G. & Nebeling, L. 2008, 'Social desirability trait influences on self-reported dietary measures among diverse participants in a multicenter multiple risk factor trial', *Journal of Nutrition*, vol. 138, no. 1, pp. 226S–234S.

Huston, S. 2010, 'Measuring financial literacy', *Journal of Consumer Affairs*, vol. 44, no. 2, pp. 296–316.

International Union of Nutrition Sciences 2005, 'The Giessen Declaration', *Public Health Nutrition*, vol. 8, no. 6A, pp. 783–786.

Keller, H., Gibbs, A., Wong, S., Vanderkooy, P. & Hedley, M. 2004, 'Men can cook!', *Journal of Nutrition for the Elderly*, vol. 24, no. 1, pp. 71–87.

Kristensen, S. & Holm, L. 2006, 'Modern meal patterns: Tensions between bodily needs and the organization of time and space', *Food and Foodways: Explorations in the History and Culture of Human Nourishment*, vol. 14, no. 3, pp. 151–173.

Lang, T. & Caraher, M. 2001, 'Is there a culinary skills transition? Data and debate from the UK about changes in cooking culture', *Journal of the Home Economics Institute of Australia*, vol. 8, no. 2, pp. 2–14.

Larson, N., Fulkerson, J., Story, M. & Neumark-Sztainer, D. 2013, 'Shared meals among young adults are associated with better diet quality and predicted by family meal patterns during adolescence', *Public Health Nutrition*, vol. 16, no. 5, pp. 883–893.

Levy, A. & Fein, S. 1998, 'Consumers' ability to perform tasks using nutrition labels', *Journal of Nutrition Education*, vol. 30, no. 4, pp. 210–217.

Levy, J. & Auld, G. 2004, 'Cooking classes outperform cooking demonstrations for college sophomores', *Journal of Nutrition Education & Behavior*, vol. 36, no. 4, pp. 197–203.

McDowell, I. 2006, *Measuring Health: A Guide to Rating Scales and Questionnaires*, 3rd edn, Oxford University Press, Oxford.

Neunschwander, L., Abbott, A. & Mobley, A. 2013, 'Comparison of a web-based vs in-person nutrition education program for low-income adults', *Journal of the Academy of Nutrition & Dietetics*, vol. 113, no. 1, pp. 120–126.

Oshaug, A. 1997, 'Evaluation of nutrition education programmes: Implications for programme planners and evaluators', Nutrition Education for the Public. Discussion papers of the FAO Expert Consultation (Rome, Italy, 18–22 September 1995), Food and Agriculture Organization of the United Nations, Rome.

O'Sullivan, T. 2015, 'Measuring food literacy in 9 and 10 year old New Zealand children: Questionnaire development, validity and reliability', Masters of Dietetics thesis, University of Otago.

Oxford Dictionary of English Parliament, 2010, 3rd edn, Oxford University Press, Oxford.

Parliament of Australia 2009, *Weighing It Up: Obesity in Australia*, House of Representatives Standing Committee, Canberra.

Parmer, S., Salisbury-Glennon, J., Shannon, D. & Struempler, B. 2009, 'School gardens: An experiential learning approach for a nutrition education program to increase fruit and vegetable knowledge, preference, and consumption among second-grade students', *Journal of Nutrition Education & Behavior*, vol. 41, no. 3, pp. 212–217.

Pollan, M. 2008, *In Defense of Food*, Penguin Press, New York.

Porter, J., Capra, S. & Watson, G. 1999, 'Food skills of people with a chronic mental illness: The need for intervention', *British Journal of Occupational Therapy*, vol. 62, no. 9, pp. 399–404.

Rustad, C. & Smith, C. 2013, 'Nutrition knowledge and associated behavior changes in a holistic, short-term nutrition education intervention with low-income women', *Journal of Nutrition Education & Behavior*, vol. 45, no. 6, pp. 490–498.

Streiner, D. & Norman, G. 2008, *Health Measurement Scales: A Practical Guide to their Development and Use*, 4th edn, Oxford University Press, Oxford.

van de Mortel, T. 2008, 'Faking it: social desirability response bias in self-report research', *Australian Journal of Advanced Nursing*, vol. 25, no. 4, pp. 40–48.

Vidgen, H. 2014, 'Food literacy: What is it and does it influence what we eat?', Doctor of Philosophy thesis, Queensland University of Technology, Brisbane.

Vidgen, H. & Gallegos, D. 2014, 'Defining food literacy and its components', *Appetite*, vol. 76, pp. 50–59.

Worsley, A. 2002, 'Nutrition knowledge and food consumption: Can nutrition knowledge change food behaviour?', *Asia Pacific Journal of Clinical Nutrition*, vol. 11, Supplement, pp. S579–585.

14 Food literacy

Key concepts and the elephants in the room

Helen Vidgen and Martin Caraher

Introduction

This book began with the Public Interest Civil Society Organizations' definition of food. Here, at its conclusion, we are reminded that:

> food is the expression of values, cultures, social relations and people's self-determination, and that the act of feeding oneself and others embodies our sovereignty, ownership and empowerment. When nourishing oneself and eating with one's family, friends, and community, we reaffirm our cultural identities, our ownership over our life course and our human dignity. Nutrition is foundational for personal development and essential for overall wellbeing.
>
> (Public Interest Civil Society Organizations 2014: 2)

In Chapter 3 food literacy is defined as:

> the scaffolding that empowers individuals, households, communities or nations to protect diet quality through change and support dietary resilience over time. It is a collection of inter-related knowledge, skills and behaviours required to plan, manage, select, prepare and eat foods to meet needs and determine food intake.

Despite this definition of food literacy being developed before the Public Interst Civil Society Organizations' definition of food, there are striking parallels. The food literacy research that underpins this book (see Chapters 3, 4 and 9) sampled food experts from diverse paradigms and perspectives – health, education, gastronomy, livelihood, industry, community; and individuals – experts in their own eating – who described what it meant to be 'good with food'. The definition of food literacy, its components and relationship to health, which come from the words of these study participants, touch on all of these elements of food and have informed the contents of this book. This book has examined social and cultural dimensions of food literacy and its role in empowerment, ownership and self-determination over food intake, particularly over the life course. In conceptualizing food literacy, not just at individual, but also at household, community and national levels, its contribution to nourishing one's self, family, friends, community and cultural identity is acknowledged.

The term appears to have emerged in response to a need to describe the totality of the knowledge, skills and behaviours needed for a healthy relationship with food. This is more than cooking, more than nutrition knowledge, more than label reading and more than having a vegetable garden; but exactly what, where to start and how to develop it remain unclear. Perhaps it is because these behaviours on their own, and the practice of linking them to obesity and chronic disease prevention, take a reductionist and simplistic view of food and the role it plays in our lives. The material presented in this book has been deliberately broad and, to a certain extent, inconclusive, to invite the reader to begin to consider the meaning of food literacy beyond the paradigm in which they practise.

The research presented by the wide range of experts in this book contributes to this developing field by providing a scope of meaning for the term, a combined understanding of its components and a conceptual model of its relationship to nutrition, ecological sustainability and health more broadly. These are critical foundations to further work in this field and help set the basis – perhaps an epistemological basis – for further development of the concept and even tools that can be used in practice. Importantly, the contributions in this book begin the development of a meaning of food literacy, even if it is not quite there yet, and the directions for further study. However, like an earlier realm of cooking and the pursuance of cooking as a way to deliver on various outcomes, this introduces problems of ownership, conceptual identity and outcomes. Is food literacy the realm of home economists, nutritionists, dietitians, environmental activists, chefs, consumer advocates, health promotion activists? The list goes on. Of course the obvious answer is that it belongs to all of them, but its application in practice may differ depending on your professional background and the source of funding to support the work. Health funding will dictate that the outcomes should be health related, environmental sustainability funders may well want to see outcomes related to changes in ecological indicators. So developing interventions and measures (see Chapter 13) requires us to work in interdisciplinary ways and put aside professional boundaries. It also requires us to start with the individuals, households and communities we are supporting to consider their motivation to develop their food literacy. This will differ between individuals and also within individuals over time, as food literacy is constantly evolving. It is useful to consider, too, what national and community food literacy might look like and what industries and partnerships would be required for its development. It is likely that national food literacy is more than the sum of individual food literacy.

Public sector practitioners typically work in settings in which they require evaluation for sustained investment of effort and funding. Similarly, for policy makers, food literacy needs to be included in monitoring and surveillance systems if it is to remain a focus. But they also need to understand the concept of food literacy and what it is possible to deliver within constrained practice. This research, represented by the chapters in this book, sets the critical groundwork needed to inform the development of a measure by describing the scope of constructs to be considered. It also sets the basis for shared conversations between practitioners and policy makers and funders (see Chapters 10 to 13 for discourses on this). Multi-disciplinary thinking often requires multi-disciplinary funding and for funders to agree on shared and differential outcomes. Some of the chapters in this book show the different contexts in which food literacy exists (see Chapters 6, 8, 10 to 12). Again we refer to lessons learned from previous experience in projects focused on the practical dimensions of everyday eating. Key issues that have restricted their success include:

- short term funding often with unreasonable outcomes;
- too much emphasis on projects as the means of delivery without sufficient policy support;
- little attention paid to the wider social determinants of food literacy including the social and economic environments;
- lack of supportive healthy environs, so we teach people about healthy consumption but the local environment is still anathema to making healthy food choices;
- a lack of food democracy embedded in projects and approaches;
- gender bias.

(based on Caraher & Cowburn 2004; Caraher & Dowler 2007, 2014; Counihan & Siniscalchi 2014; Guthman 2011)

The key to the above list of 'risks' is for food literacy not to repeat the mistakes of an earlier generation of interventions.

The term 'food literacy' emerged to describe the everyday practicalities of meeting nutrition recommendations within contemporary food environments. It may be that this needs to be extended to pick up issues raised in Chapter 12 and the discussion regarding food production. In a global world the influences on food environments are many and nefarious, what has been called 'Big Food' (Monteiro & Cannon 2012; Moodie, Stuckler & Monteiro 2013; Moss 2013). Food literacy offers the potential to deliver more food democracy by being radical and helping make people aware of the food systems and their lack of inherent democracy, the impact of the food system, and our choices on ecological sustainability (Vincenti 1997). See Figures 4.1–4.3, 5.1, 6.1 as well as 10.1 and 10.3 for graphic descriptions of these issues. The definitions and development of the concept of a dynamic food literacy set out in this book respond to evolving social, cultural and economic systems across which people navigate, over their life course, albeit within a broad health context of nutrition and food security. Those with restricted life chances are likely to be less food literate as they lack access to key assets or social determinants necessary for healthy living. Building on the work of Bourdieu and capital assets (Bourdieu & Wacquant 1992) there are five aspects that are fundamental for healthy outcomes and sustainable development.

- *Natural capital (NC)*: Any stock or flow of energy and matter that yields value in goods and services – natural environment, biodiversity, landscape features supported by sustainable food production or necessary for continued production of food.
- *Physical capital (PC)*: Assets created by economic and food production – the food economy infrastructure available to the local community or locally owned, such as shops, transport, warehouses, etc. Who controls the food system? And who owns or controls the physical capital?
- *Social capital (SC)*: The value added to any activity or economic process by human relationships and co-operation – partnerships, links, networks and communication that help individuals or organizations ensure equitable access to ecologically sustainable healthy diets.
- *Human and political capital (HC)*: Skills, training, learning and personal development needed for accessing and supporting healthy diets and sustainable food production – health gain from accessing healthy diet, influence over food policy, appropriate political frameworks and decision-making to protect and enhance healthy food production and access food policy.
- *Financial capital (FC)*: Stocks of money or other savings in liquid form, but including the physical infrastructure (shops, transport, warehouses, etc.) owned and developed by the commercial sector – the amount of money circulating in the local food economy to ensure equitable access to an adequate and healthy diet.

Food literacy needs to be radical in its attempts to influence these determinants or capitals as well as making people aware of the limits they face (Caraher & Reynolds 2005). This helps to locate work in celebrating, supporting and developing food literacy in individuals, households and communities without victim blaming. Individual responsibility and acknowledgement of broader determinants are not mutually exclusive. Chapters 7 and 8 wrestle with this balance in more detail.

Now we come to the elephants in the room, or perhaps – *not in the room*. The first of these, as we have already mentioned, is the need for a multi-disciplinary approach to food literacy and the development of multi-disciplinary policy and funding to deliver on the promise of food literacy. By doing this it is then possible to address the second and third elephants. First are social or structural determinants, one of which is culture or cultures of food. Second is the environmental impact of our food system. We have mentioned above the influence of 'Big Food' on food environments and food habits, the other related issue is local and regional food cultures, which have often arisen over millennia of practice related to local environments and ecological limitations. Some of these may seem redundant in a modern global food system but in order to meet the limits imposed by ecological sustainability there may be a need to re-address such issues. This is where the link between healthy food choice, ecological limits and food democracy overlaps. The various models presented in this book give graphical descriptions of these issues. The challenge for food literacy will be twofold in this respect: to encompass the limits of ecological sustainability with healthy eating and to help make people aware of – the politics of – the food system (Carolan 2011, 2013). This needs to work at both practice and policy levels. A key endeavour will be focused on persuading policy makers and funders to share resources and to move to a situation where they are willing to share outcomes and move beyond their disciplinary and funding silos.

Another challenge to be addressed, one that has faced home economics for generations, is gender bias; a bias in terms of its practitioner base and its targeted populations. There is an unspoken assumption running through the book that the focus is women! This is a challenge for those picking up the research cudgel following this book. Men in general seem to be less health and food literate than women, or at least they exercise less healthy and environmentally sustainable choices. So how do we get them to engage with food literacy? Conversely, is it because the knowledge and skills required for day-to-day eating have for so long been within the female domain that they have been unrecognized and under-valued such that they are now so difficult to isolate and define?

Researchers are often frustrated when their efforts are ignored by organizations that espouse a commitment to evidence based practice. Similarly, policy writers and practitioners call on researchers to better align their efforts with planning frameworks and service needs. Overlaid on all of this are the politics of research and practice which must be acknowledged and understood for research to truly be translational. Contributors across a range of sectors and countries have engaged in the ideas presented in this book. As a result, we hope they can be used in nations and jurisdictions, in government and non-government organizations, in community centres and classrooms across diverse sectors.

Now that the term 'food literacy' has been set out and its components identified, and its relationship to food intake conceptualized, practitioners, policy writers and researchers have a common language through which to begin to develop work and policy in the area. Important next stages would be the development of a measure for food literacy across varying contexts, sensitive to cultural contexts so that the models can be tested to further inform policy, practice and investment, and monitor the relationship of food literacy to nutrition over time. We are confident that the current volume and the contributions, by bringing together current thinking and research on food literacy, are the start of this process.

References

Bourdieu, P. & Wacquant, L. 1992, *An Invitation to Reflexive Sociology*, Chicago, University of Chicago Press.

Caraher, M. & Cowburn, G. 2004 'A survey of food projects in the English NHS regions', *Health Education Journal*, vol. 63, no. 3, pp. 197–219. DOI 10.1177/001789690406300302.

Caraher, M. & Dowler, E. 2007, 'Food projects in London: Lessons for policy and practice – A hidden sector and the need for "more unhealthy puddings…sometimes"', *Health Education Journal*, vol. 66, no. 2, pp. 188–205. DOI 10.1177/0017896907076762.

Caraher, M. & Dowler, E. 2014, 'Making sense of contemporary food politics', in M. Goodman & C. Sage (eds), *Food Transgressions*, Farnham, Surrey, Ashgate, pp. 227–246.

Caraher, M. & Reynolds, J. 2005, 'Sustainable food futures: Lessons for home economics pedagogy and practice', *Journal of the Home Economics Institute of Australia*, vol. 12, no. 2, pp. 2–15.

Carolan, M. 2011, *Embodied Food Politics*, Farnham, Surrey, Ashgate.

Carolan, M. 2013, *Reclaiming Food Security*, London, Routledge.

Counihan, C. & Siniscalchi, V. 2014, *Food Activism: Agency, Democracy and Economy*, London, Bloomsbury.

Guthman, J. 2011, 'Weighing', in *Obesity, Food Justice and the Limits of Capitalism*, Berkeley, University of California Press.

Monteiro, C.A. & Cannon, G. 2012, 'The impact of transnational "big food" companies on the South: A view from Brazil', *PLOS Medicine*, vol. 9, no. 7, viewed 20 December 2015, <http://journals.plos.org/plosmedicine/article?id=10.1371/journal.pmed.1001252>.

Moodie, R., Stuckler, D., Monteiro, C. et al. 2013, 'Profits and pandemics: Prevention of harmful effects of tobacco, alcohol, and ultra-processed food and drink industries', *Lancet*, vol. 381, no. 9867, pp. 670–679.

Moss, M. 2013, *Salt, Sugar, Fat: How the FOOD GIANTS Hooked Us*, London, Random House.

Public Interest Civil Society Organizations 2014, *Vision Statement for Nutrition*, viewed 8 February 2015, <http://www.fao.org/fileadmin/user_upload/faoweb/ICN2/documents/CSO_Vision_Statement_-_Final.pdf>.

Vincenti, V.B. 1997, 'Home Economics moves into the twenty-first century', in S. Stage & V.B. Vincenti (eds), *Rethinking Home Economics: Women and the History of a Profession*, Cornell, Cornell University Press, pp. 301–320.

Index

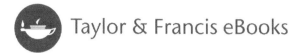

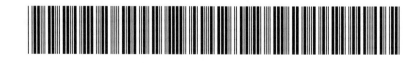